Practice-based Evidence for Healthcare

This book challenges the evidence-based practice movement to rethink its assumptions. Firmly rooted in real practice while drawing lucidly on a great breadth of theoretical frameworks, it examines afresh how clinicians use knowledge.

Evidence-based practice has recently become a key part of the training of all health professionals. Yet, despite its 'gold-standard' status, it is faltering because too much effort has gone into insisting on an idealized model of how clinicians ought to use the best evidence, while not enough has been done to understand why they so often don't.

Practice-based Evidence for Healthcare is a groundbreaking attempt to redress that imbalance. Examining how clinicians actually develop and use clinical knowledge day to day, the authors conclude that they use 'mindlines' – internalized, collectively reinforced, tacit guidelines. Mindlines embody the composite and flexible knowledge that clinicians need in practice. They are built up during training and continually updated from a wide range of formal and informal sources. Before new evidence becomes part of practitioners' mindlines, it is transformed by their interactions with colleagues and patients via their communities of practice and networks of trusted colleagues.

To explore how mindlines work Gabbay and le May draw on a wide range of disciplines to analyse their detailed observations of clinical practice in the UK and the US. Their conclusions and provocative recommendations will be of value to all practitioners, health service managers, policy makers, researchers, educators and students involved in the promotion of evidence-based practice.

John Gabbay is Emeritus Professor at the Wessex Institute for Health Research and Development, University of Southampton, UK.

Andrée le May is Professor of Nursing at the University of Southampton, UK.

Practice-based Evidence for Healthcare

Clinical mindlines

**John Gabbay and
Andrée le May**

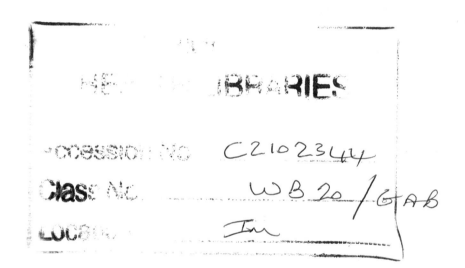
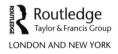

Routledge
Taylor & Francis Group

LONDON AND NEW YORK

First published 2011
by Routledge
2 Park Square, Milton Park, Abingdon, Oxon, OX14 4RN

Simultaneously published in the USA and Canada
by Routledge
270 Madison Avenue, New York, NY 10016

Routledge is an imprint of the Taylor & Francis Group, an informa business

© 2011 John Gabbay and Andrée le May

Typeset in Baskerville by Prepress Projects Ltd, Perth, UK
Printed and bound in Great Britain by CPI Antony Rowe, Chippenham,
Wiltshire

British Library Cataloguing in Publication Data
A catalogue record for this book is available from the British Library

Library of Congress Cataloging in Publication Data
Gabbay, J. (John)
Practice-based evidence for healthcare: clinical mindlines/John Gabbay
and Andrée Le May.
p. ; cm.
Includes bibliographical references.
1. Evidence-based medicine. I. Le May, Andrée. II. Title.
[DNLM: 1. Evidence-Based Practice. 2. Clinical Medicine—methods. 3.
Guideline Adherence. 4. Health Knowledge, Attitudes, Practice. WB 102.5
G112p 2011]
R723.7.G33 2011
616—dc22
2010018514

ISBN13: 978-0-415-48668-2 (hbk)
ISBN13: 978-0-415-48669-9 (pbk)
ISBN13: 978-0-203-83997-3 (ebk)

Ring the bells that still can ring
Forget your perfect offering
There is a crack in everything
That's how the light gets in

(Leonard Cohen, 'Anthem', 1992)

For each other and for Alex, Joey, Mark, Michael, Nao, Vikky, Bethan and Jonathan. Long may the family mindlines mingle and mature.

Contents

List of figures   ix
List of tables   x
List of boxes   xi
Foreword   xii
Preface   xv
Acknowledgements   xvi
Abbreviations   xviii

1   Introduction: evidence in practice   1

2   From formal knowledge to guided complexity   19

3   Clinical thinking and knowledge in practice   48

4   Growing mindlines: laying the foundations   69

5   Growing mindlines: cultivating contextual adroitness   85

6   The place of storytelling in knowledge sharing   112

7   A community of clinical practice?   127

8   Co-constructing collective mindlines   147

9   Co-constructing clinical reality   166

10 Conclusions and implications   192

Appendix 1   An example of a Lawndale practice guideline   207

Appendix 2   Practice chronic kidney disease (CKD) protocol
             (extract)   211

Notes   214
References   237
Index   261

Figures

1.1 The idealized pathway of evidence-based practice   3
1.2 Clustering data on the whiteboard   14
2.1 The Lawndale coffee room library   21
2.2 An example of a 'SOPHIE' for diabetes care   26
2.3 A schematic representation of some of the sources of mindlines   46
4.1 A schematic representation of some accumulated contents of
     mindlines   73
5.1 First line of a thumbnail   86
5.2 The SECI spiral   100
5.3 How information enters the SECI spiral and is transformed into
     knowledge-in-practice-in-context   102
7.1 A community of mindlines   131
7.2 What the multi-sectoral, multidisciplinary communities of practice
     were doing with new evidence   139
9.1 Three of the many dimensions that shape the negotiating space in a
     depression consultation   189
9.2 The emergence from two sets of social constructs of a co-constructed
     single instantiation of an illness–disease in a consultation   189

Tables

1.1	Summary of data sources from Lawndale	12
1.2	Main participants	13
1.3	Summary of main theoretical approaches	17
4.1	Organizational culture: examples of categories commonly held to comprise an organization's culture, adapted from Schein (1992) and applied to teaching hospitals	80
8.1	A précis of some of the arguments in the Lawndale GMS contract meetings for raising or lowering the threshold for defining Stage 3 CKD	155
9.1	Distinguishing different (interdependent) levels of constructs about illness and disease	184

Boxes

1.1 From data to interpretation: an example of the process of analysis 15
2.1 Some important professional contacts for GPs 37
2.2 Ways of conceptualizing mindlines using Spradley's (1979) analytical framework 45
3.1 Examples of what a GP needed to know during a typical surgery 53
5.1 Information-seeking heuristics 109
6.1 The value of narrative medicine as summarized by Hurwitz and Greenhalgh (1999: 49) 122
7.1 Features of a successful community of practice 145
7.2 General outcomes resulting from Lawndale's work following the introduction of the GP contract 146
8.1 Quality and Outcomes Framework for chronic kidney disease 152
9.1 An account, using actor-network theory, of the development of services for congestive heart failure in 'Heartshire' 178
10.1 Reflective summary points for improving practice-based evidence 198

Foreword

Common sense is, unfortunately, not always common. Such is the case, I'm afraid, in much of the academic work done over the last twenty years to understand the use of research by healthcare practitioners. For the decisions we make in our everyday lives – whom to marry, what house or car to purchase, which movies to see, where to go on holiday – we know that we're heavily influenced by our social and cultural context. It's common sense that things like the friends with whom we socialize, our access to financial and other resources, our family history, our self-image, our previous experiences in the area (negative and positive) are used to interpret whatever 'hard evidence' we collect to decide on a course of action. Why should we believe that the situation is any different for healthcare practitioners making daily clinical decisions?

Yet the academic world has largely ignored these social and cultural influences when assessing clinical guideline implementation or, more generally, the application of research evidence to decisions in healthcare. The (largely implicit) assumption seems to be that healthcare practitioners *ought* to be dispassionate, rational, probabilistic decision makers and, therefore, we will proceed as if that *is* the case. The classic confusion of *ought* with *is*. Hence researchers design interventions such as enhanced educational opportunities, more readily accessible formats for guidelines, payment incentives and even just-in-time reminders that assume there is a rational, probabilistic decision maker at the receiving end. Sometimes these interventions do actually work to squeeze the research into the decision, but more often than not they don't. When they don't we decry the practitioner's lack of commitment rather than the researcher's lack of common sense.

The problem as I see it is that most researchers have been less interested in helping the practice world do its work better and more interested in getting their own product – research – used by that world. For too long the evidence-based movement has been more about marketing research, being a shill for the academic community, than about understanding where and how research evidence can help practitioners. I do not believe that this has been a wilful misdirection of effort, just a particularly stark example of a common phenomenon – we all tend to believe that what *we* do is more important/valuable/relevant (insert your laudatory adjective of choice) than what *they* do.

How, then, do practitioners actually decide on courses of action? If they don't behave how we think they *ought* to, what *is* their modus operandi? And, given the answer to this, what kinds of interventions will therefore help them by improving the profile of research in their decisions? Note that the goal here is not for the imperial forces of research to vanquish all other inputs. Rather it is to have the role of research optimized in the context of other perfectly reasonable considerations – such as patients' preferences or local colleagues' experiences – and the cognitive processes clinicians actually use to make their decisions.

These are the issues addressed in the following pages. A text that brings common sense to the complex interaction between *ought* and *is* in healthcare practitioner behaviour. As the title makes clear – *Practice-based Evidence . . .* – the book starts from a desire to better understand the practice environment and then works those insights back to implications for the research environment, rather than the more usual reverse pathway.

At the core is the concept of mindlines. These exist at the level of an individual clinician and pragmatically 'blend formal, informal, tacit and experiential evidence' into his or her main signposts for action. They draw on collective mindlines done at the level of practices or other larger social groupings. The book uses the authors' ethnographic work as well as other literatures to describe the origins and ongoing feedstock for these mindlines, how they evolve and in response to what inputs, how they are used, how they are adapted to changing contexts and even how they relate to existing cognitive and social theory. In other words, the book provides a practical guide for how a clinician *is* making decisions and, therefore, how research might become a more relevant part of the process.

The wide range of sources that the book draws upon includes work from the business literature by Brown and Duguid (2000) which highlights 'the social life of information'. Central to the book is this emphasis on the social processes used to interpret, transform and exchange information. This approach does not start by privileging research over other sources, although it does provide insights into how this might be better accomplished. One clear implication is that if we really want to know how to create and apply clinically useful knowledge from academically produced research it is time for the social scientists to eclipse the clinical trialists. In future studies of clinical behaviour change we should be more likely to employ the tools of psychology and sociology than those of clinical epidemiology and biostatistics.

I first encountered this work through Gabbay and le May's original article on mindlines in a 2004 issue of the *British Medical Journal* (Gabbay and le May 2004). I was excited. Indeed, I immediately put pen to paper (actually, skin to keyboard) to communicate my excitement to the authors. A correspondence ensued in which I was astounded to find out that they had come up with the concept of mindlines without ever having heard of the remarkable songlines of Australian aboriginals. Upon reading their article I had felt sure they must have read the travel writer Bruce Chatwin's brilliant exposition on the topic (Chatwin 1998 [1987]).

My astonishment was because of the obvious parallels in the functions of these two kinds of 'lines'. Among other functions the songlines (also known as 'dreaming tracks') are navigation tools for the outback. They guide aboriginals from one landmark to another and, when combined with songlines 'borrowed' from other tribes, can take travellers from one end of the country to the other. Aboriginals use them as fuzzy boundaries to demarcate one territory from another in what are often ambiguously or subtly featured outback landscapes.

With a slightly less romantic turn of phrase one could imagine using a similar description to capture what Gabbay and le May have identified in this book as clinical mindlines. Indeed, in Chapter 2 they expand on this parallel, highlighting the idea of what I would call a navigation device that one might use to negotiate the lowlands and highlands, across the rivers and lakes, and between the swamps and terra firma of the clinical landscape.

By uncovering this concept of mindlines the authors have pointed the evidence-based practice movement in what should prove to be a more profitable direction. They have not only shown us the kinds of maps clinicians actually use, but also given us insights into their map-making techniques. With this in hand researchers and policy makers should be in a better position to interact meaningfully with the practice-based world.

Jonathan Lomas
Former CEO, Canadian Health Services Research Foundation
Ottawa, Canada
April 2010

Preface

It would be easy to see our concept of mindlines as undermining evidence-based practice – and indeed that has already happened judging from some of the citations of our earlier publications. Nothing could be further from the truth. We have no argument with the principle that clinicians practise better when they apply the best available evidence in their day-to-day work, nor that everything possible should be done to help them to do so. We do, however, take issue with the naïve approach that has been taken towards achieving that goal, both the over-reliance on particular types of evidence at the expense of others and the underestimation of the impact of context on the knowledge that is needed to make practice work.

We set out to examine what 'applying the best evidence' actually meant in practice because we hoped to explore why the evidence-based practice movement has had such a hard time of things. What we found was that the proponents of evidence-based practice might fare better if they used the light from many different angles that many disciplines have already shed on the problem. There are flaws in our analysis, in the work we report upon and in evidence-based practice. We hope, however, that reading this book may help you reduce those flaws. In that spirit, this book is dedicated to everyone who can transform its evidence into practice.

Acknowledgements

We have learnt from countless people along the way. Some are colleagues who we have had the good fortune to work with, some we have only conversed with, others we have only read. Many of them know who they are but many don't. We are nevertheless immensely grateful to all of them. Without them, as our work shows in more ways than one, our mindlines would not have been what they are.

We also thank Dale Webb and Harriet Jefferson for their help in the earliest stages of the project, and John Balla, Colin Coles, Lesley Degner, Mike Gill, Trish Greenhalgh, Joel Howell, Paul Little, Jane McLeod, Carl May and Nigel Watson, who took the time to read some or all of the manuscript as it neared completion. Their encouragement and friendly critiques were invaluable but they bear no responsibility for the flaws we did not manage to eradicate.

We are grateful to Maggie Haines for her support in our securing the pump-priming grant of £25,000 from the Department of Health South East Regional Research and Development Directorate, which enabled us to set out on this work.

Thanks too to Grace McInnes and Khanam Virjee from Routledge for their backing and their constant support.

The colleagues from 'Lawndale', 'Urbcester', 'Oakville' and 'Doppton' deserve our special thanks for tolerating a couple of academics lurking around them, watching their every move and asking daft questions. We hope they think it was worth it.

Finally we thank the family for giving us the time and energy that went into this work over such a long period.

We would like to thank the following for permissions to reprint their material:

1 BMJ Publishing Group Ltd. for permission to reprint Box 1.1, which appeared in the electronic version of Gabbay, J., le May, A. (2004) 'Evidence based guidelines or collectively constructed "mindlines?" Ethnographic study of knowledge management in primary care', *British Medical Journal*, 329.
2 BMJ Publishing Group Ltd. for permission to reprint Box 6.1 from Hurwitz, B., Greenhalgh, T. (1999) 'Narrative based medicine: why study narrative?', *British Medical Journal*, 318.
3 SAGE Publications, London, Los Angeles, New Delhi and Singapore, for permission to reprint Figure 7.2 from Gabbay, J., le May, A., Jefferson,

H., Webb, D., Lovelock, R., Powell, J., Lathlean, J. (2003) 'A case study of knowledge management in multi-agency consumer-informed "communities of practice": implications for evidence-based policy development in health and social services', *Health: An Interdisciplinary Journal for the Social Study of Health, Illness and Medicine*, 7.

4 Excerpt from 'Anthem' from *Stranger music: selected poems and songs by Leonard Cohen* © 1993. Reprinted with permission. All rights reserved.

John Gabbay
Andrée le May
April 2010

Abbreviations

ACE	angiotensin-converting enzyme
BMI	body mass index
BMJ	*British Medical Journal*
BTS	British Thoracic Society
CHD	coronary heart disease
CKD	chronic kidney disease
CPD	continuing professional development
CRP	C-reactive protein
CURB-65	confusion, urea, respiratory rate, blood pressure (composite score)
DVT	deep vein thrombosis
EBM	evidence-based medicine
EBP	evidence-based practice
ECG	electrocardiogram
eGFR	estimated glomerular filtration rate
ENT	ear, nose and throat
GMS	general medical services
GP	general practitioner (family physician)
GTT	glucose tolerance test
IBS	irritable bowel syndrome
ICU	intensive care unit
IT	information technology
LDL/HDL	low-density lipid to high-density lipid ratio
MI	myocardial infarction
MMR	measles, mumps and rubella
MMSE	Mini Mental State Examination
MRCGP	Membership of the RCGP (examination)
MRCP	Membership of the Royal College of Physicians (examination)
MRI	magnetic resonance imaging
NHS	National Health Service
NICE	National Institute for Health and Clinical Excellence
NSAIDs	non-steroidal anti-inflammatories
NSF	national service framework
PCT	primary care trust

PSA	prostate-specific antigen
QOF	Quality and Outcomes Framework (of new GP contract)
QPA	Quality Practice Award (by RCGP)
R&D	research and development
RCGP	Royal College of General Practitioners
rep	pharmaceutical company representative/detail
SECI	socialization, externalization, combination and internalization
SIGN	Scottish Intercollegiate Guidelines Network
SOPHIE	the term for a pop-up computerized guide in Lawndale's IT system
SSRI	selective serotonin re-uptake inhibitor (an anti-depressant)
STD	sexually transmitted disease
TB	tuberculosis

1 Introduction

Evidence in practice

The place of evidence-based practice in recent healthcare reforms

This book explores how clinicians[1] acquire and use their knowledge. They know they are expected to ensure that they adhere to the latest, preferably research-based, evidence about best practice, yet they do not always make the best use of the new sources of evidence such as clinical guidelines and systematic reviews of clinical trials (Haynes 1993; Lomas 1997; Evans and Haines 2000; Armstrong 2002; Haines *et al.* 2004; Wyer and Silva 2009). That conundrum is set against a background of health professions that are in a state of flux (Peckham and Exworthy 2003; Klein 2001; Harrison and McDonald 2008). Even by the 1990s the reput-edly omniscient senior physician, the dependably avuncular general practitioner, the handmaiden nurse and the acquiescent patient were already disappearing. Across the health professions, where the traditional hierarchies were tumbling, new relationships between professionals were emerging (see, for example, Ashburner and Birch 1999; Childs 2008) with general practitioners employing increasingly larger numbers of nurse practitioners and indeed in some rare instances doctors and nurse practitioners combining on an equal footing to form general practices. Since then multidisciplinary teams have been increasingly expected to break down the old pecking order; innovative roles such as nurse practitioners and physicians' assistants have been blurring professional boundaries. Patients – gradually becom-ing relabelled as 'clients' by some health professions to stress this very point – seem often to know a great deal about, and are ever more encouraged to have a strong say in, how their illnesses are managed. To that end they now have potential access to rich resources of knowledge and advice not only through patients' organiza-tions but through the internet. Clinicians too are faced with many more sources of knowledge that they need to take account of when practising.

As a result the professions have been described as being 'under siege' (Fish and Coles 1998: 3). As clinical freedom and authority give way to managerial-ism, the once autonomous doctor must now comply with bureaucratic norms and targets or face the consequences (e.g. Ferlie *et al.* 1996). The clinicians' employers might well constrain how they may or may not manage their patients. The shift of doctors' status from self-determining professional to regulated employee has even been described as the 'proletarianization' of medicine (e.g. Elston 1991), a term that certainly reflects the shift of power but underplays the equally important shift in education, lifelong learning and the status of clinical knowledge.

The training of clinicians has evolved hand in hand with these changes in their environment. The tradition of undergoing a fixed period of didactic clinical teaching followed by bedside apprenticeship is being phased out across the healthcare disciplines in favour of more flexible, self-directed and reflective learning. New educational principles have been transforming clinical education through problem-based learning, inter-professional learning, competencies-based training, ever more rigorously objective examinations, continuous professional development, clinical audit, appraisal and revalidation. Lifelong learning has replaced the once-and-for-all qualification. There is increasing stress on delivering and checking competencies rather than inculcating values and professional wisdom (Fish and Coles 2005). The job for life is being supplanted by mobile career paths, portfolio careers and complex private/public partnerships that undermine the traditional job security of the health professional. Moreover, the specialized knowledge that clinicians bring to their practice no longer carries the arcane mystique that it once did. The incontestability of a senior clinician's individual, autonomous knowledge has been undermined by the clinical guideline, the systematic review, the organizational target and the web-based expert system open to all, including patients. Senior doctors can be challenged by (perhaps brave) members of the clinical team who have read the latest guidance, or by patients who have had access to alternative sources of information about their disease, or by healthcare managers whose paymasters charge them with cajoling if not coercing clinicians to comply with new, more cost-effective ways of practising. As a result, the old acceptance that 'we do things this way because distinguished professors tell us we should and it's not for the likes of us to question it' is much harder to sustain. In short, the clinical knowledge base is being democratized.

And this is just as well, since the old elitism had produced unacceptable variations in practice, dependent more on the power of opinionated senior doctors than on any rational review of all the appropriate evidence. Indeed it was that very problem that provided much of the fuel for both the democratization of clinical knowledge and the proletarianization of the clinical professions in the first place. The aim of many of the reforms was precisely to expose and minimize the clinical misjudgements of a lofty elite; to replace eminence-based practice with evidence-based practice.

Evidence-based practice (EBP) took root in the medical profession in the 1990s (Sackett *et al.* 1997; Gray 1997) paralleled by other healthcare professions (Mulhall and le May 2004) and like all social movements it has had many forms and interpretations among friends and detractors alike (Harrison 1998; Timmermans and Berg 2003; Dopson *et al.* 2003; Pope 2003; Rycroft-Malone 2006). At its core, however, the EBP movement, in whatever guise it might appear, has urged clinicians to use the available research evidence either by finding, appraising and applying the best evidence themselves or through using evidence-based guidelines and treatment protocols (Figure 1.1).

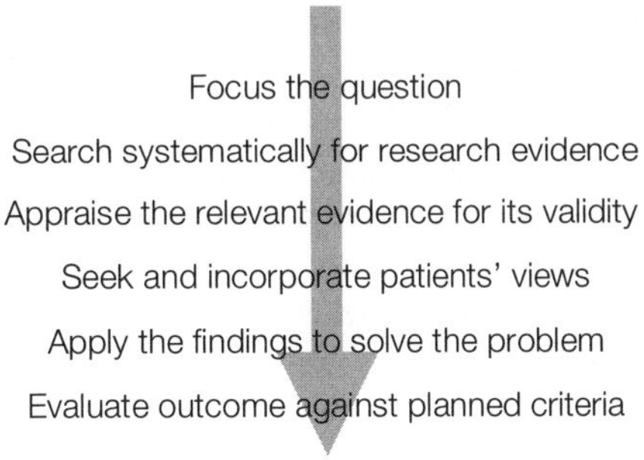

Focus the question
Search systematically for research evidence
Appraise the relevant evidence for its validity
Seek and incorporate patients' views
Apply the findings to solve the problem
Evaluate outcome against planned criteria

Figure 1.1 The idealized pathway of evidence-based practice.

When David Sackett and his colleagues, who spearheaded the movement, defined evidence-based medicine as 'the conscientious, explicit and judicious use of current best evidence in making decisions about the care of individual patients' (Sackett *et al.* 1996: 71; Straus and Sackett 1998; Haynes 2002), they were being more sophisticated than many who joined them to create the EBP bandwagon (Trinder and Reynolds 2000).[2] Sackett and colleagues' definition recognizes the importance of clinical judgement when applying the best evidence in any given set of circumstances. In contrast, however, much of the organizational change linked to the EBP movement seems to have been about applying research evidence overzealously and unthinkingly in clinically inappropriate ways. Clinicians find themselves urged, for example, to apply the results of clinical trials that might have been carried out in selected minorities of patients who are quite different from the majority that they themselves treat. Or, worse, they find themselves under pressure to use clinical guidelines that are not always as explicit as they should be about the sources and the limitations of the evidence on which they are based (e.g. Grol *et al.* 1998; Lugtenberg *et al.* 2009).

EBP has led to a host of reforms across healthcare. They include the mass of guidelines now available to clinicians, many of which are now prepared to the very highest standards of evidence and practical relevance, even though – much to the dismay of those who carefully prepare the guidelines – clinicians are notorious for ignoring or rejecting them unless they are somehow coaxed or coerced into using them. EBP has also grown in tandem with the Cochrane Collaboration in which colleagues from around the world sign up to a lifelong mission to systematically review all the available research evidence using meticulously controlled and scrupulous techniques in order to inform best practice in their chosen area.[3] This has been revolutionary not only in the way it has critically collated huge quantities of research information that was previously ignored, misinterpreted or used inappropriately, but also in the way it has inspired an almost evangelical fervour to pursue high-quality evidence and discard bad science (CRAP writing group 2002). Excellent as it is, however, the Cochrane Collaboration still relies heavily on the randomized controlled trial as the chief arbiter of truth, playing down other forms of legitimate knowledge and still largely ignoring the social and economic aspects of healthcare. Moreover, on close examination the detail often seems to favour scientific pedantry over the needs of clinical practice. EBP has also fostered a welcome emphasis on applied health sciences (as characterized, for example, by the rise of pragmatic and complex trials, of health services research and of health technology assessment). A parallel development has been the growing industry of research on the implementation of research, little of which, paradoxically, is widely implemented.[4] Finally, we see the growing influence of the National Institute for Health and Clinical Excellence (NICE) not only in its native UK, but in countries the world over that are also experiencing pressures to deliver more cost-effective care. NICE issues both general guidelines and specific directives about new treatments; both are rooted in detailed and rigorous assessments of the evidence on cost-effectiveness. But, like many of NICE's counterparts that are springing up around the world, its work is also accompanied by unprecedented levels of bureaucratization and organizational accountability in healthcare, designed to encourage if not enforce conformity to 'best practice'.

Such changes have given reformers the opportunity to try to alter clinicians' behaviour by using change management techniques to introduce more evidence into practice. In the UK, for example, the government has encouraged the 'modernization' of health services not only by injecting more cash into the NHS, but also by relentlessly changing the contractual relationship with health service providers in ways that are designed to encourage evidence-based practice and hence reduce variation in practice. A wide range of schemes have been aimed at the individual practitioner, from training and education programmes to revalidation of their competence to practise, in order to try and corral clinicians and ensure conformity to current best evidence (e.g. Mulhall and le May 1999; Grimshaw *et al.* 2001, 2004). Such activity has been complemented by measures designed to improve the available knowledge base; these include new resources for applied research and new tools (e.g. the development of care pathways) to foster compliance, and national service frameworks (NSFs) that set out best practice, evidence based as far as possible. Whether that has succeeded in improving standards of care – which it almost certainly has done, if patchily – or has been as distressing and disruptive to practice as some complain, is not the point here. The fact is that such measures are transforming the professional basis of healthcare.

The result of this sea change is that practitioners are nowadays more likely to be exposed to the best evidence either directly or – more usually – through widely promulgated guidance. And few would now dispute the principle that clinical practice should be based on the best available evidence, or that the basic principle of EBP is potentially beneficial to practice and hence to patient outcomes. (What can be wrong with systematically and explicitly reviewing and using all the available evidence about the likely effects of alternative courses of action before making a clinical decision? Moreover, can increasingly cash-strapped health systems afford the waste that occurs when clinicians act idiosyncratically?) But there have been many barriers to overcome, not least the defiance of clinicians, and especially those who argue that the evidence is often impracticable, irrelevant or absent, and takes too long to find (Grol 1997; Newman *et al.* 1998; Dopson and Fitzgerald 2005). Knowledge, attitudes and beliefs have all played their part in that resistance (le May *et al.* 1998; Ferlie *et al.* 2001; Dopson *et al.* 2010 [2002]), as have the complexities of organizational behaviour (Ferlie *et al.* 2000). The knowledge base both of individual clinicians and of the relevant sciences in general has often been inadequate to sustain EBP; the attitude of clinicians has often been one of wariness of the motives and competence of those producing guidance or advocating changes to practice; and strongly held beliefs have undermined the use of evidence. In one study of the implementation of EBP, for example (Dawson *et al.* 1998), the senior hospital doctors believed that the guidelines on asthma and glue ear did not apply to their specialized and complicated patients, while the general practitioners believed that the guidelines did not apply to their mostly atypical patients, and the junior doctors said they really didn't have time to practise evidence-based medicine (EBM) and anyway had to do as their bosses told them. In short – at least in the 1990s when EBM was relatively new – all parties believed that the guidelines applied to someone else but not to them. Catch-22. Yet the direction of central policy is tending inexorably towards more protocol-driven systems of care, exacerbating the potential tensions between clinical autonomy and rationalist bureaucracy (Gray and Harrison 2004).

Even where there has been a willingness to adopt evidence and try to change practice, organizational barriers such as inadequate resources or inappropriate systems have provided further obstacles. For example, one might accept the importance of scanning all patients who have had strokes, but what if the magnetic resonance imaging (MRI) scanners are not available (CSAG 1998)? Perhaps above all, practitioners have found that the science base is often not there when they need it; that there are still large shadows of uncertainty where the evidence is too insubstantial to justify a change in practice. That, indeed, is why there has been such an increase in needs-led, service-oriented research whose aim is to produce answers to the *practical* questions facing clinicians (Baker and Kirk 2001). Yet, despite that increase, the landscape still seems full of grey areas and unresolved questions (Chalmers 2008; James Lind Alliance 2010). In sum, for all these reasons and more, while there has been a reform in the way evidence is applied to practice, the change is not nearly as radical or fundamental as the proponents of EBP might wish.

How this study arose

The work leading to this book arose out of the authors' concern about the persistent mismatch between the rational, linear, scientistic approach that the EBP movement demands and the pragmatic, workable approach demanded by the messy world of practice. As senior health service academics both of us had spent our university careers trying to bridge the gap between academic research and practical healthcare, promoting evidence-based practice and researching its practicalities for many years. ACLM in the twenty years since leaving the NHS for a university career had put most of her academic efforts into promoting evidence-based nursing and trying to close the gap between nursing research and practice. JG, who ended up running a university department devoted mainly to producing health technology assessments as evidence for the NHS and NICE on the cost-effectiveness of healthcare interventions, had always striven to narrow the gap between academic and practical public health. So it should be very clear that both of us were, and remain, strongly in favour of evidence-based practice. But over the years we had both become increasingly frustrated by the naïvety of the views that the proponents of EBP promulgated about the nature of evidence and how it should be implemented. Because of our desire to understand better how clinicians might put theoretical knowledge to practical use, both of us had independently developed an interest in organizational behaviour, and in particular the current trends in 'knowledge management' and 'communities of practice' – of which much more later. As a result we began working together to research these questions and quickly came to the conclusion that we needed to explore two crucial discrepancies.

First there was the gap between research and practice, encapsulated in the persistent problem that, despite the massive efforts by the establishment – health professions, research funders, educators, patient organizations, governments, health commissioners, insurers and other payers – to promote EBP, clinicians still so often seem to ignore research evidence in their daily practice. Second there was the glaring disparity between the policy makers' methods for trying to promote EBP and what social scientists, philosophers, psychologists – and just about anyone who studied such things – have long told us about the nature of knowledge and how it gets used in the real world. The approach to knowledge management in health services has generally been to try and deliver better-researched facts to clinicians and to try and help them to make good use of such facts. But this strategy assumes a rational and individualistic approach to knowledge acquisition that flies in the face of all the evidence about what some have called 'the social life' of knowledge – the intricate, convoluted and confusing pathways by which people in an organization negotiate, adapt and transform new knowledge that is often far from factual. Maybe, we surmised, clinical knowledge also had a 'social life' that could be the key to overcoming the persistent frustrations of evidence-based practice. The task we set ourselves, therefore, was to look afresh at how clinicians actually acquire and use their knowledge in practice. Perhaps, we reasoned, the insights from such a study might help to overcome the frustration and failure dogging our own efforts and those of our colleagues to strengthen the use of evidence in practice.

Introducing ethnography

We decided to begin that fresh look with doctors and nurses in primary care; to try to get 'inside' the way that they actually put their knowledge to daily use. The best way to do this, we decided, was to approach it as anthropologists do when they are trying to understand a different culture: by using ethnography to study one or more groups of clinicians (Bloor 2001).[5] Ethnography has been described as 'the art and science of describing a group or culture' (Fetterman 1998: 1) where one is trying to understand their way of life from their point of view. 'One . . . makes contacts, finds a trail into a research site, hangs around and asks questions, struggles to figure out how to analyse the uncontrolled material, and worries about the generalizability of the results' (Agar 1996: 7). Our 'hanging around' had a clear purpose: to understand what is *really* going on when clinicians use knowledge in practice. It entailed spending a lot of time watching them, chatting, learning from them, engaging with them, standing back, commenting, questioning, interviewing and doing more proactive and specific data gathering (e.g. checking documents, delving into particular kinds of practice activity, going to other sites to cross-check findings) when the need arose. Ethnography involves no interference or experimentation, nor any fixed pattern of data gathering (Hammersley and Atkinson 1983). It boils down, as Agar (1996: 2) has put it, 'to the same old problem of one human trying to figure out what other humans are up to.' The aim is to use whatever means one can to build up a 'thick description' (Geertz 2000) of the actions and events one is observing, to get below the surface and interpret the subtleties and meanings that the actors themselves might attribute to them.

And yet the ethnographer is not learning how to be one of the people under study. The aim is also to compare and contextualize the findings in such a way as to produce an interpretation that furthers the ethnographer's own theories of how the world works (Sanjek 1996). Such an exercise is therefore not mere observation, but involves a lot of intense analysis that runs alongside and interacts with the fieldwork. This is true of any science − it has long been known that it is impossible even for scientists to completely strip away their own thinking from what they are observing (Hanson 1958) − but ethnographers tend to be particularly self-conscious about it. As one standard textbook puts it (Fetterman 1998: 1), 'the ethnographer enters the field with an open mind, not an empty head', and we were no different. We were not coming to this task with a blank slate; on the contrary we were undertaking this fieldwork precisely because we had done a lot of thinking, reading and writing about the way research, practice and health policy interact, and about the nature of knowledge in practice. We had already, as the anthropologists' methodological jargon calls it, 'foreshadowed' the problem we were investigating. Indeed, as will become obvious later, one of our prior views was that all knowledge, including clinical knowledge, is a social construction and all observations, including scientific ones, are theory laden. So we had no illusions that our observations would inevitably be coloured by our theoretical framework.[6] Moreover, a major part of our analysis, which we developed alongside our fieldwork, entailed reading widely about knowledge management, the sociology of knowledge, and related social sciences that seemed relevant (notwithstanding the fact that the world of evidence-based clinical policy making and practice had remained steadfastly impervious to them). This would all inevitably, indeed intentionally, shape our analysis.

The potential for one's own background and theoretical assumptions to bias the findings is a central problem for ethnographers. Part of the solution is to make a virtue of explicitly reflecting on that problem as an integral part of their method, which is why, perhaps to the surprise of readers trained in the natural sciences, we will sometimes be quite explicit and personal in this book about the way we as researchers were reacting to what we found. Not only is such explicit subjectivity necessary to allow the reader to assess how far our interpretations may have been influenced by our prior concepts, but being 'reflexive' is actually part of the ethnographic research process; it was a crucial way to guard against our perceptions being unduly distorted by our prior thinking. The more one lays bare the thinking behind one's observations, the more one can judge – and allow others to judge (Hammersley 1990) – what the observations in the field really mean, which is, after all, the purpose of the ethnographic exercise.[7]

We also had to deal with another common methodological problem. The ethnographer has to maintain a crucial balance between getting close enough to the culture to really understand what is happening and remaining distant enough to remain detached. Both of us, having originally trained as clinicians, had been members of the 'tribes' we were proposing to study,[8] so we knew that it would probably be all too easy to get close to the practitioners. On the other hand we would have to be particularly careful to see their practice with fresh eyes rather than slipping back into the 'tribal' mindset. We would need, in other words, to be extra cautious about 'going native', and it did indeed often prove difficult to avoid adopting the role of a clinical colleague and to constantly remind ourselves that, as the cliché has it, we were there to make the familiar strange (Agar 1996). (See also p. 196.)

The stated aim of our ethnography was to find out how practitioners use knowledge to shape their individual and collective healthcare decisions, and to see how this was related to their organizational context. We wanted to describe the day-to-day activities of practice, focusing on how clinicians used knowledge in their interactions with patients and carers, and with their colleagues. We hoped to find key areas where they were formulating changes in their policies and protocols so that we could follow how those changes were actually brought about. We expected these to include not only modifications, small and large, in the way clinicians treat patients, but also how they reacted to the plethora of central guidance, not to say pressure, to change the way care was organized and delivered. These, we reasoned, would allow us to explore the ways in which different sources of knowledge and evidence – such as new treatments or research findings, new guidance, or changes in local or national NHS policy – might be put into practice.

These may seem rather complex questions to lay on one study of one set of clinicians, but ethnographic research has to trade off the breadth provided by, say, a survey or a series of case studies against the narrower but potentially more profound insights achieved from studying one location in great depth: 'small places, large issues', as one author has tellingly phrased it (Eriksen 2001). So we decided to begin by looking in depth at just one primary care group practice. We had also considered looking at several GP practices but in the end we were persuaded that the best approach was to concentrate on one site and then to briefly check out our findings elsewhere. However, the problem remained that general practice in the UK is enormously varied. There was no question of any one practice being representative of general practice any more than the Trobriand Islanders, from whom Malinowski was able to deduce so much about human behaviour in the 1910s when he was developing ethnography as a scientific method, are representative of New Guinea, let alone the whole human race (Malinowski 1922). How, then, should we choose a single primary care team for the first study?

We wanted to look at relatively mainstream doctors and nurses, so we steered clear of university or other atypical practices. On the other hand, given that our overarching aim was to understand how practitioners underpin their practice by using the best available evidence, there was no point in studying doctors and nurses who don't do so. We reasoned, therefore, that we needed an ordinary practice that practised extraordinarily high-quality healthcare. First, that would be where we were most likely to see how good, run-of-the-mill clinicians keep up to date and make use of the various available sources of knowledge, including scientific and other evidence, to inform their practice. Second, if really good doctors and nurses were not using the scientific evidence in the manner prescribed by the evidence-based practice movement, then it was unlikely that lesser practitioners were doing so. (Furthermore, if we were to pick a mediocre practice and find that they were not making good use of the available evidence, all we would show was that mediocre clinicians are also mediocre knowledge managers – hardly surprising.) Third, a detailed account of the ways that good practitioners did manage to practise in an evidence-based way might be a useful exemplar for others who would like to improve the way they acquire, share and use reliable knowledge to help raise their standards. And fourth, if such top-quality practitioners were not using the methods, guidelines and protocols that they are being enjoined to use, then we would be onto something because, by finding out the methods they do use successfully, we might have important lessons for the evidence-based practice movement.

Introduction to Lawndale

The next problem was to find such an exemplary site and gain access to it. We tried to discern the best local practice by using the publicly accessible data but this was relatively unhelpful. And anyway, even if we found a practice by such measures, we could not, even as clinical academics, just walk in and observe it. However, we had university colleagues who worked part-time for local primary care groups – the organizations then responsible for managing primary care services – and who were therefore intimately acquainted with all the local group practices. They could point us in the right direction and arrange an introduction. They were also able to give us the local angle on the swirling morass of policy changes and organizational restructurings that were going on in the NHS (Glendinning and Dowling 2003; Peckham and Exworthy 2003; Sheaff 2008), and this had helped us to clarify our research questions. The more they told us, the more we felt that it was important to choose a practice that was not only clinically of a high quality, but also coping well with the maelstrom of primary care reorganization (some called it re-disorganization) at that time. We were likely otherwise to find ourselves doing an ethnography of clinicians' organizational coping strategies rather than their use of varied knowledge sources to affect their practice.[9] So it was by these two major criteria – high-quality practice and organizational competence – that we chose a practice we shall here call 'Lawndale'.

'Lawndale' is in 'Woodsea', a largely blue-collar coastal town in a semi-rural area of the south of England, some fifteen miles from the city of 'Westchurch', where the local hospital is. (There is another one nearby: 'Northton General'.) When we started our ethnography there in 2001 there were seven partner GPs – two women and five men whose ages ranged from about thirty-five to about sixty – plus three salaried sessional GPs and at any given time one or two GP registrars (trainees). Other key clinicians included three practice nurses and a phlebotomist. They were responsible for the care of around 12,500 patients, of whom around a third were over retirement age, but which also included many young families. Fully computerized, Lawndale was exceptionally well organized. It had recently moved to a very well-appointed modern, purpose-built, two-storey building on the edge of Woodsea towards the end of a broad, bustling high street. Next door was a pharmacy. Not only did the practice have an excellent reputation with the local population, but – which was of course why we had chosen it – the higher echelons of the local health service saw it as a leading-edge practice, fully engaged in the 'modernization' that the NHS was encouraging. When we first walked into the smart practice premises we immediately felt an air of quiet, tidy, warm efficiency. Lawndale seemed to have a vibrant atmosphere with motivated and smiling front-desk staff who greeted the patients with respectful familiarity. The facilities were first rate and the clinical staff seemed to work well together and provide an excellent service. We were soon to also find a good deal of objective external recognition of Lawndale's success as a practice: we learned that nearly half of the senior partners had recently earned the prestigious Royal College of General Practitioners 'Fellowship by Assessment', and three years into our study the College also awarded Lawndale the coveted Quality Practice Award (QPA). One year later Lawndale was among only two of some twenty practices in the area to obtain the maximum points in the first year of the new GP contract, showing that the practice met all the required standards, bar none.[10] Later, the practice manager also gained Fellowship by Assessment from the Institute of Healthcare Management and was, unusually, made a full partner in the practice. All of this amply confirmed that our primary care colleagues had been right in recommending Lawndale. Whether or not the clinicians there practised according to the tenets of the evidence-based practice movement we did not yet know. But they clearly represented English general practice at its best both clinically and organizationally.[11]

Our work there led us also to other sites (see p. 11) to check and expand our findings with much shorter periods of observation and participant observations in another general practice and in US and UK teaching hospitals.[12] As we developed our ideas and analysis, we were also able to draw on what might be called 'retrospective auto-ethnography', an attempt to rethink our own experiences as clinical student, trainee, teacher, trainer and policy maker. We also took the opportunity to reanalyse data from the many research and development projects in which we had been involved over more than two decades, where the main focus of study had been attempts to bring research evidence into clinical practice.

Observation and analysis

Before describing our findings it behoves us to explain two more things: how we obtained and analysed our findings and what theoretical approaches informed that analysis. Some readers may prefer by this stage to dispense with all these preliminaries and skip to the next chapter. But, if they do so, they should consider coming back to this and the next section at some stage so that they can make a fair assessment of the way we obtained and interpreted our findings since, as we have already suggested, those findings will inevitably be steeped in the methods and the conceptual framework that underpinned them.

We started in 2001 with participant and non-participant observation of around seven days' worth of GP surgeries, home visits and nursing clinics during which we would briefly explore wherever possible – either immediately afterwards or later in more convenient informal settings – why the clinician believed he or she had acted in particular ways. Such exchanges were helped by the fact that we, the ethnographers, were both clinically trained.

We also attended well over fifty formal practice meetings of various types and had innumerable unstructured informal individual and group interviews and chats (Table 1.1). We noted our findings during (or immediately following) our observations or conversations. (At some of the early meetings we piloted the use of tape recording but this proved an inefficient method for most of what we needed. Some key interviews, however, were taped.)[13] Where appropriate we supplemented our field notes by reviewing written work such as the relevant NHS documentation (e.g. about the NHS's new GP contract[14]), practice literature, circulars, professional magazines and guidelines. All of this took place intermittently over a period of nearly eight years, during which we came to know the practice very well and were even described as 'part of the furniture'.

To see if Lawndale was in any way atypical, in the autumn of 2001 JG also did fieldwork (three surgeries, a practice meeting, three semi-structured one-to-one interviews, several short discussions with the GPs and occasional email contact) in a very different practice, 'Urbcester'. This was a highly regarded inner-city, university-linked practice in the north of England dealing with a high proportion of unemployed and immigrant patients as well as students. Besides having informal interviews with many ex-colleagues in practice around the UK while developing our analysis, JG also had the opportunity in 2004–5 to closely observe approximately ninety hours of the work of internal-medicine teams in a major US teaching hospital in 'Oakville'. To explore the extent to which our emerging model might be developed in the hospital context, JG observed emergency takes, 'attending rounds', 'morning reports' and the individual work of the residents, interns and students as they admitted and investigated patients. Finally, in 2009, JG observed four days of teaching and learning by a group of third-year UK medical students who were getting to grips for the first time with psychiatry at 'Doppton' Hospital. The examples that we use throughout the book to illustrate our argument will be taken from all these sources but the main focus will be Lawndale. We will sometimes use examples from among doctors, sometimes nurses (Table

Table 1.1   Summary of data sources from Lawndale

Observations of clinical work – often involving informal interviews (2001–2)

---

*10 GP surgeries
*6 sets of home visits by GPs
*4 nurse-led surgeries
(plus 1 half-day observation and formal interview of practice manager)

Participant observations of meetings (2002–9)

---

1 lunchtime executive meeting
*3 routine partners' meetings, including executive and clinical meetings
*6 continuing professional development meetings/education meetings/training sessions
1 meeting of administrative staff
1 awayday of all practice staff
1 awayday of partners and practice manager
*1 practice meeting on coronary heart disease audit
*1 audit meeting
*1 critical incident meeting
~40 informal coffee room gatherings and one-to-one and informal group discussions
*10 Quality Practice Award 'QPA Meetings' of practice staff (= all QPA meetings over one year, of
which three were recorded and transcribed)
*1 QPA-related nurse team meeting
*1 meeting of GP representatives from all local practices to discuss primary care trust-wide
coronary heart disease audit
*26 'GP contract' meetings of practice staff
*1 QPA inspection day
*1 GP contract inspection visit

Formal (taped) interviews (2001–9)

---

*8 interviews with GPs (3 conducted in 2002 by Dale Webb)
*1 group interview with clinic staff (practice nurses and phlebotomist)

Documentary sources

---

*Practice guidelines, manuals, and protocols
*One partner's 'Fellowship by Assessment' portfolio
*One partner's continuing professional development portfolio
*Quality Practice Award (QPA) submission drafts and related paperwork
*'GP contract' (general medical services; GMS) documentation

(Items marked * were principally concerned with clinical matters)

1.2), but unless indicated otherwise it should not be concluded that any particular
finding was confined to the group or profession that we have used as an exemplar.

The principal analysis used our field notes from the observations and informal interviews, which included detailed observations of both individual clinical
encounters and collective formal and informal policy making. At first we transferred all relevant statements in the field notes and interview transcripts onto
around 500 'Post-it' notes and clustered these into emerging themes (Figure 1.2).
As we went along we noted incidents atypical of our emerging model and used
these to test and develop the analysis. Our analysis was not simple induction but
was informed by several theoretical frameworks, which we briefly outline in the
next section. However, we were not testing any hypothesis or preconceived models.

As the study continued, we discussed after each of the observation sessions

Table 1.2 Main participants

Pseudonym	Position
Lawndale	
Clive	Senior GP partner (1980*)
Nick	Senior GP partner (1970)
Jean	GP partner (1980)
Peter	GP partner (1990)
Barry	GP partner (1990)
Tony	GP partner (1990)
Audrey	Part-time GP partner (1980)
Vivienne	Part-time GP (1980)
Janet	Practice manager
Shellie	Trainee, subsequently new part-time GP partner (2000)
Rachel	Trainee, subsequently new part-time GP partner (2000)
Angela	Senior practice nurse
Rose	Practice nurse
Heather	Practice nurse
Marge	Phlebotomist
Adam	Trainee GP
Tamsin	Trainee GP
Jason	Trainee GP
Urbcester	
Lara	Senior GP partner
Ben	GP partner
Frances	GP partner
Other UK GPs	
Jim	Senior GP partner (1970)
Phil	Senior GP partner (1970)
Sue	Senior GP partner (1970)
David	Senior GP academic (1980)
Oakville	
Craig	Third-year postgraduate resident
Chrissie	First-year postgraduate resident
Surinder	Fourth-year medical student
Josh	Attending physician
Sita	Hospitalist
Doppton	
Becky	Third-year medical student
Hitesh	Third-year medical student

* Qualification year rounded to nearest decade

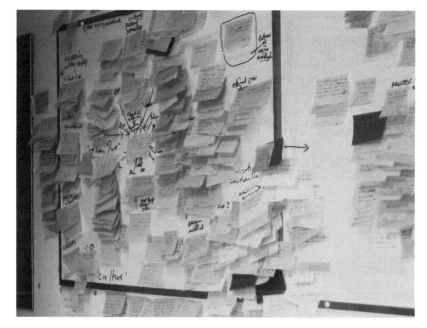

Figure 1.2   Clustering data on the whiteboard.

> I have never followed a science, rich or poor, hard or soft, hot or cold, whose
> moment of truth was not found on a one- or two-meter-square flat surface that
> a researcher with a pen in hand could carefully inspect.
>
> (Latour 1999a: 53)

what seemed to be the main emerging themes and subsequently independently
read several times through all our recent field notes, marking out the themes and
categories of events and exchanges that we had observed (Box 1.1). We critically
shared, reviewed and developed the analysis and as we began to write up the
work we undertook specific observations and interviews to check our emerging
themes. To help validate our analysis we tested the credibility and face validity of
our findings with the participants at our main study site – a technique often used
in such research. But maybe the best 'reality check' has been not so much the
affirmations from Lawndale nor the similarity of the picture at Urbcester, but the
way so many other clinicians who have heard or read about our study have told us
they recognize the picture that emerged.

Conveying the theoretical underpinnings

We have written this book not as a conventional ethnography, but rather as a
developing argument about 'what was really going on'. Our explicit aim for the
book is to relate our findings to our reflections on the relevant theoretical literature
so as to develop an accessible and usable model of the routes by which clinical

Box 1.1 From data to interpretation: an example of the process of analysis

During a conversation about the way the partners learn from each other, a Lawndale GP had told JG that they tended to use 'anecdotes with a purpose'. This comment was noted on a Post-it sticker, together with the date and field-book reference. We placed the sticker on the whiteboard among a growing cluster of around thirty similar notes in a section labelled 'Meetings'. Other items there included 'I'm generally OK about it if a partner later disagrees with my diagnosis or my actions' which had been noted six months earlier in a chat about the extent to which GPs discussed their cases; another, five months earlier, noted that the senior partner had smilingly admitted that his 'younger partners would gently point out' where his practice was not up to date. We felt that these data seemed to relate to another note about how the practice policy on statins had developed from the practitioners' individual decisions, which they had shared through informal chats, eventually leading to a formal meeting where one partner led an audit on statins use; this, they said, had been followed by argument/ discussion and someone agreeing to read up some detail and report back. So perhaps the relevant heading wasn't only 'Meetings', we decided, but broader than that: so we added the label 'Each other'. Near to this cluster was a note of an ironic joke – made in the coffee room when a local consultant was visiting – about how GPs 'always keep up with all the research literature [ha ha]!' and we recalled, on returning to the field notes, how avidly the partners capitalized on the consultant's visit to find out about the latest developments in his field and to ask him – both through the coffee room chat and a lunchtime seminar – about some recent difficult cases. Was this not, we asked ourselves, an example of the importance of 'Meetings', rather an 'Each other'? Or was it 'Education/CPD'? We also linked it to a nearby cluster called 'Opinion leaders' and then realized that while many opinion leaders were external to the practice, some were internal – as in the example of statins policy development. This was amply confirmed when we later saw how partners took leading roles – e.g. on asthma or diabetes – at formal practice meetings. Moreover it became clear as this train of analysis developed that once the group had entrusted themselves to the expertise of an external or internal opinion leader, they would not then question the evidence source. Moreover they often vaguely referred to those self-same 'meetings with each other' when we asked them to reflect on the reasons for decisions about individual patients. So was this indicative of collective mindline development?

(Reproduced from Gabbay and le May 2004 full text version, with permission from BMJ Publishing) knowledge passes into everyday clinical practice. Unfortunately, some of that theoretical literature can be quite perplexing to the very audiences that we believe most need to understand its message: clinicians, clinical students and trainees; health service policy makers, managers, 'change agents', information scientists and 'knowledge officers'. They, after all, are the ones who need to grapple with the practicalities and consequences of introducing evidence-based practice and we have therefore done our utmost to make the ideas accessible to them. Many years of teaching complex philosophical and sociological concepts to initially reluctant clinical students and trainees have emboldened us to write the book not only as an account of our research findings, but also as an introduction to a very wide range of important intellectual fields that ought to be highly relevant to that audience. Readers will therefore find that from time to time we devote space to a relatively straightforward exegesis of the matters listed in Table 1.3, illustrated with material from the ethnography. We recognize the dangers of drawing on such a disparate and sometimes mutually contradictory theoretical base, but all of these strands of thinking have helped us to develop our argument. We hope our treatment of them will not be seen as oversimplification of (or by) the organizational theorists, social scientists and philosophers upon whose work we draw. Our eclecticism is meant to alert our audience to the wealth of illuminative analyses that can help explain how clinicians use information, not to suggest that we think all the approaches are true, still less that we think we have done them justice. However we hope to make a modest contribution not only by synthesizing some of the ideas from these disparate disciplines but also by applying them, often for the first time, to the world of healthcare.

In the following chapters we will draw principally on these bodies of work to illuminate our ethnographic findings. Each chapter contains one or more prologues consisting of vignettes drawn from our observations of key findings that are relevant to the main topics to be dealt with. These by no means represent the full database that informed our analysis. The prologues are designed merely to provide a context for our analysis, to help illuminate the developing argument, and to provide material for further reflection. Some of the vignettes are descriptions of observations, some are quotations from interviews and others are edited extracts from our field notes or reflective comments written shortly after the event. Although every event mentioned is typical of what we observed or heard discussed, they have sometimes been woven into an artificial narrative, for example grouping disparate events or even occasionally weaving together two episodes with two different clinicians into one consultation if that accurately but more efficiently conveys the kind of occurrence that we wish to highlight.[15] Although intended to be read as a narrative (which can be done at any stage before, during or after reading the rest of the chapter) the vignettes are a fragmented series of small episodes. If they seem disjointed, it is partly because of the way we have chosen to present the illustrative material but it also, it must be said, reflects life in primary care.

A word, too, about our citation of references. This is not the place for systematic reviews of literature, which would be an unrealistically massive undertaking across so many broad fields. For that reason we do not intend the references to represent

Table 1.3 Summary of main theoretical approaches

Theme	Main theoretical approach
Multiple roles (Chapter 2)	People play a wide range of often simultaneous, often conflicting roles in their day-to-day practice and clinicians are no exception.
Patterns of thinking and knowledge-in-practice-in-context (Chapter 3)	Clinicians' thinking usually takes the form of pattern recognition explained by psychological theories of schemata, frame theory and illness scripts, working to heuristics and rules of thumb. Professional knowledge as 'knowledge-in-practice-in-context' is quite different from textbook knowledge.
Educational foundations of mindlines (Chapter 4)	Biomedical sciences, practical skills and soft skills are acquired through various forms of learning, including apprenticeship, which, crucially, are linked to socialization.
Developing expertise (Chapter 5)	Clinicians gradually achieve expertise and 'contextual adroitness' that involve different skills at different stages of their development. New knowledge is processed by an organizational knowledge spiral/cycle before being internalized.
The role of storytelling (narrative) in knowledge exchange (Chapter 6)	Although a scientific approach would dictate otherwise, a good deal of what professions learn is by bricolage through anecdotes and personal stories, which are then melded with more formal knowledge.
Communities of practice as a means of learning and developing knowledge (Chapter 7)	Clinicians learn a great deal from their informal interactions with each other, focusing less on the science than on practical knowledge of what works best in what circumstances, and what it means to practice acceptably.
Collective sensemaking (Chapter 8)	By making sense of complex sets of problems through collective, often tacit 'negotiations' clinicians arrive at concepts of illness and disease that go far beyond simple clinical considerations and are continually collectively refined.
Social origins of clinical knowledge (Chapter 9)	Clinical knowledge, which has been ingrained over a lifetime of socialization, is shaped by its inherent context, which can be elucidated through such theoretical approaches as the 'habitus', structuration, actor-network theory and social constructivism.

the full range of evidence for (and against) our arguments. (See also Chapter 4 note 4.) Rather they should be regarded as work, including work we ourselves have published, that helped to shape our thinking; they are what musicians might call 'our main influences'. The references are also intended to help the reader become more familiar with the topic under discussion. To paraphrase a well-used bookselling website, our references often mean 'Readers who have been intrigued (or incensed) by this idea might also like to look at (Reference XYZ)'. To make it easier for readers to see where we have included them, each of the references at the end of the book cites additionally where they appear in the book.[16]

Each chapter ends with a 100-word summary, but here we outline the contents even more briefly. Chapter 2 describes the complex nature of the clinicians' work and the place of formal evidence sources such as research and guidelines in helping to deal with that complexity. We will suggest that clinician's internalized guidelines, which we call their mindlines, are better suited as the means to inform clinical decisions. Mindlines, we assert, are an inevitable part of how and why clinicians think and act as they do. Chapter 3 discusses the nature of mindlines in relation to established psychological concepts such as 'scripts', 'rules of thumb' and 'heuristics', before exploring the nature of knowledge as used by practitioners. In Chapters 4 and 5, we outline how mindlines are laid down in clinical training and are continually reconstructed and collectively refined in the clinical organizational setting, often through 'storytelling', as we describe in Chapter 6. Chapter 7 details the role of communities of practice in developing 'collective mindlines', discussed more fully in Chapter 8, which not only guide clinical thought and action but embody and reinforce the roles of clinicians working in a health system. This will lead us to begin to explore in Chapter 9 some deeper sociological ramifications about the ways in which mindlines imply a reappraisal of the very nature of clinical knowledge. Finally, in Chapter 10, where we summarize our analysis and consider its implications for practitioners, educators, policy makers, academics and researchers (not forgetting patients), we suggest that the evidence-based practice movement needs to understand and take account of the pivotal influence of mindlines if it is to avoid being doomed to continuing disappointment. Good practice should be based on reliable evidence; but the useful evidence that clinicians embody in their mindlines usually turns out to be practice-based evidence.

Chapter 1: Summary

Despite the organizational, economic and cultural pressure on clinicians to adopt evidence-based practice there is still controversy and frustration on all sides about the way it is or is not used. We set out to study how top-quality clinicians use knowledge in practice, to try and understand better the part played by the formal evidence base. To do this we conducted a long-term ethnography in one UK primary care practice, supplemented by other observational studies. We will present the results in the context of a wide literature that should, but unfortunately rarely does, inform the implementation of evidence-based practice.

2 From formal knowledge to guided complexity

Our first prologue focuses on the extent to which formal sources of knowledge such as guidelines and protocols are used in day-to-day clinical practice, and if not, why not. An underlying theme throughout this chapter is also the way clinicians rely on internalized guidelines that they carry in their heads. We start one morning at Lawndale.

❖ *Tony's first patient announces archly 'I can't get it up, I can't keep it up and I'm going on holiday next week with my new lady. Can I have a handful of Viagra, please?' A very thorough history elicits a clear psychological explanation stemming from a recent bereavement, but Tony goes meticulously through his routine of checking for possible physical causes of impotence. He also goes through the full routine of explanation including admonishments about alcohol, even though the patient has said he doesn't drink. The doctor needs to be sure to cover everything even while tailoring what he says as he goes along. After giving a private prescription, because the patient isn't eligible for Viagra on the NHS, Tony feels the need to explain to me why he did not follow the usual protocol but negotiated the quick fix that the patient wanted. 'I know I should have done a hormone profile and waited but with this being his first holiday since his wife died, I think this is what he wanted and needed to get him over the hurdle. It will work for him. The guideline says I should check out all the causes but I'm not following it. I use it as a tester but the thing is that as a GP, I can always see the patient again soon.'*

❖ *Meanwhile towards the end of a long consultation with Peter, when a woman has asked him if she should try a new treatment she's heard about, Peter admits his ignorance about it and says he'll ask around to see if it's likely to help. He tells me later that sometimes you get a run of people who have heard about some information he hasn't come across. Emerging problems with clopidogrel had been one example. There had been letters from the Department of Health and/or the drug company (he couldn't recall which) but it was the local pharmaceutical adviser who had been the most helpful in succinctly summarizing the issues and reliably sorting out a way forward with the drug. Did he look at the NICE (National Institute for Health and Clinical Excellence) website? Sometimes the summary pages; but most of it wasn't relevant to GPs – the pharmaceutical adviser was much more useful, he said. (A point confirmed by many other discussions with GPs who asserted that very little of what they read in NICE guidelines was of direct relevance to them.)*

❖   *The GPs are discussing their frustration about being deluged with guidance, most of which is irrelevant to them, but in amongst which are very important new treatment pathways that they only heard about through other sources but would like to have been alerted to more promptly. 'The other thing', adds Shellie, 'is that you have to wade through* fifteen pages' *(she grimaces and they laugh approvingly) 'of common sense before you get to the* one sentence *that actually changes anything.'*

❖   *Clive's patient has brought a hospital letter that mentions an abstruse condition. 'Never heard of it!' says Clive to the patient and looks it up. He finds nothing of any help and the treatment prescribed for it at the hospital isn't on his IT system. He makes a mental note to find out more.*

❖   *The GPs tell us about many different places where they can go for information. Clive says he uses centrally issued guidelines to check things occasionally and quite likes Prodigy (now NHS Clinical Knowledge Summaries [CKS]), which is accessible from his practice computer, but he admits he's in a minority there. Tony says: 'I'd probably start with the Internet. Clinnix, for example, is an excellent place to look. I also like Doctor on Line, which I use to get patient information. But I often think I must come back to look at the information that's provided for doctors [as opposed to patients] in those things.' Similar questioning of all the GPs at Lawndale, Urbcester and elsewhere elicits a long list of sources, including Mentor, SIGN (Scottish Intercollegiate Guidelines Network), local guidelines from the hospital and the pharmaceutical adviser, GP Update, Pulse, Clinical Evidence, the National Prescribing Centre's* MeReC Bulletin, *the* Drug and Therapeutics Bulletin, *GP Notebook, Doctor, the online National Library for Health, Patient UK, NICE, drug datasheets, a wide range of favourite books such as the* Oxford Handbooks, *and – probably the most widely used – the* British National Formulary. *What's noticeable is the variety and the fact that they so rarely look at any of them while we observe them.*

❖   *During our first week we are impressed by the well-organized library in the coffee room full of what appear to be useful books, journals, guidelines, circulars etc. (Figure 2.1). Four years later we walk in one morning to find it has gone. No one used it much, they tell us; they wanted the space to accommodate more easy chairs and a small table for clinical meetings flanked by a desk with two computers.*

❖   *David, an academic GP who has published widely about evidence-based practice, has emailed a reply to my query as to where he looks for guidance during his surgeries. His reply reads: 'it's the inbuilt Mentor [expert system] that I would refer to (probably an average of once a day at least – say around 1:20 to 1:25 patient contacts) and quite often I'll visit the other sites with patients to show them in real time what to explore at their leisure later. I use the BNF about 1:4 patient contacts . . . I think there are other clever GPs that access all sorts of things like Cochrane and Medline and NICE on their handheld Blackberries etc. and they keep telling me there's other resources on the PC at work, but I've no bloody idea how to find them . . . I will scour journals and Medline and even books for general education, and look at NICE printouts (I think they're on our practice intranet which I can't use properly).'*

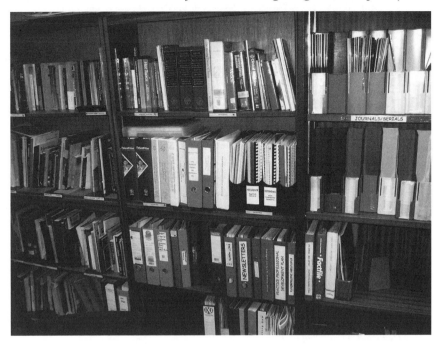

Figure 2.1 The Lawndale coffee room library.

❖ *Invited to use Barry's room while he is away, I spot thirty or so laminated guideline charts stacked on Barry's bookshelf among all the textbooks and folders. I peruse his notice board. There are two pages cut from a GP magazine about travel vaccinations, one with an article about St John's wort for depression, a laminated chart on managing duodenal ulcers that Peter had helped a local working party to compile and that (unusually for guidelines) seems to be on nearly every partner's wall, and a guideline on meningitis. (I recall how the fear of missing a case of meningitis is a GP's worst nightmare.)*

❖ *Vivienne – a part-time GP on a 'back to work' scheme – has several guideline charts on her notice board including one for anaphylactic shock. She tells me she put it up there after she had had someone go into shock while in her surgery, when she had to call her more senior colleagues to help deal with a rapidly evolving emergency. She'd realized it would have helped her to have a quick guide to hand. Fortunately she hasn't ever had to use it since.*

❖ *Extract from transcript of taped interview with Jean: 'I mean you can't say, "Oh yes Mrs Bloggs I'll just have a look in here and see what it says", but I mean, you know, I think really probably most doctors in all honesty probably work to their own little guidelines anyway, don't they? I mean how do you know what you're going to prescribe? It's probably from your own little formulary of medication. So I think, well I would like to think, most of us probably do stick to the vast majority or the main thrusts of some of those guidelines, so the GP sees somebody who's had a myocardial infarction . . . I mean certainly I would look and make sure that they're on a statin and look and see what their cholesterol was and make sure it was below five, and try and do that fairly opportunistically. That's not always obviously possible depending upon the situation but yeah.'*

❖ *Extract from transcript of taped interview with Peter: Do you have a sense of how much the GPs and nurses are actually using formal guidelines in their day-to-day work with patients? 'I think the nurses are good at using them and I think the doctors tend to put them on the shelf. It's not practical to open up a protocol while you're in consultation, that's what I find, so the protocols that I use are the ones that are stored in my head and unless I'm going over them frequently then bits may disappear so it needs to be ingrained I think on my brain to be a good protocol and I suppose what these [QPA] meetings are doing is reinforcing the good practice. So although we're not actually going line by line through the protocols we're going over the things that we really think are important and that actually form the basis of the protocol. The nurses do adhere to them much better and if the protocol in some way can be incorporated into one the intranet systems then it gets done even better. I find them a bit unwieldy trying to open it up in the middle of consultation.' And after the patient's gone? 'Sometimes yeah if there's something that rings a bell and I'm not quite sure about it and, particularly if you've got the opportunity for getting them back, if you're sending them off for a blood test you can say okay we'll discuss that when you come back and you can brush up on what you're going to say.'*

❖ *Clive tells how he was in discussion with a senior academic GP who has helped produce national guidelines for the management of mild to moderate depression in primary care. Clive had teased him about how dogmatic academics can be about such things, for example about not restricting the number of repeat prescriptions for antidepressants (part of the guideline). 'I have about fifteen patients', Clive had told him, 'who I keep on repeats because they are stable and always relapse if they come off the pills. I know it's against your published guidelines so I just say "come and see me every three months or so" and I give them another prescription.' The professor had replied that – contrary to his own guidelines – he would do exactly the same.*

❖ *At a (tape recorded) planning meeting for a research project on primary care commissioning an experienced GP spontaneously says: 'In the end the decision that GPs make, which generally is based on individual patients in the consulting room, is done on a kind of an intuition basis . . . It is really rare, I think, to explicitly use knowledge that comes from a guideline or a protocol. It does happen but the nature of the illness that is brought to GPs is such that most of the time the guideline and protocol are irrelevant. You have to fall back on a kind of intuition which is generated from all sorts of sources and I think most of the time you can't say where you got it from . . . The other thing is that GPs have been relatively independent and not doing what they're told as PCTs had to do what they're told and they had to follow guidelines and protocols.'*

❖ *An independent software developer for NHS clinical pathways tells us: 'Every time you speak to a clinician and ask them what their pathway is for any condition they look blank and then maybe a few minutes later remember there is one somewhere. And then if they do find it, it's usually out of date and not fit for purpose for one reason or another. We were finally given a decent one the other day and within five minutes we'd found two fundamental logical flaws that made it impossible for us to use it in our software.'*

❖ *Rose and Angela are chatting in the treatment room about yesterday's work and a patient Rose is expecting later for a dressing. Heather starts a session of telephone triage before seeing her own list of patients. She quickly moves through six telephone calls ranging from the concerns of an elderly lady's daughter about her mother's falls to a mother worried about medication for her twenty-month-old child. Some calls result in appointments to see her later that day or referral to a doctor for a consultation or home visit, some result in advice about treatment, and others end with reassurances that she will be there all day and could be contacted again. At the end of the session I ask Heather how she developed her knowledge about triage. A course is the first thing to spring to mind, then her experience, which she says 'just built up' coupled with some feedback on her early calls and their outcomes from the doctors in the practice. She shows me a file from her triage course, which also contains aides-memoires that she made up for herself in the early days of triage. The information for these she says came from the course material, a minor injuries manual produced by a leading pharmaceutical company, some papers and flash cards from journals, information leaflets, patient fact sheets, surgery protocols for home visits, guidelines from the local hospital about asthma and articles from women's and other popular magazines – these she says are useful because of their lay language, which helped her to know what to say on the phone. Although she says she doesn't use them now – 'it's all sort of in my head' – she keeps adding bits to the file; she likes bits of paper!*

❖ *Later in the treatment room Marge the phlebotomist is taking blood from her last patient of the afternoon, chatting sympathetically about the problems of the hospital outpatients waiting system. Rose treats a leg ulcer with Iodosorb. I ask her why she uses that. She has used it for a long time and (unlike a new one she tried recently, which went badly wrong and which she'll never use again) it usually seems to work fine. Anyway, patients come out of hospital with it on, so it's probably still the one to use. I ask if she ever reads up such things. She mentions* Nursing Times *and* Wound Care *but admits she rarely reads such articles there unless she really needs to. She is more likely to ask the community nurses who treat a lot of these.*

❖ *That evening in one of the first QPA meetings Nick is explaining to the nurses that we need to show we are treating patients because it is proven to work, not because we have always done it that way. Tony adds that evidence-based practice also requires us to audit and check that we are doing what is needed, but that does not mean we have to follow the evidence-based protocols slavishly. Janet agrees and adds that indeed the QPA requires us to take account of the patients' views as well. That moot point of tension between protocol and pragmatism remains unresolved as they go on to try and allay the nurses' worries about audit, confidentiality and the need to avoid a blame culture.*

❖ *In Lara's surgery at Urbcester, a fourth-year pharmacy student is asking for a repeat pre-scription for a drug that he has found helps prevent his migraine. He has been to see an eminent neurologist who is an acknowledged migraine expert. They read the consultant's long letter together. ('You can tell it was private consultation by the length of the letter', Lara jokes.) The specialist has written that he does not give preventive treatment for more than six months at a time. Lara notes that, although he states this quite dogmatically, he gives no reason. She cannot think of a good reason for his view and she can see that the patient – who is after all almost a fully trained pharmacist – is very keen to continue. She prescribes it.*

❖   *In the office next door Ben is typing his notes, one-fingered, after saying goodbye to an Afghan patient with a young baby that is not thriving. Communication with her had been almost impossible, although despite her lack of English it had become clear that her husband had gone missing in the fighting there. He shows me the pop-up that has just appeared on the computer screen and feigns a look of horror. 'Oh dear. I didn't do anything to tick the prevention box.' He launches into a mocking rant at some guidance he has just had from the RCGP. 'We're supposed to provide videos, all in English, to show how we elicit patient concerns. We have to record smoking habits, but I didn't notice anything about chewing betel nuts [common among Urbcester's immigrants] . . . Nothing on domestic violence either', he snorts. 'And we're supposed to summarize 90 per cent of all our notes if we want to be trainers. With our patient turnover?! We can hardly keep up with registering them so that they appear on screen! And here we are, struggling to provide continuity of care while patients and doctors come and go at a rate of knots.' He laughs ironically. I notice that after the next woman – an eighty-two-year-old covered with bruises from yet another fall after yet another night on the drink – he records 'precontemplative' in the prevention section of her notes on screen. It is a moot point whether this is an ironic protest or a genuine note to back up his later discussion with her regular GP to see what else can be done to help her. Perhaps it is both.*

Research-based evidence, expert systems and guidelines

There are many sources of evidence that primary care clinicians can make use of to guide their decisions and which we were expecting to see in use at Lawndale (M.B. Gabbay 1999; le May 1999; Cullum *et al.* 2008). Yet throughout our observations there it was clear that although clinicians might occasionally browse through journals they rarely directly consulted research articles or systematic reviews of evidence even when seeking out answers to specific questions. Nor did they ever show signs of having gone through the steps of accessing and critically appraising evidence that are advocated by the proponents of evidence-based healthcare (Figure 1.1), not once in the whole time we were observing them. Why should they, they reasoned, when they could rely on others who were trained to do just that? And yet we were studying the Lawndale clinicians because they were top-notch clinicians. The authorities had recommended them as being among the very best in the area, trainees in the region were falling over themselves to be trained there, the recent Fellowships by Assessment had confirmed that at least three of them were practising to the highest standards of UK primary care, and their audits generally confirmed that all the partners practised at a similar standard, which stood up well against criteria based on current evidence-based guidance.[1] So, to see how research evidence was being used in this indisputably good primary care practice, we had to widen our focus to include other routes by which research evidence might move into practice, such as guidelines, expert systems and contractual targets.[2]

There was no shortage of evidence-based clinical guidelines; a well-intentioned plethora of guidance unendingly arrived on the practitioner's desk by post, in journals, or through the internet. Almost daily there was a reminder from some authority or other about the proper way to deal with some given clinical problem.[3] Yet, during nearly forty hours that we spent observing the Lawndale clinicians with their patients, we never saw them consult a guideline to help with a decision, although on a couple of occasions they pointed to a laminated guideline on their walls in order to explain something to the patient or to one of us. At the Urbcester practice likewise we saw no one using a guideline to help them during the surgery. The Lawndale nurses told us they would turn to a guideline only when (rarely) faced with an unfamiliar problem, and that once they were familiar with the procedure – for example nurse triage of patients with an unusual condition – they would never need to look at it again. So we had to conclude that, if formal, research-based knowledge was entering the practice of these exemplary frontline clinicians through the kind of guidelines that we were expecting them to use, it was certainly not doing so in 'real time'.

That is not at all to say that the clinicians ignored guidelines. Indeed, as we shall see, they had (indirectly) internalized much of the content.[4] The doctors told us (and our observations confirmed it) that they might look at guidelines in their own time – perhaps to check on a query that they had made a note to come back to, or more generally to ensure that their own practice was generally up to standard, or perhaps in preparation for a practice meeting where they were being expected to review the practice policy for a given clinical condition.[5] These were incorporated into formal practice protocols for many conditions, which were sometimes the basis also for pop-up reminders that they themselves designed ('SOPHIEs') to ensure that staff did not forget to carry out appropriate actions for patients with any given condition (Figure 2.2). But in general they tended not to need these. As for guidelines that they received from other agencies, Peter, for example, told us that when a new one arrived in the post he would leaf through it as a way of keeping up to date – as long as it looked authoritative, impartial and well produced[6] – reassuring himself that there was nothing major that needed changing in his practice. 'But', he said (despite having a couple of guidelines pinned on his surgery wall, one of which he had helped to write), 'to be honest I don't find them very helpful'. If a guideline was too far out of line with what he already did, he told us, there was usually good reason to dismiss it as irrelevant or biased; but if something new struck him as sensible and worthy of consideration, he would follow it up, often by discussing it with colleagues before deciding how to handle the discrepancy. (See Chapters 5–7.) But generally, he said, 'they [guidelines] sit on the shelf'. This was a typical response, even from those who said that guidelines could sometimes be helpful. There was indeed plenty of guidance to be seen on the bookshelves of their surgeries alongside the textbooks and other general sources that they might consult when they had to and in the practice

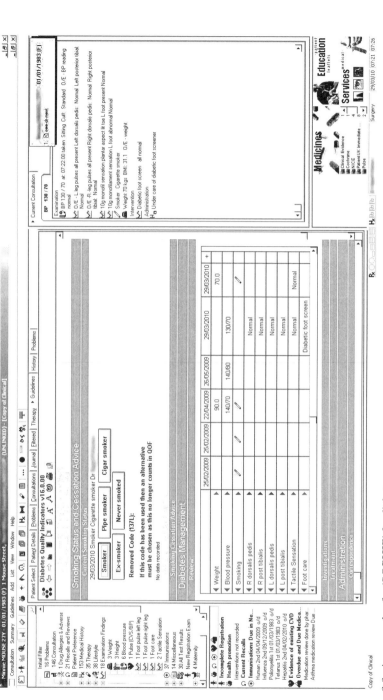

Figure 2.2 An example of a 'SOPHIE' for diabetes care.

library. So guidelines played their part in helping clinicians know whether they were in line with current guidance or not, by casually browsing them (as others besides Peter had told us), or by specifically using them to check points of doubt, or – more likely – by joining discussions about them and as a result being able to reassure themselves that their practice was up to date.

As for expert systems, although Lawndale's IT system allowed easy direct access to a number of them – and more generally to the internet – it was very rare for the Lawndale doctors to use them during their surgeries.[7] Clive was an enthusiast for an expert system (Prodigy) but admitted that none of his partners liked it. By their own average estimates in 2001 they might use such facilities less than once a week when with a patient, mostly to download information to give to the patient. This usage has generally increased a little since then to perhaps once a day,[8] but during our observations of clinical activity (2001) we *never* saw them use such systems to guide their actions in real time and, although we did see Clive occasionally use the system to look something up that he was unfamiliar with, even he was more prone to turn to a book than to the IT system. The generally low usage was not confined to Lawndale. At Urbcester in 2001, after we had had a conversation with Ben about using their in-house expert system and his favourite internet sources, he grinned when he realized he had just left his computer to go to the bookshelf to try and identify a rash. 'Oh dear, I've gone to a textbook and not the internet!' Yet his Urbcester colleagues had tipped Ben as being the keenest user of their bespoke in-house system. It turned out that he hardly ever used it. Trainees were usually a different story. Those at Lawndale, several others that we talked to elsewhere, and likewise some relatively recently qualified GPs, none of whom we observed in practice, told us that they used the internet-based expert systems quite often – perhaps up to a handful of times a day – during their surgeries and that they learnt a lot from them.[9] However, even they conducted the vast majority of their consultations without relying on the explicit use of guidelines or other formal sources.

Guidelines have been the main channel through which the evidence base has been transmitted to clinicians in the UK.[10] Surveys of GPs (Newton *et al.* 1996; Siriwardena 1995; Watkins *et al.* 1999) have suggested that they are generally quite well disposed towards them, a finding confirmed internationally in a systematic review of thirty surveys worldwide (Farquhar *et al.* 2002).[11] A recent UK survey of 800 GPs, of whom half responded, suggests that, whereas awareness of hypertension guidelines was high, agreement and adherence were much lower (Heneghan *et al.* 2007). But surveys, often with relatively low response rates and usually based on hypothetical questions, may not give the whole story. A qualitative study in England, for example, showed that GPs' largely positive attitudes towards guidelines did little to ensure their uptake (Dowswell *et al.* 2001). An interview-based study with twenty GPs in the West of England revealed broadly similar attitudes to those that we found (Langley *et al.* 1998; Lipman *et al.* 2004), but a more recent interview-based study in Norway suggested a much more overtly sceptical attitude (Carlsen and Norheim 2008); Grol *et al.* (1998), who audited the decisions of Dutch GPs against guideline recommendations, found that 'compliance' depended largely on the attributes of the guidelines. More recently, Dutch GP focus groups gave a variety of reasons for not complying, chief of which were that they disagreed with them, had organizational constraints, were unaware of specifics or found them ambiguous or unclear (Lugtenberg *et al.* 2009). The great majority of 14,000 Australian GPs declined when offered free external expert system guidance (*BMJ Clinical Evidence*) as part of an implementation research project (Buchan *et al.* 2009).

Certainly the attitudes at Lawndale to guidelines and to searching the 'evidence base' varied; Jean and Barry (p. 141), for example, were more prone to turn to published guidance than some of the other partners. Our discussions with other GPs around the UK confirm that some of them do look up such sources, mainly on the internet. Our observations and discussions allowed us to speculate that the differences, regardless of discipline, may perhaps be related to, among other factors, the clinician's age, stage of training and experience, with younger clinicians in training being more likely to turn to such sources, but such questions will require further and different kinds of research (see p. 197). Although our study was not designed to investigate variability in the use of guidelines, what we can corroborate is the fact that clinicians' attitudes towards, and use of, guidelines do vary. Moreover they were ambivalent; one of the GPs' frequent complaints about all the guidelines made available to them was that was no efficient way to separate the useful (sometimes essential) wheat from the deluge of chaff that was irrelevant because it was either too obvious or too abstruse. We cannot and do not claim that our observations were typical, but we can say with confidence that the excellent and experienced clinicians that we observed at Lawndale and Urbcester normally found it neither necessary nor helpful to refer to guidelines or other sources of evidence directly during their day-to-day practice. Clearly we needed to find out why that was.

Was it because they already knew what these sources would say (Freeman and Sweeney 2001)? They did claim, as one put it, to 'already have a pretty good inkling of what was in most of the national guidance', but no one could be expected to know the detail of the relevant evidence across the wide range of conditions that the clinicians were dealing with. There was no suggestion that the established GPs assiduously read and committed guidelines to memory. On the contrary, they treated them somewhat askance, at best browsing them or consulting them to check specific questions – sometimes specifically because they had heard about a new guideline that they should take note of. Yet when they audited their practice on any aspect of care, as they frequently did, it generally conformed well to criteria based on the available guidelines (see, e.g., p. 148), and when they discussed their practice among themselves they appeared to be well aware of the main content of the relevant guidelines (see Chapter 8). Clive, for example, when asked without warning, was able to rehearse the British Hypertension Society thresholds for treatment (albeit with some scepticism about their feasibility; and, as we usually found, such formal knowledge was being called upon to help prove a point, not to inform practice). So, in general they justifiably believed that they were doing more or less what the guidelines recommended and if not that there was good reason for the differences. But they were not, and would never claim to be, omniscient about the latest evidence or guidance. During consultations there were inevitably moments of uncertainty, doubt and lack of knowledge. Even then, however, they did not turn immediately to guidelines, expert systems or other formal sources of evidence.

Did they avoid using guidelines when practising because they were reluctant to be seen looking something up and revealing their ignorance? Probably not, as they did sometimes look up drug doses or side effects before prescribing a drug; their *British National Formularies* often looked well thumbed. Nor were they afraid to openly call a colleague in to help solve a problem when they were with a patient. Moreover, when we asked them, they professed that in front of most patients there was no shame in openly doing such things. But still we did not see them consult the expert systems, guidelines or similar sources of evidence during a surgery or clinic.

Was it because consultations were so swift that there was no time to look things up? Probably not, since if that were the case one might have expected them to quickly check a guideline or other formal source while waiting for the next patient and we did not see them do this. They told us that they sometimes made a note to check something later, but we saw this being done only a couple of times during our forty or so hours of observing their clinical work. As we will see in Chapters 6–8 such subsequent checking was more likely to take the form of an informal discussion with colleagues than looking up a guideline, a book or other 'evidence-based' sources. So we concluded that neither professional pride nor lack of time was the reason to eschew guidelines during their day-to-day practice.

Was it that they didn't trust or believe the guidelines? Here the answer was more variable. It was clear that some sources of guidance were regarded as more helpful and reliable than others and that some were derided as being quite unrealistic for general practice (see, for example, Graham *et al.* 2000). A typical comment about the latter might be that the guidance was far too complex and/or lengthy to be of any real use (see p. 20), or – often relatedly – that it was obviously written by some 'expert' (a term often used sneeringly in this context to imply that the authors had no understanding of the realities of general practice) or that there was an underlying motive behind the guideline (e.g. to save money or to promote a particular commercial, bureaucratic or political interest) that cut across the GPs' own ethos of care (Links 2006). But they did not simply ignore the content of guidelines; indeed, where there was continuing doubt about some aspect of their practice, they might well turn to guidelines and other evidence sources to inform their deliberations, when they would interpret them selectively. In general much of the content of the guidance was, when reflected upon and discussed, in line with what they already did and where it was not then – as we shall see in Chapters 5 and 8 – they might selectively incorporate it into their practice or after due consideration might actively decide to reject it. So a blanket lack of credibility or trust was not the reason why guidelines were so infrequently consulted.

Clinicians are 'science-using, information-sorting interpreters of timebound circumstances', so they always need to use judgement to 'particularize' their knowledge (Montgomery 2006: 174), and to do so in a wider organizational context (May 2007). So, did guidelines have such a marginal role because they rarely matched the exact circumstances of an individual patient (Oswald and Bateman 1998, 2000; Summerskill 2005; Rothwell 2005; May *et al.* 2006a)? After all, guidelines are usually about typical, straightforward cases, which many patients are not. However, we found no evidence that this was a major reason. Quite apart from the fact that most of their patients did follow the normal patterns of illness, it is most unlikely that competent practitioners would ignore science-based guidance simply because patients vary. After all, clinical practice, as many have observed, is very much about marrying the generalities of science to the specifics of individual care.[12] Were guidelines unhelpful because they are based on clinical trials that inevitably rely on statistical odds and yet one never knows how those odds will work out for a given patient (Byrne 2004)? Again, good clinicians know that their job entails matching general probabilities with the individual prognostic probability of each idiosyncratic patient whilst having only a very limited comprehension of either. As Hunter stresses at the outset of her seminal study of 'doctors' stories', '[t]he practice of medicine is an interpretive activity' (Hunter 1991: i).[13] In fact most GPs and practice nurses are unlikely even to be aware of, let alone fully understand, the statistical inferences on which guidance is based (usually of the form that X per cent of Y patients recovered compared with Z per cent of the control group within a statistical confidence of *P*). Perhaps recognizing this, most guidelines tend simply to state that in cases of A, all things being equal, one should do B. But all things rarely are equal, as only the most naïve proselytizers of evidence-based practice would deny, and guideline writers expect full well that their users will modulate them in the light of individual circumstances. Since practitioners know that guidelines are *intended* to be used with clinical judgement, not as a fixed protocol, we concluded that discrepancies between patients were not the reason for forgoing their use when faced with a problem case.

A related but simpler explanation might be that in specific situations, as Peter had suggested, guidelines were just not much help.[14] This was closer to what most of the Lawndale clinicians seemed to think. (Guidelines, like research knowledge and formal education, decontextualize knowledge [Lave 1996: 22] but practitioners inevitably had to contextualize it.) Catch-22 again:[15] guidelines could overcomplicate the obvious and yet not be detailed enough to deal with the actual problem. Where a patient's condition was straightforward, then a competent clinician would find a guideline superfluous; they knew how to deal with routine cases. And if the case were unusually complicated, then no guideline would cover that particular eventuality. The lack of adequately specific guidance for any given clinical situation echoed something we had repeatedly found over the years in our previous studies of the implementation of research evidence in practice (Dopson and Gabbay 1995; Mulhall *et al.* 1996; CSAG 1998; Dopson *et al.* 2001; Surender *et al.* 2002). Even in clinical areas chosen precisely because there was good evidence that practice needed to change, the clinicians and policy makers that we had studied had time and again run into the problem that research evidence from trials and systematic reviews was simply not available at the level of detail they needed for key aspects of care. In most instances, as soon as the practitioners had begun delving into the specifics, the strength of available evidence had seemed to evanesce – either because the scientific results of the trials (even if they *were* robust and valid) did not reliably transfer across to the population of local patients or because the research questions did not focus on the clinical problem facing the practitioner. An example at Lawndale, dealt with in more detail in Chapter 8, was the evidence about screening patients for early kidney failure, where national NHS guidance turned out to be based on a population of Americans very unlike the elderly folk of Woodside, and there was no evidence available to guide many of the practical details of undertaking such a programme of screening. So part of the reason for the failure to refer explicitly to formal sources of research and guidance does indeed seem to be a lack of formal, research-based guidance for a great deal of what clinicians actually do.[16]

A complexity of roles and goals

The prologue to this section highlights the multiple roles that clinicians play, requiring them to balance often conflicting goals within the same clinical decision.

❖ *Clive's working day begins as usual at 7.30, and before he's seen his first patient he has had an email correspondence about a local cost-effectiveness committee he's on, spent fifteen minutes sorting out a problem with Peter's computer, discussed a personnel matter with Janet (practice manager) and checked a new patient health promotion leaflet. He also begins to work through a pile of mostly patient-related paperwork (repeat prescriptions, laboratory results, hospital letters etc.) and reviews the applicants for their trainee registrar post. Jean, meanwhile, sitting in her surgery, is taking time out from her paperwork to look at last week's* British Medical Journal (BMJ) *– she likes to keep up – but is interrupted by a phone call from a patient.*

❖ *The 'cholesterol consultation': Nick sees an overweight patient whom he knows well, whose high blood pressure is well controlled but who has not been able to lose weight and has now had a blood result showing a high cholesterol level. The patient – a non-smoker – is clearly at increased risk and Nick prescribes a statin. He also spends three or four minutes explaining and reassuring – a mixture of pop science and pop psychology. A lot of what he says sounds routine and some of it frankly seems irrelevant to this particular person (I am reminded of Tony's routine spiel about Viagra) but nevertheless he is subtly beginning the job of persuading the man that he will need to adapt his lifestyle. Nick bends over backwards not to sound censorious (a joke and a smile about not having to give up all the good things of life, not to be too austere about it all). He is trying to educate and advise, even persuade, whilst at the same time also avoiding alienating him. Otherwise the goal of gradually helping him to manage what will now become a lifelong chronic condition may become much harder to achieve. Nick must now assess the patient's needs (which seem to be very different from what the patient wants) and negotiate a workable and acceptable path forward.*

Explaining and advising and counselling, which might entail supporting the patient through difficult decisions, life events, behaviour change or coming to terms with a difficult situation, has taken a substantial proportion of the allotted ten minutes, not least because there has been an element of negotiation and compromise. I ask him afterwards whether he has any coronary heart disease (CHD) prevention guidelines. 'Maybe' he grins wickedly, glancing up towards his bookshelf with a look that says he has no idea where. He says it's 'in my head' and 'down to experience'. When I check online later it seems that the clinical matters dealt with in, say, the 'Joint British recommendations on prevention of coronary heart disease in clinical practice: summary' (British Cardiac Society et al. *2000) seem relevant to only a tiny part of what Nick has done today for this patient. (Tony, with a similar case later, does very similar things, but also shows the patient the 'Sheffield risk chart' to help explain the best way to reduce risk.)*

❖   *Clive prescribes a statin to a woman at moderate risk of CHD. He sits on a committee to review cost-effectiveness of medicines, but says he tries very hard not to think in that mode when faced with a patient; not to 'mix the roles'. Yet while talking about how he has weighed up the risks and benefits of statins for cholesterol in this woman, while showing me the Sheffield tables, he says that he has to 'make decisions in the interests of the country as well as the patient'.*

❖   *Nick spends a long time explaining and dissuading an elderly woman who wants to change her diuretic because of a (probably spurious) low potassium reading. Nick wins the day and the diuretic stays. Immediately afterwards the woman, still a little disgruntled, mentions an unrelated skin problem and asks for a particular ointment. Nick would not normally use it but he immediately concedes. The compromise to 'clinical correctness' seems justified since by giving her that favour he is keeping her on side in order to manage her more vital heart failure.*

❖   *Clive is called to an elderly patient's home. Complaining of 'ice in my chest', she looks unwell. Should she be admitted immediately or could the practice, together with community services, manage her? She is receiving care from various local authority and community services and has been regularly attending a clinic run by one of the practice nurses. Clive weighs up the clinical and social pros and cons from the patient's perspective, following which he phones the hospital and arranges admission. But a great deal more has gone into that decision. The practice is under pressure: from the local trust to try and limit, in principle, the number of referrals to hospital; from the pharmaceutical budget to monitor and minimise its prescription costs; from the university to teach best practice to the students; from the community services to liaise closely over the home care of chronically ill patients; and so on. Clive also knows the strengths and limitations of the community nursing services and his own practice nurses, not least because he has played his part in organizing the ways in which they would operate and inter-relate to deal with the patient if she stays out of hospital. This includes everything from the way they delegate and carry out clinical work, to how they use the IT system, to how they deal with the call when she phones from home. Clive knows there is a new bed manager at Westchurch Hospital who could make life difficult over a marginal decision to admit such as this one (because they not only have a new admissions referral policy, but are running into a financial crisis), but the patient would prefer Westchurch to the*

Northton General. The Westchurch physician on take that day is technically excellent but brusque, whereas Clive would prefer her to be under a geriatrician at Northton who may be more sympathetic to this patient's psychosocial needs. As Clive phones a few key people – all on first name terms – to ensure admission, I am left wondering how helpful the new referral guidelines from Westchurch are going to be in practice.

❖ *Janet, the practice manager, receives a public health notice requesting the recall of all patients under the age of eighteen who had had a particular batch of Hepatitis A vaccination, which had been suboptimal, and who required revaccination. The problem of using the information system to retrieve the names and addresses of those patients proves thorny. As she goes through the process of trying to solve it, we note that she requires over twenty items of knowledge, few of which have a 'formal' source one can just look up. They range from how urgent this is, to the age at which boosters are given, to who prescribed it when, to how to run a query on the software system, to whether they were paid per dose or per patient, to how to write to patients without causing alarm. Most of them she already knows, but several require her to ask others such as Nick about the clinical urgency of the problem, Angela (senior practice nurse) about other clinical and procedural details, the practice's finance person about contractual payments, and someone that Nick has met through a software users group on a national network, and whom she emails for a final solution. An hour (and several interruptions) later the task is all but completed and the recall letters can be sent to the right patients.*

❖ *In the midst of a later meeting about how to code blood results in the computer, Peter asks in passing how he should have coded a certain anaesthetic cream 'without dressing' (which costs £1) as opposed to the same cream 'with dressing' (which costs £10), which the local cottage hospital had prescribed. Gasps of horror at the price. Nick says 'Surely we should all use the simple cream. Can't we just use cling-film for the dressing?' Tony adds that it would be better, actually, than the tiny bio-occlusive dressing that is supplied. Audrey says that Westchurch Hospital does use cling-film. That settles it: a two-minute dialogue that includes a mixture of economics, 'common sense', experience, local expert example and colleague assent, all sparked by an anomaly in computer coding, has clearly changed several people's minds about the management of painful skin lesions. They joke that they should send a tube of the plain cream to the local cottage hospital so it doesn't happen again.*

❖ *In a clinical meeting devoted to coronary heart disease that Lawndale let us tape record, the following are the main topics discussed by the seven GPs, three nurses and a phlebotomist during the first forty-five minutes, before they go on to discuss Jean's proposed protocol for heart failure patients (pp. 141, 148) for a further fifteen minutes:*

- *the role of the national service framework and its targets;*
- *local population statistics and case load;*
- *local services (quantity and quality of various hospital and community rehabilitation arrangements, and how to make best use of them);*
- *how to 'run lists' on the computer;*
- *call and recall systems;*
- *grey areas of interpreting cholesterol tests;*

- *'numbers needed to treat';*
- *review of most cost-effective treatments (done on PowerPoint as a spoof Who Wants to Be a Millionaire? quiz);*
- *personal reflections on practice patterns, reviewed and debated;*
- *cost comparisons;*
- *problems of computer coding;*
- *value of BMI (body mass index) measurement;*
- *health promotion payments to GPs;*
- *prevention of diabetes;*
- *the place of diet in the care of CHF;*
- *indications for statins and beta blockers;*
- *use of echocardiography services (ideal and actual);*
- *blood pressure control (feasibility of target readings);*
- *problems of polypharmacy;*
- *how to get the message across to patients;*
- *how hard to push if they are unwilling;*
- *setting up systems in a clinic;*
- *training staff;*
- *a local scheme for reviewing and improving care;*
- *how and when they order LDL/HDL (low-density lipid to high-density lipid) ratios/ cholesterol/triglycerides (i.e. what best to write on the form and why) and how they interpret them;*
- *should these tests be done fasting or not?;*
- *what local consultants suggest and why;*
- *risk tables and their pros and cons;*
- *published trial results;*
- *funding available from the PCT;*
- *problems with the database;*
- *work allocation;*
- *the problems of getting locums;*
- *delegation/referral to nurses;*
- *whether to adopt another locally successful scheme for recording and following up patients.*

By the end of even the first day's observation at Lawndale we were already struck by the fact that the doctors in their surgeries, and to a lesser extent the nurses in their clinics, were doing far more than the technical medical or nursing care of patients. We had expected that they would have to adapt and personalize clinical science to suit individual circumstances, and to balance their clinical and administrative roles, but there was much more to it than that. In the course of a few minutes, if not simultaneously, we might see them slip effortlessly and instinctively between several roles, each aimed towards different goals that could never be the focus of mere clinical evidence. An example was the vexed question of prostate cancer screening. The best available scientific evidence was clear: screening a symptomless patient not only was cost-ineffective but might be damaging to the patient. Yet if an elderly, symptomless but worried man asked for a prostate cancer (prostate-specific antigen; PSA) test, there was a balance to be struck between conflicting goals coming from clinical care, rational screening policy, managerial targets and professional standards. No guideline would take account of this constellation of concerns when advising whether to order the test or not. Or, in the case of a child with a sore throat, while a GP may be treating the infection (which might well be the subject of a guideline) she might also be educating the parent, meeting prescribing targets, saving time, delegating tasks, gaining trust, anticipating contractual audits and so on (which were not part of any guideline and yet were an integral part of the transactions we were observing). At the heart of this dilemma was the conflict of roles between the GP as medical technician, educator, contractor, manager and much more, and any role conflict inevitably impacts on performance (Jaén *et al.* 1994; Presseau *et al.* 2009).

Hage and Powers (1992) have suggested that one of the key features of our epoch is the 'complexification' of roles.[17] People in all parts of society need to contend with ever more complicated and diverse roles in order to satisfy ever more inconsistent demands. The old 'role scripts' are inadequate, roles are redefined, new kinds of knowledge and skills are needed to fulfil them, and this in turn impacts on one's sense of identity. For clinicians, for example, the tensions are quite explicit between making the consultation as long as necessary to help the patient, but as short as possible to help those still waiting to be seen and to help the smooth running of the clinic. Yet in the 1970s JG worked briefly with a world-renowned specialist in a major London teaching hospital who would often take a whole morning to see just three or four outpatients in painstaking detail. Nowadays, the old-fashioned, erudite, unworldly doctor who can spend as much time as is needed with a patient to indulge in the science and ensure that all angles are fully covered has been replaced by the multitasking, some would say harassed and embattled, modern consultant with efficiency targets to be met, managerial responsibilities to be fulfilled, multidisciplinary training obligations to be honoured and so on. The necessary skills have changed accordingly. Similar transformations in the identity of the practitioner – both doctor and nurse – have occurred in primary care, even if they are disguised by what appear to be relatively routine clinical encounters that appear smooth and straightforward.

It was clear that, in meeting the conflicting goals that were required of them, the Lawndale clinicians were inherently and constantly playing a wide range of roles. The fact that consultations were short[18] and apparently routine with very little ostensible decision making did not mean that contradictions brought about by role complexification were absent. Rather, they had been sorted out on so many previous occasions that they required little or no fresh resolution. So, for example, each GP seemed to have arrived at their own routines and thresholds for whether or not to prescribe an antibiotic to a child with a sore throat. Our probing suggested that, although such decisions might appear instantaneous and untroubled, they nevertheless entailed the resolution of many of the tensions between, among many things, likely clinical benefit, long-term risk, costs, and maintaining credibility with the patient, with professional colleagues and with potential future auditors.

Each clinician had already developed their own solution for a very large range of such situations. Over time they had built up their own individual ways of deal-ing with the many tensions and pressures, leaving them able to decide relatively quickly how to deal with the many dilemmas that they routinely faced, but which eluded the guidelines and other formal sources of clinical knowledge. Following Fondas and Stewart (1994), we suggest that four main factors had contributed to the particular balance that each clinician had developed between the con-trary demands of their roles. First there are the personal characteristics that the individual in question brought to their work: the kind of person they were and the influences they had had during their training. Were they, for example, more inclined to take a preventive or curative approach and, if so, did they lean towards being directive, simply telling patients what to do, or participative, explaining or negotiating at length? Did they tend to worry about cost-effectiveness or regard that as relatively unimportant? Lawndale clinicians each tended towards one or other of these approaches, and the variation between them was a matter of (edu-cated) personal style.

The second factor was the 'role set' – i.e. the colleagues with whom they came into contact day to day. We will discuss the crucial influence of the immediate group of colleagues in Chapters 5–8, but a glance at the list of people with whom each GP needed to maintain a working relationship (Box 2.1) suggests that a great deal would depend on how influential that 'role set' was and how much sway those key players had over what the clinician did. Role theorists have applied the term 'role sending' to the way in which one's colleagues signal in various ways their expectations of one's behaviour (Fondas and Stewart 1994). This is particularly important when one begins a new job. So, for example, when Adam came bound-ing into the practice as an enthusiastic and bright GP trainee fresh from hospital, a great deal of the time and effort from his trainers and colleagues, who otherwise admired and learnt from his up-to-date knowledge, was spent in gently but firmly showing him how in primary care one needed to limit the number of investiga-tions and take a 'less obsessive' approach than he was used to in hospital. Every time they teased him about his zeal they were conveying to him their views of the roles they expected him to play and, over time, his balance between his clinical and managerial roles visibly changed. But third, wider organizational influences were affecting both him and his role set – such as the way the RCGP structured his training requirements, the way the GP contract was changed, the increasing muscle of organizations such as NICE and the PCT – all of which could help tip the balance of his decision to order a PSA for that elderly gentleman worried about his prostate, or to prescribe an antibiotic for that child with the sore throat.

The fourth factor is the nature of relationships between those other three influences, the person, the role set and the organization. Just how influential can each be and how much leverage can they assert over each other? Primary care in the UK has traditionally been built around the GP as an independent provider of care, but the foundations of that arrangement have been shifting markedly over the past two or three decades, with an inexorable increase in the control exerted over individual practice by both the immediate role set (the primary care team and other local healthcare providers) and the higher echelons of the NHS

***Box 2.1* Some important professional contacts for GPs**

- partners and clinical staff (GP colleagues, practice nurses, physiothera-pists, counsellors etc.)
- support staff such as the practice manager and receptionists
- GP trainees
- patients and their families
- patient organizations
- local charities
- local hospital specialists
- the local public health department
- neighbouring practices
- community nurses
- laboratory services
- the primary care trust
- the local medical committee
- the Royal College of General Practitioners
- the local pharmaceutical adviser
- the local pharmacists
- the local drug company representatives
- the suppliers (and other users) of the computer system
- the manufacturers of (e.g.) the sterilization equipment
- medical students
- the local university and its academic doctors
- the local postgraduate deanery and others responsible for training
- local authority social services, housing and environmental health
- privately run nursing homes
- the local chamber of commerce

(Glendinning and Dowling 2003; Peckham and Exworthy 2003). In Chapters 8 and 9 we will touch upon the way in which power relations between the key actors in the various sections of the NHS influence knowledge in practice, but simply note here that this is not a one-way event. Clinicians are not passive recipients of external influences from, say, the NHS hierarchy or the evidence-based practice movement. They themselves, as we observed, were always having to actively balance the different pulls and contradictory goals that different players expected them to meet. So, for example, when a patient wanted Jean to spend longer with him or to prescribe a proprietary drug, while the practice team generally would prefer her to keep the surgery to time or to meet the primary care trust's targets for generic prescribing in the Medicines Review, it was Jean who made her own balanced decision in each case, often to give the patient the time (and forgo her coffee break) or to prescribe what *she* felt was appropriate. Even Adam, who as a trainee naturally responded much more than Jean to the pressure from the Lawndale partners to reduce his overzealous investigations, remained more likely to order investigations than his colleagues, and this was accepted by the team. In short, the eventual balance of forces between the various expected roles was 'negotiated'[19] through each individual's interactions with those around them.

Clinical decisions owed a lot to a practitioner's relationships with key people (Box 2.1). Few of the clinical decisions that we observed could be said when analysed retrospectively to be completely free from knowledge of the local health system. Even though the clinicians themselves might take for granted the importance of what one might call local know-how, know-where and know-who, they were implicitly using that knowledge to the benefit of the patient and the practice in all but the simplest cases. Sometimes, as when Clive sent the lady with 'ice in my chest' to Westchurch Hospital, the decision relied not just on the patient's situation, but also on a close knowledge of the demands of, and on, local people and organizations, and the GP's good relations with them. Such knowledge was also very frequently an important part of the advice given to patients so that they could make the most of services both locally and further afield. We saw GPs making the necessary links, opening the right doors, ensuring with other services that things went smoothly, following up on the actions of others, checking and interpreting information for the patient, acting as patient advocate – even sometimes as a lightning rod for patients' frustrations with the health, social services or legal systems. And there were instances when the same knowledge and skills, coupled with a knowledge of the patient, were used to protect the system from the patient, as when a patient was known for consistently making unreasonable or aggressive demands.

In sum, a thorough knowledge of local circumstances was integral to many clinical decisions. It will come as no surprise that published clinical research evidence, expert systems and guidelines cannot take that into account. The evidence-based practice movement accepts, of course, that clinicians need to harness the evidence judiciously according to individual circumstances; guidelines are not directives. However, such an approach – stick to the evidence but tweak its application a little here and there – ignores the sheer breadth and variability of the multifarious considerations the clinician needs to take into account when deciding what to do. The reality of practice means that guidelines do not even come close to dealing with all the considerations that a clinician needs to weigh up not as a mere add-on but as an *inherent* part of dealing with clinical problems.[20]

Differing roles and goals

When we reflected on what we had observed in the surgery and the clinics, where possible also discussing it with the practitioners, it became apparent that even seemingly quick and simple decisions and actions usually concealed quite difficult and complex balances between what we identified as four overarching categories of roles: clinician, health promoter, manager, and guardian of professional standing. Each category had many subroles and goals of which we were quickly able to count at least fifty, but that depended on what we chose to include. There would be little point in trying to produce a catalogue since not only could they have been subdivided in infinitely different ways but their number could also have been augmented, for example, by looking more deeply into the clinicians' inner psychology (e.g. what motivated them as practitioners, how they achieved a work–life balance, how they handled interpersonal tensions or responded to 'role senders') and more broadly into wider matters of healthcare policy (e.g. the political economy of state-imposed healthcare reforms, the role of the consumer movement, the power of the pharmaceutical industry), which impacted on how they played out the roles and goals that they had to juggle. So we have limited ourselves to the more immediate aspects of the clinicians' professional activity, and give only illustrative examples in an attempt both to draw attention to the sheer variety of the shifting roles and goals and also to begin elucidating how the practitioners had learnt to cope with them in providing the excellent care that Lawndale was known for.[21] We do not suggest that their goals were always met or the roles properly fulfilled. Indeed the point is that they could not be, since the clinicians' decisions were often a compromise between their incompatible demands (see also, for example, McDonald and Harrison 2004; Hannes *et al.* 2005).

Clinician[22]

Even the role of pure clinician, providing technical care to individual patients who are ill, is not just a matter of applying clinical science, but a host of sometimes inconsistent goals. The first goal might be to establish – or re-establish – rapport sufficiently to understand what the patient (or their relatives or carers) wanted from the encounter and to assess how best to handle the discussion.[23] So, while they were welcoming the patient, their role was already one of gauging the required degree of empathy (perhaps affability for the shy or familiar patient, or aloofness for the garrulous) and achieving whatever common ground was needed to quickly and politely get to the important point without seeming rushed or off-putting. This – which we might call the first stage of a facilitation role – inevitably used up some of the allotted time and every clinician had his or her own style of doing so and tended to accord it more or less time. Some also used it as an opportunity to try and elicit some local news and views with the goal of gaining a better general understanding of local issues and currents of concern. Establishing rapport could be time well spent, and was often combined with beginning the main business of making sense of what was wrong with the patient and what to do about it. In most consultations, the role of facilitation was not only important for setting the tone of communication, but also the key to the way the clinician managed the duration and course of the consultation and subsequently negotiated the management of any illness. They often made a great deal of effort to create the space and ease that the patients needed to express their concerns and their views. But when, for example, a patient moved to a topic the clinician did not want to discuss, we might see the practitioner turn away or start to type something into the computer:

the patient usually got the message. We often observed clear tactics by which the clinicians would either empower or disempower a patient by the way they used verbal (including tone of voice) and non-verbal cues. Finally, whether or not the consultation, as it sometimes did, ended with an 'anything else I can do for you?' (the role of proactive problem seeker, perhaps) would depend on whether, for example, the clinician suspected an undeclared problem, whether the surgery was running late, or there was a need to strengthen the relationship with this patient for the future (as in Nick's prescription for the unrelated ointment that in effect was part of the longer-term goal of keeping the patient on side in managing her heart failure.)

So much for the roles and skills necessary to shape the process of the consultation. (See also Pendleton *et al.* 1984; Stewart *et al.* 1995). We will not dwell on the core content of the clinical roles, such as diagnosing, investigating and deciding on the patient's treatment, since those may be taken as read. They are the main focus of most of a clinician's formal training and of the updating and guidance that they continually receive, and we will see much more of them throughout the book. However, the 'cholesterol consultation' (see also pp. 150, 162) allows us to unpack some of the many aspects of those apparently core roles of care provision that interact with, are informed by and may conflict with other roles and goals, such as health promoter or (especially for the GP partners) manager.[24] As the consultation proceeds, Nick is undertaking a large number of activities that are not covered by the guidelines but seem nevertheless entirely necessary and appropriate. In doing so he is dealing with the conflicting goals of trying to persuade the patient to change his lifestyle while avoiding alienating him. Explaining and educating can be at several levels, which again reflect the different roles that GPs play, for instance spelling out the pathophysiology and anatomy, the likely progress and prognosis, the consequent desired actions by the relevant parties, practice organization and the relevant parts of the health and social services system. Moreover 'explaining' may be driven by different goals, for example to persuade rather than inform (as in another instance when Clive gave a very clear and logical explanation to cajole a patient to try a particular pragmatic treatment, but later admitted to us that he actually had no idea why the treatment might work – it just did – but he knew that was not enough to persuade the patient to use it.)

Health promoter/disease preventer

The clinical roles and goals make up the first of our four categories, but in the 'cholesterol consultation' one can already see elements of the others such as Nick's attempt at disease prevention by trying to minimize the further consequences of the high cholesterol. Within even short consultations, the GPs sometimes took the opportunity to check blood pressure, ask about smoking habits, suggest vaccinations, discuss lifestyle and so on. Disease prevention and the promotion of health for individual patients have in the past few decades been increasingly encouraged as a vital part of primary care.[25] The commitment of GPs to this preventive role varied, and hence the default balance between the efforts expended on such activities as opposed to dealing with existing illnesses would also vary, as would the perceived likely receptiveness of the patient, which was also a major factor.[26]

On many occasions the GP would pass up what appeared to us to be an obvious opportunity to convey some health message; if we subsequently challenged them about it, explanations included the diminishing returns of repeatedly giving the same old message or a clear desire to avoid eroding the relationship by preaching at the patient. To follow the evidence-based guidance about, say, the effectiveness of brief opportunistic counselling for smoking cessation (e.g. Stead *et al.* 2008) might mean that other crucial aspects of the doctor–patient relationship were damaged – even to the extent that the patient would prefer in future to avoid seeing that GP. On the other hand, there were good reasons to ask the patient about their smoking habits; it might indeed help the patient quit, and also it might help the practice to reach contractual targets that would increase the income and the general standing of the practice.[27] So, while GPs were being pushed to give that advice through their managerial role to meet contractual targets, their main motivation was the underlying ethos to uphold the standards of good practice that would help improve the patient's health – and the two did not always coincide. This became explicit at an early QPA meeting, where there was a lively discussion about the choice of health promotion topic to work on. Jean leapt on the opportunity to use the preparation for the award as an occasion to improve primary prevention. Clive seems to be concerned about the cost and resource consequences of doing so with little return on health. Nick wanted to compromise with something pragmatic and achievable. All agreed on making best use of their time with patients by checking things that really will make a difference, and not wasting time on those that won't. What was harder was knowing which those were. Even if they had a general default position, there would always be the chance of some clinical or other reason that overwhelmed other considerations, as betrayed by a telling quote in the title of Summerskill and Pope's (2002) article on barriers to secondary prevention in primary care: 'I saw the panic rise in her eyes and evidence-based medicine went out of the door'.

Manager

GPs, especially those with partnership status, had to contend with strong managerial and organizational pulls that could impact upon their clinical decisions. The partners, because they were in effect running a small business, felt a keen edge to their managerial roles, which included responsibility for the overall clinical, organizational and financial success of their practice. (This was despite none of them having formal management training and their being therefore very reliant for guidance on Janet, the practice manager.) These responsibilities introduced additional tensions. During the 'cholesterol consultation', Nick naturally wanted, in his clinical and preventive roles, to reduce the high cholesterol and hence the risk of heart attack or stroke by using a statin drug that is known to be effective. But in his managerial role he was also required to ensure that what he did was relatively cost-effective. He also wanted to help meet the practice's contractual targets for the management of ischaemic heart disease, to lead his colleagues by example and to ensure that he would be able to demonstrate his good standing in a forthcoming audit of the way this group of patients have been treated. His choice of which statin to use was further related to the conflict between the managerial demands of cost containment and his personal clinical preferences based on experience with similar patients. When, some months later, the patient might show little improvement and the question might arise whether Nick should change the prescription, his decision might well be to make the switch to the relatively expensive statin that he would actually have preferred to use in the first place. But Clive, who was on a local committee that reviewed and gave advice about high GP spending and therefore had a more explicit awareness both of the evidence about the relative efficacy of the two drugs and of his role as custodian of the public purse, would almost certainly have a different decision threshold for switching from the cheaper to the more expensive statin. The trainee GP, Adam, would act differently again because, besides wanting the best for the patient, he had to take account of another set of goals such as meeting training requirements by building up an appropriate portfolio of demonstrably well-managed patients to help him achieve specialist registration, and impressing partners with his up-to-date knowledge so that he would get a good reference for future jobs. For each clinician, any clinical action was a resolution to their own particular set of motivators and inhibitors, linked in turn to the cascade of goals they found themselves juggling, often unconsciously, in which each GP had their own, different point of comfortable equilibrium that was rarely amenable to the linear dictates of written guidelines.

Guardian of professional standing

There remains one further set of roles and goals to explore here, namely that of upholding professional standing. This has a number of components, the first of which is maintaining and developing the quality of one's own work. It was not unusual to find that a health professional's individual decisions about the care of patients involved:

- ensuring one was up to date and was seen to be so;
- preserving one's credibility (with patients and internal and external colleagues);
- reviewing one's own practice, for example as part of reflective continuing professional development (CPD);
- ensuring good record keeping so that an audit or other review of one's performance would be a fair reflection of the quality of practice;
- seeking to further one's reputation by demonstrating expertise;
- improving one's workload and the simple self-preservation of managing one's workload, which might entail not only time management but controlling one's exposure to problem situations and patients.

Not just the individual but the collective quality of the whole team's practice entailed such goals. As we will show later (Chapters 5–8) much of the discussion at team meetings was about confirming best practice, developing auditable practice guidelines and protocols, reviewing and auditing care, interrogating others (e.g. local experts, partners, trainees, other health service personnel and pharmaceutical reps) to check out new developments in care, controlling external demands on time and activity, and dealing with complaints. They were very proud of Lawndale's reputation and showed more than a hint of competitiveness with other practices in the area; some partners wanted Lawndale to be the best and to be seen as such. This drive, as well as the simple desire to practise good care or to reap financial rewards, helped impel them to continually try and improve the service. When Clive first announced that the target was to achieve 1049 out of 1050 points in the GP contract's 'Quality and Outcomes Framework' there was much ironic laughter about the missing point. Rose quipped that when she was doing a cervical screening she'd better say 'Never mind that, let's review your epilepsy to get the points.' There was always an undercurrent of continuing tension between what they considered to be actions aimed primarily at good clinical care and those aimed at maximizing Lawndale's standing in respect of 'the points'.[28]

Finally it is worth mentioning the desire to uphold the overall standing of general practice and primary care (not always the same thing, as for example when there was a discussion about whether a given service were best done by the practice or by other community primary care services) and to a much lesser extent of the medical profession as a whole, in an environment where the GPs sometimes felt their autonomy and reputations to be under attack from politicians and the media. There were decisions when such considerations seemed to be at the back of their minds, especially for those who were actively engaged in medical politics, but also to a lesser extent for all of them as members of their profession. For example, in his discussions with GPs at other practices, Clive was always urging them not to refuse point blank to do infeasible things that the government was pushing for as part of the new contract, but to constructively suggest clinically more sensible solutions to the impasses, otherwise the GPs' position would become politically untenable. It was not hard to see that attitude pervading many of the contract discussions – as for example over the reformulation of the meaning of early renal disease (Chapter 8).[29]

Clinical mindlines

Guidelines, like most of the research that they are based on, almost always dealt just with the *clinical* aspects of the practitioners' roles, perhaps occasionally adding some aspects of prevention and health promotion or a managerial component such as cost-effectiveness. That, though, is a very slim set of considerations when set against the complex subjective judgements that were implicit in so many of the clinical and practice policy decisions we observed. Textbooks, expert systems and guidelines cannot help very much when a busy clinician is making decisions that need to resolve conflicting goals such as weighing financial costs against health benefits against managerial targets, all while applying probabilistic science to individuals and simultaneously handling all the people, with their differing needs and demands, who are involved in optimally managing an illness. That, we suggest, is the key to why guidelines were not used during clinical practice; they simply did not live up to being directly applied to the multifaceted blend of knowledge and reasoning that stems from the complex and often incompatible roles and goals that inform clinical decision making.

What we saw instead, from very early in our Lawndale ethnography, was that the clinicians were relying on what we came to call their 'clinical mindlines' (Box 2.2). We use this term to refer to internalized, collectively reinforced and often tacit guidelines that are informed by clinicians' training, by their own and each other's experience, by their interactions with their role sets, by their reading, by the way they have learnt to handle the conflicting demands, by their understanding of local circumstances and systems, and by a host of other sources (Gabbay and le May 2004). Mindlines are not only much more flexible and complex than guidelines could ever be, but are also much better adapted to combining the many roles that we saw the clinicians undertaking. They accommodate the vagueness and fuzzy logic that are part of professional as well as everyday life (van Deemter 2010). Unlike guidelines and expert systems, mindlines are sufficiently broad and malleable to deal both with individual patients' needs and the multifarious factors that come into the reckoning when making decisions. Clinicians build up mindlines as a bank of personalized, flexible syntheses of all the different types of theoretical and experiential knowledge that they need to be able to call upon instantaneously. But because, as we have seen, practitioners each develop their own particular balance between the demands of their roles and because their clinical decisions also involve values, ethics and a whole set of other principles, it is inevitable that mindlines will vary between practitioners. Mindlines allow considerable plasticity and elasticity for adaptation to individual patients and circumstances, but nevertheless, as we shall show, 'collective mindlines' are shared and developed with colleagues through their 'communities of practice', which draw the boundaries around what is acceptable with regard to both the knowledge and the values that the clinician brings to bear on every decision they make.

As we shall describe, mindlines are rooted in early training and then adapted, reinforced or refined by the clinician's own and others' experience, by seeing how local opinion leaders work, by hearing of recent developments at educational meetings and courses, by 'grazing' many types of professional, scientific and commercial literature and guidance, including the general media, and by the available organizational infrastructure and resources (Figure 2.3). By taking account of a very wide range of different types of evidence, mindlines give the clinician what has been called their 'capability' – 'the extent to which individuals can adapt to change, generate new knowledge, and continue to improve their performance' (Fraser and Greenhalgh 2001: 799) – which goes well beyond mere technical competence. Through being indirectly and implicitly discussed and shared with colleagues, often involving storytelling, mindlines are continually checked, honed and if necessary revised. They are capable of absorbing change: they tend to revert to the 'default setting' when challenged, but as the challenges mount up mindlines

---

Box 2.2 **Ways of conceptualizing mindlines using Spradley's (1979) analytical framework**

Mindlines are 'kinds of':

- experiential knowledge in practice;
- prior knowledge 'in my head';
- 'grit in the brain';
- personalized mental checklists;
- elastic practical routines;
- amalgams of different kinds of knowledge;
- flexible pathways that encompass all the practical roles;
- adaptable, fuzzy logic that accommodates conflicting goals;
- socially constructed patient pathways;
- triggers for different strategies of care.

They are also:

- bounded areas of acceptable practice;
- rooted in early training;
- developed through 'grazing' many types of professional, scientific and commercial literature, including published guidelines;
- discussed and shared at relevant meetings;
- modified by exchange with colleagues and experience with patients;
- collectively as well as individually held;
- adapted – but also reinforced or entrenched – by continuing education;
- checked against trusted sources of expertise;
- flexibly adapted to individual patients;
- open to plasticity of performance;
- capable of absorbing change but tending to revert to the 'default setting';
- affected by social, economic and organizational demands;
- shaped by local factors;
- ways to change practice.

---

can become a vehicle for changing practice. They are affected by organizational demands (e.g. the need to meet standards and targets set by the Department of Health or to ensure maximum income for the practice), and can be enabled and constrained by local organizational factors (e.g. the availability or lack of local specialist hospital services or of community-based therapists). They are reinterpreted – often following implicit negotiation with patients – for each instance of

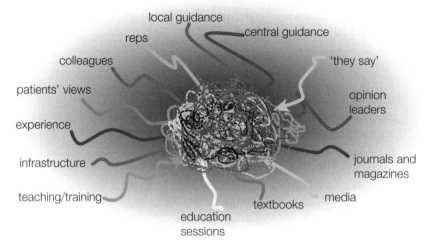

Figure 2.3 A schematic representation of some of the sources of mindlines.

the clinical problem in question. In short, clinical mindlines are a complex social construction, linked to a web of sources that not only build and reinforce the embedded knowledge and values that allow the clinicians to function, but give them their sense of who they are and where they fit into the scheme of things.

The term 'mindlines' arose from a quip about the mind as the real locus of guidelines while we were doing the initial analysis and taking note of comments made *en passant* by several of the GPs and others. Whilst it has become a memorable encapsulation of the concept, it has a disadvantage that has been pointed out to us by several practitioners who have recognized this description of knowledge in practice but have been worried that the term mind*lines* may make clinical thinking sound too *linear*. As one GP colleague put it: ' "Lines" suggests an enclosed system with definite influences that you can measure and be aware of reliably. [Isn't it] more like variable diffuse, often bending sets of influences which vary on different days in their impact depending on what else is going on and which sometimes go in different directions?' Our intention is to convey just that. As will become apparent, mindlines are much more complex than mere lines, or even outlines, of clinical thought. If anything, they resemble more the 'songlines'[30] of indigenous Australians – the 'labyrinth of invisible pathways' that are best visualized in the form of 'spaghetti . . . writhing this way and that', consisting of stories that guide a person's wanderings across the Outback where every episode explains how the land came to be as it is, and that must be continually sung in order to keep the land in existence (Chatwin 1998: 13–14). In fact even something as fanciful as a labyrinth of wriggling, world-creating spaghetti is too concrete and too linear a metaphor. The constantly performed labyrinth of mindlines may be what keeps clinical practice alive, but the problem is that mindlines are not a *thing* at all. They are more of a collective *process* that provides not only a flexible set of propensities to act in optimal ways in different circumstances, but also a large range of well-tried modulators for all likely occasions. But we are getting ahead of ourselves. We should begin by trying to explain more basically how mindlines allow clinicians to use evidence to make complex decisions quickly.

Chapter 2: Summary

Practitioners absorb knowledge from many disparate sources including some guidelines and expert systems but rarely access them during actual practice. Instead, clinicians follow internalized guidelines, 'clinical mindlines', which they have built up over their entire careers and which are more suitable than formal sources to handle the complexities of practice-in-context. Practitioners continuously face dilemmas posed by many competing goals that stem from their roles not merely as clinician but, for example, as manager, health promoter or guardian of professional standing. Mindlines blend formal, informal, tacit and experiential evidence, and unlike guidelines are sufficiently broad and malleable to resolve the resultant tensions.

3 Clinical thinking and knowledge in practice

Chapter 3 begins by exploring the way that clinicians can arrive at their decisions so quickly.

❖ *8.30 a.m. on my very first day of observation at Lawndale and it's Clive's first patient of the morning: a man breathless with an exacerbation of his chronic bronchitis. My first set of field notes say 'He [Clive] seems to be carrying out a mental protocol. Where did it come from?' When the patient leaves, Clive reels off for me his routine approach to this condition. I keep trying to ask him but it is frustratingly difficult to pin him down. He just calls it his 'mental guideline' and says it comes from reading and experience. 'Not all partners would do quite the same', he says, 'but there is a vague consensus'.*

❖ *In a supervision session with Tamsin, his trainee, Barry tries to explain to her how he would have dealt with one of her patients with erectile dysfunction. There is a great deal of careful detail as he tries to reconstruct the logic and all the caveats and considerations that would have led him to choose one or other of the many treatment options he lists and discusses. His explication of just that one aspect of treatment takes nearly half an hour, having raised many still unanswered questions.*

❖ *Extract from taped interview with Tamsin (Tamsin speaking): 'You automatically start thinking in the same pattern don't you when you see something and get to a diagnosis and get to the management.'*

❖ *Extract from transcribed tape recording with Peter (he is trying to reconstruct his decision process for us about a patient with high blood pressure, whom he had dealt with quite rapidly in the surgery): 'I have to say the blood pressure was actually slightly better, not ideal, I've got to say last time I converted the propranolol to atenolol because I thought it would give a smoother protection curve if you like and was a little bit more specific than propranolol and blood pressure was slightly better I don't think particularly because of the change to atenolol, but I wanted to do that as a starting point and then I would look at the other two medications and we'd agreed that we won't make any changes because she's been so well on these old treatments, but if on review next time blood pressure hadn't come down any further, it was 150/90 today and was 160/95 the time before and 170/100 when the nurse tested it. The nurse had done the initial blood pressure follow up, referred to the GP as part of her protocol cause it was outside the range, our accepted range, so 150/90 is really just at the limit of what I'm expecting for her and if it's that level again or if it's higher than that then I would think that I would probably stop one of her old treatments or even both hydralazine and bendrofluazide and perhaps add in a different medication, something like an ACE [angiotensin-converting enzyme] inhibitor. I'm not sure yet.'*

❖ *Barry on a visit to an old people's nursing home prescribes antibiotics to one lady with Alzheimer's disease who has a chest infection, but not to another. I ask him why. 'It's a rule of thumb: all things being equal, if I sense that they are bothered or agitated by the infection then I give them antibiotics.'*

❖ *Clive visits a child with suspected measles. He diagnoses roseola. 'I did that', he tells me in the car, 'because when I was an SHO in paeds I had it drummed into me that before you ever diagnose measles you should consider roseola especially if the child isn't very ill. And this one wasn't.'*

❖ *The psychiatry tutor at Doppton is taking the students through a case. 'When you see dementia always think delirium and if you think it's delirium always think dementia', he says twice as he writes it on the whiteboard. The way he has made his presentation around a case where this was crucial, and the way he stresses this lesson, I get the feeling they shouldn't ever forget that dictum. But the rest of the discussion of the case reveals how little certainty there can be about anything in terms of how to manage the patient in question, and how much relies on judgement. Is she at sufficient risk to be sectioned (compulsorily admitted to hospital)? Is she depressed as well as demented? Is there an acute component or a chronic steady state? None of this, I reflect, is remotely amenable to simple dictums or even simple guidelines.*

❖ *Jean prescribes amoxicillin for a child with sinusitis. 'They say', she says to me, 'that that's the one to use.' I ask who 'they' are. 'The pharmaceutical adviser, for one, the local ENT surgeons for another. But we're under a lot of pressure not to use antibiotics.' I ask from whom. 'From the government, the pharmaceutical adviser, the journals, everyone really. But it's a grey area. And mum obviously wanted her daughter to have them.' The next patient is a lady in her late forties with an upper respiratory tract infection. It's been going on for a month, the voice sounds nasal, and the patient says her sputum is green. Jean examines her carefully, but she tells me afterwards that from those three signs she already knew she was going to prescribe an antibiotic. (I recall from my own training being told years ago that green sputum is usually a sign of bacterial infection and suggests the need for antibiotics.)*

❖ *Vivienne's patient, who has had many chest infections, says immediately 'My phlegm's been lime green!', and the way he says it with a flourish suggests he assumes he will now get an antibiotic. But, being on the back-to-work GP scheme, she has been having tutorials about the management of chest infections. She examines him very carefully and persuades him he doesn't need them. She successfully takes a similar line with three more patients in the same surgery.*

❖   *Tony after seeing a young man with epididymitis says he usually sends a urine sample to check for infection, tries anti-inflammatories for two weeks and then, if that doesn't work and/or the tests come back positive, antibiotics. I ask how he arrived at that routine. 'A lot of that is extrapolation of a practical approach rather than something from a book', he says and can add little more even when pressed. This is quite a contrast with the detailed account he had given me earlier that morning about cholesterol testing and management, when he was able to give more detail because he had recently been involved in debates about it with other GPs.*

❖   *Clive jokes that he has often reached a diagnosis before examining the patient, which he then does just for show. 'In fact I am often of the opinion when I go to visit a patient with a trainee or student that by the time we have gone through the differential diagnosis on the way there, we have usually actually made the diagnosis before we get there.' He says it in jest, but it is an illustration of his view that GPs start with the likeliest diagnosis or action and then set out to check it.*

❖   *Vivienne seems to have a richly nuanced routine for how she deals with back pain, including things to ask and examine, a graded series of drugs, and clear views about radiography, physiotherapy, early manipulation, mobilization, exercise, sick leave and so on. When asked where it came from she immediately says 'a back pain day' at Westchurch Hospital. But, when pressed, it turns out that what really stayed with her from that course was the need to refer patients early to the hospital because that demonstrably leads to better outcomes, whereas by 'protecting' Westchurch Hospital by trying to look after the patients at the surgery she was more likely to have them unable ever to return to work. Little else, on closer questioning, had changed that day in her intricate and subtle routine for back pain patients.*

❖   *Attending a (very practical) refresher course on resuscitation is a requirement for all staff. As we walk to the room, Peter says he can never remember the ratio of compressions to respirations and always reverts to the first one he learnt (7:2), which he knows has since been amended. He is reminded on the course that the recommended ratio these days is four times that rate, 30:2, but afterwards is not confident he will recall that in the flurry of an actual event. Jean says after the course that, although there was nothing new, it is vital to refresh it and that actually she had had to resuscitate a neighbour shortly after last year's refresher and it had given her 'bags more confidence' to deal with it.*

❖   *An elderly Urbcester Pakistani man with multiple chronic illnesses hobbles in to Frances with a swollen, painful foot. 'Just pop your foot on the couch for me', she says. As she examines it she gives a running commentary. 'Gosh it really is quite swollen and the skin's very tense isn't it? And very red. Quite hot and . . .' (he winces) 'painful too!' As I watch and listen to her I find myself involuntarily recalling my pathology lectures:* tumor, rubor, calor, dolor *(swelling, redness, heat, pain), the classic signs of inflammation drummed into us at medical school. 'It's obviously an infection', she concludes, there being no other obvious cause after she does a few routine checks. She prescribes flucloxacillin, an antibiotic. When he is gone I ask her why she decided on that prescription. She explains how she had checked it was not a thrombosis. 'No', I say, 'I could see that. I meant: "Why flucloxacillin?"' 'It just comes immediately to mind' she answers, 'I just think "Skin. Fluclox." I guess your next question is why 500 mg? Because I wanted maximum benefit. If it had been a question of "Hmmm . . . does he need an antibiotic or not?", then I would have given him 250. But he clearly needed one, so it was 500. I dunno – it's just how your mind works. I'm sure there's no evidence.'*

❖   *Tony tells me that Barry has seen a partially wheelchair-bound patient who has recently begun a new relationship and whom he was going to start on a progesterone-only contraceptive pill. But she says she is worried because the information leaflet about the pill mentions the possible side effect of a deep vein thrombosis (DVT). Barry was pretty sure it is not really a risk, but because she is relatively immobile (which is itself a risk for DVT) he is nevertheless, because the patient is so insistent, concerned enough to discuss her case with Tony, who knows the patient and went out to see her at home. Tony found that she is actually getting in and out of her chair quite a lot, and the two GPs agree that with such evident mobility the risk is probably minimal but they still are not convinced. He is discussing this with me on our way to coffee, where – as it happens – a pharmaceutical rep is making a short presentation to the assembled partners about a contraceptive. He and Barry raise the question and the rep explains that the mention in the patient information leaflet etc. of the risk of DVT is part of the industry's defensiveness and the risk is actually minuscule (and of course the risk from any pregnancy would be much, much higher). The assembled partners – who have as usual been in ostentatiously sceptical mode when receiving the rep's 'spiel' about her products – discuss the general worry that they have about giving reassurances that turn out to be wrong. Tony later tells me that he and Barry, still not feeling secure enough to reassure the patient, then went to see Jean, who is the Lawndale partner with lead responsibility for gynaecology, and whom the partners have come to regard as being reliably the practice's most knowledgeable GP in that field. The three of them discussed the matter and she agreed that even a small risk might need to be checked. So she turned to a large standard textbook which states categorically that there is no risk of DVT from the progesterone-only pill. Only then was Barry sufficiently confident to go back to the patient and explain why she should stay on that pill. I hear later that the patient agreed to do so.*

Knowing decisions?

'But do we ever actually *make* decisions?' Nick laughingly, but only half jokingly, asked us about our observations of the practice. What he meant was that most of the clinical work was fairly routine and did not require a great deal of conscious reasoning to determine the next step to be taken.[1] And he was also perhaps trying to defend why he and his colleagues were frequently unable to explain properly why they had decided to act as they had with any particular patient. As has been repeatedly found in other sectors (e.g. Boden 1994), clinicians often had to deal with fuzzy, incomplete and flexible information that continually needed to be clarified, refocused or even occasionally completely realigned, often through talking with other people involved. Thus they might inch forward step by step, layer by layer – arriving at reasonable and 'satisficing'[2] ways to act that never quite looked like a decision. Yet clearly at some level they *were* making decisions all the time, if only through a series of fine-grained and fluid interactions that took account of the multifarious considerations discussed in Chapter 2. Whereas the evidence-based practice movement appears to be based on the premise that clinical practice is a series of decisions, in reality the process is often one of weaving one's way through complex and often intangible negotiations that both react to and impact upon the task in hand (Greenhalgh *et al.* 2009).[3]

Accomplishing that task required the practitioners to know a great deal, even if they were unaware of how much knowledge was involved and how they were using it. To try and gain some idea of just what that meant, we analysed two typical surgeries early in the study – some twenty patients seen by two GPs – to find out what kinds of things they needed to know. The result, which is abbreviated in Box 3.1, was enough to show us that our initial research question about the ways that clinicians manage knowledge was not going to be as simple to answer as we had hoped.[4] We had naïvely assumed that we would be looking mostly at the management of technical clinical knowledge, such as how best to diagnose and treat diseases, but we quickly realized that this was only a very small part of the story. Although we had of course known that there was much more to practice than technical knowledge and skills, we really had not expected to find quite so many factors playing their part in even the most routine of clinical decisions. We were aware, for example, that the MRCGP (Membership of the RCGP) curriculum requires its members to have a very wide range of competencies, skills and knowledge, which appear at first sight to cover many of the matters illustrated in Box 3.1. Yet even this turned out to be pitched at a general level that went nowhere near the actual knowledge used in practice. Compare, for instance, the Lawndale GPs' specific, local 'soft' knowledge items under section 12 of Box 3.1 (e.g. 'What different local consultants want from you', 'What the local hospitals are like in terms of waiting times, convenience, accessibility, and how much that matters to this patient') with the RCGP's 'Knowledge of the structure of the healthcare system and the function of primary care within the wider NHS' or 'Understanding the processes of referral into secondary care and other care pathways'. The MRCGP curriculum could only be the starting point; it was quite clear that without the practitioners carrying in their heads an enormously broad range of different types of knowledge, general and specific to the local context, even the simplest clinical task would be protracted and clumsy. How, then, did they manage to do this and to bring it all to bear, and so quickly, in everyday practice?

One interpretation (Greenhalgh 2002) is that this is a form of intuition, 'a decision-making method that is used unconsciously by experienced practitioners but is inaccessible to the novice. It is rapid, subtle, contextual, and does not follow simple, cause-and-effect logic' (ibid.: 395). What she is alluding to is Clive's hunch when he said his 'nose' or 'acumen' told him something was seriously wrong as soon as he saw the woman with 'ice in my chest', who did indeed subsequently turn out to require admission to hospital even though there was nothing at first that he could conventionally pin down to justify it. Far from being irrational, 'intuition' has been called 'analysis frozen into habit' (Herbert Simon, quoted in Patton 2003: 989). As we shall explore further in Chapter 5, it is born of hard-won

***Box 3.1* Examples of what a GP needed to know during a typical surgery**

1   What the patient wants and needs
2   What the patient already knows/believes and the care they have received in the past
3   What is likely to be the best way of establishing rapport with the patient, so as to best negotiate care
4   How patients perceive you
5   When a patient's condition is serious and needs extra care even if there is as yet no obvious reason
6   What is the accepted way to manage any given condition
       Why that is the agreed practice, i.e. scientific rationale
    a   How reliable is the science?
    b   What are the local deviations from the accepted best practice and why?
    c   How realistic/practicable any guidelines are and why
7   Risks *vs* benefits *vs* costs of various options of treatments
8   The costs of key treatments (money, likely staff time, other resources)
9   What treatments are likely or not to be approved of by the local NHS commissioners
10   When 'stuck', where to find expert help (in person, in print or online)
11   When you are getting out of your depth (and what you need to do about it in any given circumstance)
12   About local consultants and services
    a   Who the best person is to refer questions or patients to
    b   What consultants' special interests and skills (and defects) are
    c   How they are likely to practice (e.g. new drugs)
    d   What different local consultants want from you
    e   How to get the best out of consultants for your patients
    f   Who the local opinion leaders are and in what fields and how reliable they are
    g   What the local hospitals are like in terms of waiting times, convenience, accessibility, and how much that matters to this patient
13   About your practice colleagues (especially when seeing each other's patients)
    a   What the skills and qualifications are of others in the practice
    b   What their capacity for work is, and how they organize it
    c   To whom you can delegate what

---

      d How each partner would like their patients to be handled in their absence

      e How to handle each partner if you disagree with how they have managed a patient

14 How to communicate many different types of things to many different types of people

15 How to use the computer system

      a How to record and to find out what you need to deal with a given patient

      b How the IT system works and how best to use it

          i   for this patient

         ii to trace groups of patients, e.g. for recall

        iii to maximize administrative efficiency and income generation

16 How the practice is operating

      a Activity data (own; other partners; nurses; practice as a whole)

      b How colleagues feel about own and each other's activities

      c How your time is being managed/used (cf. others)

17 Administration skills for running practice – personnel, finance, employment law, infection control, risk assessment, health and safety, item of service payment schedules etc., how to manage the interface/boundary with the practice manager

18 Ground rules of how the practice runs (organizational/logistical/cultural)

19 The practice profile – kinds of patients – demography; culture; local events; prevalence of similar illnesses (*is* there 'a lot of it about'?)

20 How other local practices and out of hours colleagues operate

      a Communicating with them

      b Knowing when and when not to rely on them

21 What is happening nationally about aspects of practice organization (e.g. national service frameworks, organizational changes, IT, media awareness of new treatments)

22 'News' – e.g. health scares, when a drug is being recalled, when a treatment is being advocated or criticized in the press, health-related events in popular soap operas . . .

---

expertise; indeed Karl Weick (1995) describes intuition as 'compressed expertise'. Greenhalgh argues that intuition is not in opposition to deductive, scientific thinking, but is combined with it in ways we do not yet understand. There is a need to dig deeper and develop, she suggests, 'a science of intuition' (Greenhalgh 2002: 399). But to call it intuition is merely to describe its existence, not to explain it. Our own view goes further: we contend that 'intuition' is merely a word for tacit (i.e.

unspoken, hard to express) or implicit knowledge that the clinician can instantly access but has not yet been able to explain. The 'science of intuition' should therefore be a much broader science that also includes tacit knowledge that *is* subsequently explained since they are different not in kind, but merely in how well they have so far been expressed. For consistency we therefore generally prefer not to use the term 'intuition'.

It is notoriously difficult to unpack clinicians' thought processes.[5] Higgs and Jones (2000) describe how 'clinical reasoning', which is not necessarily logical and deductive, deals with the unique, multifaceted specificity of a person's clinical problems in the wider context of the knowledge explosion, the healthcare environment and the clinician's own professional framework. A great deal of research over nearly four decades has aimed at understanding the nature of that reasoning. (For overviews see, for example, Dowie and Elstein 1988; Higgs and Jones 2000; Norman 2005; Eva 2005; Thompson and Dowding 2009.) Some of that research (e.g. Elstein and Schwarz 2002) has suggested that clinicians faced with a clinical puzzle do indeed follow a logical line of reasoning based on the (supposed)[6] hypothetico-deductive methods of science. Arguably at some level this sometimes does happen, as when a GP posits an hypothesis – for example that the patient has angina – and then tests it by first asking the right questions and then ordering an exercise electrocardiogram (ECG). Are they, though, really undertaking a process of logical deductive investigation? The research evidence suggests that whereas students and trainees may go through such a conscious stepwise process – and there is evidence that even they tend not to (Norman *et al.* 2007) – experienced practitioners do not normally do so (see Chapter 5). At Lawndale, where most consultations seemed to proceed almost instantaneously, it was certainly not easy to detect conscious hypothetico-deductive reasoning as the practitioners followed their mindlines. Anyway, even if the clinicians were deliberatively testing hypotheses, how did they so rapidly formulate the hypotheses in the first place?

Psychologists of various traditions have shed light on the problem. The renowned cognitive scientist Marvin Minsky, for example, posited in an influential essay over thirty years ago a 'frame theory' suggesting that:

> [w]hen one encounters a new situation (or makes a substantial change in one's view of the present problem) one selects from memory a structure called a frame. This is a remembered framework to be adapted to fit reality by changing details as necessary. A frame is a data-structure for representing a stereotyped situation, like being in a certain kind of living room, or going to a child's birthday party. Attached to each frame are several kinds of information. Some of this information is about how to use the frame. Some is about what one can expect to happen next. Some is about what to do if these expectations are not confirmed.
>
> (Minsky 1975)

In grasping such situations, Minsky's frame theory suggests, one fills in crucial parts of the pattern (especially where the given situation does not quite match the remembered framework) by further checks and investigations or perhaps just by interpolation or imagination (like the fabled 'eye of faith' that allows doctors to 'see' things in radiographs that may or may not be there). Or one ignores the anomalies and goes with the overall picture despite them. The concept of the 'frame' is similar to that of the 'schema' (Fiske and Linville 1980), which has been influential among psychologists since the 1960s. Schemata are mental patterns ('cognitive frameworks') built up largely through our experience of the world. They enable us to interpret everyday situations rapidly, effortlessly and perhaps automatically (though not always accurately!) without having to think about them. Schema and frame theory have, directly or indirectly, inspired experimental work across many fields and it is not difficult to see how such a model might apply to the way in which clinicians think not only when diagnosing their patients (which has been extensively researched) but also when treating them (which has not).

Illness scripts, heuristics and rules of thumb

Early experimental work in the medical field echoed this view, suggesting that expert diagnosticians use 'domain knowledge' (Patel and Kaufman 2000), whereby they organize their knowledge around principles (domains) that allow them to swiftly get to the nub of a problem. A more recent, similar model ('categorization') suggests that, as clinicians gather information about a patient, they quickly recognize the emerging picture as an instance of a prototype or of something remembered ('this is just like that case of X') and assign it to that category (Hayes and Adams 2000). The key seems to be pattern recognition. Psychologists using experimental and reflective methods (where for example students and clinicians are asked to think aloud when considering carefully chosen clinical problems) have revealed that most of the decisions of an expert clinician are based on almost instantaneous recognition of sets of typical patterns. Boshuizen and Schmidt, for example, showed in the late 1980s that clinicians develop 'illness scripts' that enable the practitioner to activate at once the whole clinical picture, which can then be matched to any further information that is then elicited from the patient (Boshuizen and Schmidt 2000; Charlin *et al.* 2007). Their work, which has been widely used to inform medical education (e.g. Bowen 2006), suggests that a script has three components: the predisposing conditions, the pathophysiology and the consequent signs and symptoms. As practitioners acquire more information about a patient, they usually 'instantiate' one of several alternative competing scripts that almost literally spring to mind (even more quickly if the story is related by another who shares the scripts and hence gives the most pertinent information in an expected sequence – see Chapters 5 and 6).[7]

   The notion of illness scripts, which has arisen from empirical experiments, is compatible with what we observed at Lawndale, Urbcester and elsewhere, but is specific and narrow in that it is limited only to technical clinical knowledge.[8] Mindlines encompassed a far wider range of variables and factors than the illness scripts described in the literature. Recognizing a pattern of symptoms and signs was only a very small part of the decision making we were observing. What 'springs to mind' with an illness script is a medical diagnosis that gets one to the nub of the pathology. However, it also entails other factors not only about the patient's individual circumstances but also about the range of options and competing goals that the treatment decisions may have to contend with (Chapter 2). In addition, the evidence being adduced in making the decision could include a wide range of sources of information (the experience of previous cases, dimly recalled undergraduate textbooks, the research summarized in articles read since, guidelines recently discussed, stories of the experiences of colleagues and so on) that all go far beyond the illness script but still have a bearing on the outcome of the consultation. And yet the decision still appeared to 'spring to mind' just as illness scripts are said to do.

Schmidt's group suggested that, having moved from the logic of basic biomedical mechanisms to amassing a fund of illness scripts, experienced clinicians go one step further and make mental use of 'exemplars' based on prior instances of similar cases that act as their diagnostic hypotheses (Schmidt *et al.* 1990). Practitioners using illness scripts and exemplars do not require conscious reasoning to arrive at their decisions (just as most people, already knowing that 12×12 is 144, don't need to use long multiplication to work out 120×12: they just add a zero). It is in complex, unfamiliar or anomalous cases, where the patterns don't fit, that one might expect inductive or hypothetico-deductive reasoning to kick in. (Following the pattern of the ten times table is no longer helpful when seeking the answer to 11.847×12.563.) So, when clinicians are stumped by unusual, difficult cases, they may test hypotheses, but even then it seems that the process of matching the unfolding information to the 'hypothesis' being tested (say, a possible diagnosis) is much more complex and iterative than the simple hypothetico-deductive model based on (idealized) scientific method would suggest.[9] Doctors do not just gather appropriate new data and use it to test an hypothesis; there is good evidence that they select and weigh up new data, inflate, minimize or discard the information it provides, classify it according to other knowledge and ideas, alter their categories for organizing it and reinterpret both the hypothesis *and* the new findings as they are going along (Hayes and Adams 2000).[10] Indeed Ridderikhoff has suggested, based on a study of problem solving among sixty-eight doctors, that they inductively collected hypotheses (patterns), not data, showed very few signs of testing those hypotheses, and hence did not learn from the experience (Ridderikhoff 1991, 1993). Most clinicians would like to think that they do learn, especially from an unusual or unexpected case, and especially if they actively, better still collectively, reflect on it. But then most clinicians like to think they think logically.

Studies of doctors thinking aloud about clinical cases reveal how easily their hypothetico-deductive reasoning is prone to failures such as not thinking of the right hypothesis or missing, misconstruing or misinterpreting the clues being collected (Elstein and Schwarz 2000). Often these errors result from the necessary short cuts that we all take in our thinking, which the psychologists who first described them in the 1970s called heuristics. Heuristics are the tried and tested thought patterns that people rely on when called on to make a judgement in circumstances where fully rational decisions are not possible because of lack of time or lack of information (i.e. almost always!). The originators of the term argued that heuristics may be 'highly economical and usually effective, but they lead to systematic and predictable errors' (Tversky and Kahneman 1974).[11]

There are two ways to view heuristics in clinical thinking. On the one hand (e.g. Klein 2005) it can be seen as a flaw that needs to be remedied; on the other (e.g. Eva and Norman 2005) an elegant evolutionary adaptation that allows us to deal efficiently with the reality of imperfect decision making (a view reinforced by the fact that it is novices rather than experts who think and act with deliberate logical thoroughness – see Chapter 5). Those who tend towards the former extreme would like to reinvigorate the rationality of medical thinking by eliminating the 'heuristics and biases' that they believe undermine clinical thinking. Those sources of bias have been shown to include easily recalled events that crowd out important but forgotten ones, poor estimates of probability, dismissing negative evidence, inaccurate extrapolation, cherished myths, unrealistic expectations or the sheer momentum of repeated experience and confirmation bias (Elstein 1999).[12] Others, such as researchers in adaptive behaviour and cognition at the Max Planck Institute, have taken quite the opposite view, promoting the development of heuristics as a 'fast and frugal' way to make one's thinking more proficient. That group's research suggests that heuristics are often at least as accurate as complex statistics in pointing to the right decision (Gigerenzer *et al.* 1999). Indeed their influential book opens with a medical example – a paean to the pre-eminence of a simple three-stage decision tree to assess the level of risk in a patient admitted with a heart attack, as opposed to the standard twenty or so investigation results that are used in a typical large US hospital. Despite the biases and errors described by opponents such as Elstein, they regard it as self-evident that such heuristics have advantages for practice (Gigerenzer 2007). Torn between the pragmatic efficiency and the inherent unreliability of such short cuts, one medical writer has averred that 'the heuristics of medicine should be discussed, criticized, refined, and then taught. More uniform use of explicit and better heuristics could lead to less practice variation and more efficient medical care' (McDonald 1996: 56). He and others have concurred that there is no avoiding that this is how clinicians think, and therefore we have to take a middle road and understand and overcome the way that rapid clinical reasoning can be misguided by the heuristics they inevitably use. (We return to this question in Chapter 10.)

One type of heuristic in clinical practice has been dubbed the 'rule of thumb'. Following on from work done among nurses (e.g. O'Neill 1995) and UK GPs (Essex 1994; Essex and Healy 1994), Malin André has studied the use of 'rules of thumb' through her research, which is based on questionnaires and focus groups, and has found that doctors use them for much of their routine clinical work (André *et al.* 2002, 2003). She takes the view that rules of thumb are 'well adapted for decisions in defined contexts' (André 2004: 5). The GPs she studied immediately recognized that statements such as her own 'when a patient can bear weight on a leg it isn't broken' (ibid.: 19) were familiar guides to action, and they were able to articulate many more. Each focus group she worked with came up with between forty and sixty statements such as 'Pains in the chest described as prick, cut or that a knife is stabbed in the chest – that's definitely not the heart anyway'; 'CRP less than 10, then it's a virus'; 'If a patient made an appointment for pain in the neck . . . [or] shoulders and then is totally unaffected . . . then I think . . . stress or depression?'; 'Fall on the hip – X-ray' (André *et al.* 2003: 515–516). Her GPs made such statements rapidly, with little conscious deliberation, yet in a manner that suggested to her that the rules actually represented a good deal of quite complex prior thought and experience. She describes them as resembling 'verbalized pattern descriptions' that 'could be considered to be a link between theoretical knowledge and practical experience' (André 2004: 38–39), which allowed swift, stepwise progress in the consultation. When specifically asked for their rules of thumb about, say, diagnosing sinusitis all fifty-two GPs mentioned a combination of symptoms and signs such as purulent drainage, fever, unilateral maxillary pain; and a typical rule of thumb for prescribing antibiotics for such patients included lack of response to decongestants and the length of time the symptoms had persisted. However, they varied markedly as to which variables tipped their decision one way or another (ibid.). André also notes two important features of rules of thumb that were echoed in our findings at Lawndale. First, part of the variation between the different GPs' rules of thumb depended on their different styles (e.g. whether they had patient- or doctor-oriented consultation styles – see p. 190). Second, the GPs appeared to learn a lot of their rules of thumb from word of mouth rather than the written word; indeed she even suggests that, judging from their rules of thumb, those who had little discussion with other GPs were more in danger of 'loose' thinking (ibid.: 41). We will return to both of these findings in Chapters 5–8.

There has also been work in this vein by Kathryn Montgomery in the USA, who moreover suggests that doctors' 'maxims, aphorisms and old saws' are often mutually contradictory (raising the question of when to use which). Her examples include 'Occam's Razor: look for a diagnosis that can explain all the findings' versus 'Hickam's dictum: it's parsimonious but it may not be right' or 'always do everything for every patient' versus 'don't just do something, stand there' (Montgomery 2006: ch. 7). Montgomery, who found many such examples during her observations in a major US teaching hospital, argues that such contradictions illustrate why 'clinical reasoning is far more situated and flexible than even the most complex clinical algorithm can express [. . .] Counterweighted situational rules embody the tension inherent in clinical knowing' she argues. 'The maxims work in the real-life care of patients and in clinical education precisely because of their contradiction . . . [T]hey are situational wisdom that has arisen out of (and proven useful in) circumstances very like those identified in a particular case' (Montgomery 2006: 117–119). The contradictory maxims, she suggests, show that there is more to clinical reasoning than mere pattern recognition: there is also the need for situation-based interpretation that cannot follow straightforward decision rules. In saying this, Montgomery is, of course, considering only the clinical aspect of doctors' thinking; how much less apt must clinical algorithms be when one takes account of the wider range of roles and goals that also need to be considered?

In summary the evidence from a wide range of studies suggests that very few clinical decisions are based on overt, step-by-step deductive reasoning while the decision is being made. What appeared to be the instantaneous decisions that we saw in the majority of consultations at Lawndale were the result of psychological processes that may have involved scripts, heuristics and rules of thumb, but also complex but equally instantaneous patterns of thinking that took account of the complex and competing goals, demands and local circumstances and systems – the mindlines. When a decision was not instantaneous, it was because something out of the ordinary needed to be thought through before the clinician could make sense of it or act with confidence. An example might be the wheelchair-bound woman who was extremely concerned and insistent about the risk of thrombosis from the contraceptive pill. Such an unusual set of circumstances took this beyond the usual consultation and Barry needed to seek advice, read and think things through. The fact that examples of explicitly methodical thinking were unusual should, however, not imply that clinicians' work is not based on deductive logic. Even in routine cases where no such deductive processes were detectable, the practitioner was sometimes able retrospectively to impute such logic when asked to try and unpack their rationale for a given action (see also, for example, Balla *et al.* 2009). This was clear, for example, when Barry's logical reconstruction for his trainee of just one small aspect of a patient's care took over twice as long as he would normally have spent on the entire consultation (p. 48). We would suggest therefore that there is indeed a deeply embedded logic founded in rational deductive investigation and thinking that has, over the years, informed the development of the practitioners' mindlines. Seldom does that logic need to be unpacked, which is why they seldom displayed overt hypothetico-deductive reasoning. Clinicians were using a wealth of well-trodden but buried paths built on an accumulation of (more or less) logical patterns of reasoning mixed with comparable past scenarios that are rapidly accessed in their minds. This rich mixture is far more suited to practice than guidelines or protocols or the clear steps that are traditionally associated with the linear model of evidence-based practice (Figure 1.1). It is also far more complex than the schemata, pattern recognition, domain knowledge, illness scripts, heuristics or rules of thumb described above.

The big difference between what we observed in Lawndale and all of these psychological models is that the latter are all narrowly limited to just the clinical aspect of the work of the clinician whereas the rapid way in which Lawndale GPs arrived at their decisions took account of a far broader picture than that.[13] What we observed entailed a means of instantly and flexibly grasping a pattern that encompassed all the multiple roles and goals and the wide spectrum of types of knowledge (Box 3.1) that were involved in even the most everyday clinical decisions. To recognize that green sputum points towards bacterial infection needing antibiotics is to recognize the illness script, or use a rule of thumb. However, to decide to admit the lady with 'ice in my chest' to hospital was an almost equally instantaneous decision that not only took account of the clinical picture and usual care, but also embraced the unusual psychosocial ramifications and the local managerial, financial, professional, ethical and other considerations. It is for that reason that the decision, replete with hard-won tacit knowledge, required the clinician's mindlines and not a simple rule of thumb or heuristic. The distinction is as important as the difference between car drivers being able to change gears and brake before cornering at any given speed, and their knowing, without having to think about it, when to do so depending on who is in the car and how much of a hurry they are in, and with different loads, tyres, road surfaces, traffic and weather conditions.

Knowledge in practice

Using one's mindlines may entail not just the immediate grasp of a complex set of circumstances but also the need to continuously modify the action that the clinician has initiated. The original logic (or heuristic) often has to be adapted, modified or even subverted by the specific circumstances that develop. (Whoops. Better slow down, this has the feel of black ice.) Such modifications usually involve an element of *craft*, which cannot succeed without some degree of skilled improvisation that builds on any original theory-based plan of action. Nor is it always clear until the task is complete what knowledge might be needed to complete it (Keller and Keller 1996). Moreover, we would add, it is only after the task is complete that the post-hoc knowledge gained from that experience becomes 'compressed' as 'intuition' or tacit knowledge that has by then become a modification to the clinician's mindlines for possible use in similar future instances.

The finding that clinicians use many types of knowledge going far beyond the confines of textbooks and guidelines will come as no surprise to anyone familiar with the literature on professional knowledge. Many writers have argued, particularly when considering the best way to educate professionals (e.g. Fish and Coles 1998; Jenkins and Thomas 2005; de Camargo and Coeli 2006), that there is a big difference between on the one hand the technical-rational, theoretical 'codified' knowledge that is explicit, written, taught and examined and on the other hand the craft or 'artistry' of the practical, often tacit knowledge that is implicit, absorbed, learnt and practised.[14] In this section we explore some of the features of the latter type of knowledge, which is what we mainly observed in use at Lawndale, since if research evidence, which is part of the codified canon of knowledge, is to be incorporated into the clinician's practical knowledge then it behoves the exponents of evidence-based practice to understand how the two are related.

Donald Schön, following a number of authors[15] who had already distinguished a 'gap between formal professional knowledge and the demands of real-world practice' (Schön 1991 [1983]: 45), analysed a range of professional practice in great detail, including clinical work, science, engineering, management, town planning and especially architecture. Developing this work from the earlier idea of theory-in-use (Argyris and Schön 1974)[16] Schön showed in his very widely quoted (and misquoted) book *The Reflective Practitioner* that, whereas many professionals may prefer to work on (and were formally trained for) 'the high ground' of solidly rigorous technical knowledge, the reality was usually the 'swampy lowlands' of messy problems that are incapable of simple technical solution because they need experience, 'intuition' and sheer muddling through (Schön 1991: 42–43). He suggested that handling the swampy lowlands required a form of 'knowing-in-action', a tacit form of knowledge that relies on continuing interactive reflection implicitly linked to the task in hand (ibid.: 49) Thus when Jean decides whether or not to prescribe an antibiotic for the child with sinusitis she is not simply applying the algorithm suggested by textbooks or guidelines, but is weighing up and reflecting on the likely outcome of prescribing this drug to this child in these circumstances at this time, reflecting not only on the 'facts' but also on her previous experience and understanding of the family and her feel for how the child (and mother) will respond and how the consultation is going. This is not just a matter, Schön would contend, of applying knowledge 'A' (the place of antibiotics in paediatric sinusitis) to situation 'B' (this child); it is using a different kind of knowledge, and moreover one that is very hard if not impossible to put into words. It is this 'knowing more than we can say' (ibid.: 51) that may explain Nick's embarrassment, quoted at the beginning of this chapter, at rarely being able to fully explain his decisions. Using such reflective knowledge-in-action, argues Schön, is akin to knowing how to hit a golf ball accurately, how to bring a difficult meeting successfully to an end, or how to improvise a jazz solo. Although these all involve rules or schemata previously absorbed (perhaps unconsciously), an experienced practitioner just does them spontaneously, just 'acts his mind' (ibid.: 51) with a 'feel' for the action that cannot be explained. Moreover, Schön maintains, professionals need to rely above all else on this 'knowing-in-action' since a very high proportion of the tasks confronting them do not conform to the textbook picture or, as we have seen, to the available research and guidelines. (He quotes an ophthalmologist's claim [ibid.: 64] that 80–85 per cent of cases fall outside the familiar patterns of diagnosis and treatment – a figure remarkably similar to the [mythical?] one often quoted concerning the proportion of decisions for which there is no solid research evidence.[17]) However, when Schön concludes that this 'knowing-in-action' or 'reflective practice' entails a very deliberate logic of purposeful, premeditated experiments to deal with anomalous situations, his evidence for that claim is less than convincing and moreover we were unable to find any evidence that Lawndale GPs or practice nurses worked in the deliberately experimenting way he postulates.

Another widely quoted writer on professional knowledge, Michael Eraut, despite being critical of Schön's concept of reflection-in-action, enthusiastically shares the underlying idea that professionals use not only 'propositional' knowledge, which is his term for the codified, canonical knowledge of textbooks and guidelines, but also what he calls procedural, practical and tacit knowledge and skills that are 'constructed through experience and [whose] nature depends on cumulative acquisition, selection and interpretation of that experience' (Eraut 2004: 20). Indeed he draws a parallel between formal teaching and a fifteenth-century map: just as the map does not even begin to depict the reality of the world beyond the confines of the restricted culture of the map maker, formal teaching merely reflects the limited world of the textbook. Writing mainly about the training of teachers, Eraut's work suggests that, unless they are beginners, practitioners of that (or any) profession do not merely imitate what a book or a person tells them; on the contrary, it is a part of a mature professional ethos to interpret and adapt new learning through one's own experience and context. He found learning to be so deeply dependent on context that something learnt in one situation *could not* be simply transferred to another (ibid.: 20). Eraut observed that what was learnt quickly on a teacher training course, for example, could take days to implement successfully in a classroom full of individual children. (We contend – see Chapter 4 – that the same applies to what most clinicians learn, despite their widespread sardonic quip 'see one, do one, teach one'.) His findings, which were also typical of what we found at Lawndale, moreover suggested that people pick up knowledge from many piecemeal sources and blend them with their own and others' experience, which makes it impossible for them to identify how any one piece of knowledge is put into practice or how many sorts of knowledge (e.g. implicit and reactive on-the-spot learning) go into making a decision (Eraut 2000). Drawing also on Schön and on Schutz's phenomenological sociology, Eraut concluded that even schemes of knowledge that are

> consciously and directly attributable to codified, canonical, propositional knowledge become at least partly personalized through the process of being used. The personal meaning of a public idea is influenced both by the personal cognitive framework in which it is set . . . and by the history of its personal use.
>
> (Eraut 2004: 106)

This theme is taken up by Fish and Coles (1998), who contrast two views of professional practice that they call 'technical rational' and 'professional artistry'. Among the many differences that they describe, the technical rational approach follows rules and norms, applies theory to practice, and emphasizes the known. In contrast, professional artistry 'starts where rules fade', derives theory from practice, and embraces uncertainty. Their analysis focuses on the implications that this has not only for the way clinicians practice (e.g. reductively or holistically) but also for the way in which we educate professionals (or 'train' them, as the technical rationalists would say!). They stress the place of critical reflection, 'critical appreciation' and collective professional judgement. We will return to this and to their call for a different approach to research into practice at (pp. 202, 204).

It is not just educationists who have grappled with the question of differences between propositional, canonical, textbook knowledge and personalized, practical knowledge – what Montgomery (2006: 8) calls 'practical reasoning'. In his classic analysis *Profession of Medicine*, the sociologist Eliot Freidson (1988) included a chapter on 'the clinical mentality' in which he drew attention to the action-oriented, as opposed to theory-oriented, nature of medical expertise. He found that doctors, responding to the often uncertain nature of their work, needed to be pragmatic in dealing with 'the complexity of the concrete', and were 'prone in time to trust [their] own accumulation of personal, *first hand experience* [his emphasis] in preference to abstract principles or "book knowledge", particularly in assessing and managing those aspects of [their] work that cannot be treated routinely' (ibid.: 169). This, he found, leads them to develop a self-reliance based on cases they themselves have dealt with. Freidson was quick to point out that the medical profession's claim that there is no substitute for real clinical experience (whether that claim be inescapably true or a self-deceiving myth) conveniently gives doctors a powerful edge over non-doctors. After all, how can armchair scientists or others compete when they are not in a position to have the clinical experience, and hence the practical knowledge, that the medical profession jealously guards for its own members (Jamous and Pelloile 1970)? Whether or not one agrees with Freidson's implication about the self-serving mystique of tacit knowledge-in-action, there can be no doubt that Lawndale clinicians would occasionally criticize unhelpful guidance precisely on the grounds that the authors (those 'experts' they sometimes derided) clearly didn't have the relevant primary care experience to make the guidance credible. Perhaps, to see it as Freidson might suggest, this was a way by which GPs could reassert their status relative to their academic and hospital colleagues.

The health professions may indeed gain status, including economic and social benefit, from their reliance on practical knowledge not obtainable from a book, guideline or web page. Then again, practical knowledge is inescapably a part of practice even in areas of human activity where there is no such secondary gain. For example, Jean Lave, a social anthropologist and learning theorist, has demonstrated that housewives and children also rely on practical rather than theoretical knowledge (Lave 1986). Shoppers whom she carefully observed in a supermarket computed, on average, the comparative prices per unit weight of products 90 per cent correctly when standing in the aisles compared with 57 per cent when given the same problems as a formal exercise. They were unable to remember or articulate the mathematical method of proportional division that they were taught at school (is six for $3.40 a better deal than five for $2.80?), but nevertheless accurately (after fumbling with different makeshift approaches) dealt competently with the problem in the shop (ibid.: 92). She quotes also the memorable example of a teacher who found that a high school kid who could not be persuaded to grasp the principles of arithmetic and was 'the dumbest kid in the class' (ibid.: 93) turned out to be the faultless scorer for the local bowling league (a phenomenon paralleled among many UK darts teams). On the other hand, young Liberian apprentice tailors whom she studied were able successfully to use arithmetical knowledge they had learnt both in school and also in the tailor's workshop, but not to transfer the learning between the two (a feeling, we might add, that many clinical students recognize when they move between, say, conducting pharmacology class practicals and calculating drug doses on the ward). These and many other examples, she argues, undermine our cherished dichotomy between rarefied theoretical knowledge and day-to-day practice. It is not that people do or do not apply the theoretical knowledge. Rather, as we shall see, they use a different kind of knowledge: 'knowledge-in-practice'. Nor do they use knowledge in a linear way; they move iteratively, dialectically, between the problem, the knowledge used to solve it and the *context* (ibid.: 100).

Knowledge-in-practice-in-context

When Barry correctly adjusts the dose of statins in a familiar patient without referring to a systematic review of cholesterol and the risk of heart disease or even referring to the widely used 'Sheffield tables' (Rabindranath *et al.* 2002) that were to be found in most of the GPs' offices, he may not be failing to follow the theory, as some would suggest. Rather, he may be demonstrating a different way of arriving at the correct solution to the clinical problem. Why, then, does he feel the need to apologize to us about it? Jean Lave would argue that the only reason that he feels (albeit mildly) embarrassed is the weight of the received ideology that formal theory is somehow better than practical knowledge; whereas, she suggests, maybe the dichotomy between the two – and the implied value judgement – is false.

Lave would go even further; Barry, she would say, is not a person just using knowledge-in-practice. He is also a 'person-acting-in-setting' (ibid.: 99) – an experienced GP in a busy surgery with a familiar patient and a familiar condition which he has treated many times before with this statin. The immediate setting or context actually structures the way in which people solve problems. Thus in one of Lave's ethnographies a weight-watcher who was asked while preparing her lunch to calculate $^2/_3$ of $^3/_4$ of a cup of cottage cheese pondered for a while and then took a cup $^2/_3$ full of cheese, poured it onto a chopping board in the shape of a disc which she divided into four and used three of the quarters. (Never did she calculate arithmetically that $^2/_3 \times ^3/_4 = ^1/_2$.) Had there been no cups or chopping boards, only pencil and paper, that improvised knowledge-in-practice would not have been possible. The setting is what makes this use of practical knowledge possible or not. At a simpler level, we all understand how a certain setting makes it easier to recall a fact related to the context. (How much easier it is to recollect the names of old neighbours when you are actually visiting the street where you once lived.) What matters, therefore, is *knowledge-in-practice-in-context.*

More importantly, Lave argues, not only does the setting help to shape the practical knowledge but the need for that knowledge also helps to shape the setting: they are mutually constitutive. A clinical example may illustrate this point: monitoring and understanding the oxygen levels in a patient's blood is an integral part of the whole process of working on an intensive care unit (ICU). Such activity entails a form of practical knowledge ('craft') that is made as foolproof as possible and becomes almost automatic after long experience of working there. If there were not the need to understand how blood oxygen levels are varying, however, intensive care units would not be structured so as to provide the cues, technologies and techniques that not only help monitor oxygen levels, but make it almost inevitable that the staff respond appropriately to them (Carmel 2003).[18] The context and the practice both shape each other – or, perhaps more accurately, the practitioners construct both in tandem over time.

More recent work has shed further light on how people solve the same problems differently in different contexts. One elegant study of Swedish schoolchildren who were asked to work out the cost of sending parcels of varied weights showed that in a maths lesson they were twice as likely to use sums as in the social skills lesson, where, given the same task, they tended just to look it up in a postage table. And, as the authors point out, in real life when we neither have the table to hand nor a set of scales nor the time to go to the post office, we might just add some extra stamps and hope. The way we solve problems depends on our perception of the circumstances and of the possible consequences. Indeed, most of the actions people undertake are so deeply contextual that neither meaning nor learning can be properly attributed to them without also taking full account of the situation in which they happen (Säljö and Wyndhamn 1996) – an inference shared by most of the contributors to the volume where that study is reported. As the editor concludes: 'scientific understanding of individuals engaged in a practice must include some analysis of the socio-historical context in which the practice develops and proceeds' (Chaiklin 1996: 378).

It does not take a leap of imagination to see parallels between such observations and the different ways in which clinicians approach a given clinical challenge depending on whether it occurs in surgery, in the patient's home, on a hospital ward, at a PCT meeting, in an examination hall or in a guidelines development group. Nor is it difficult to see that there is every chance that those differences will lead to different actions, as when Tony (p. 19) decides perfectly reasonably to forgo the full hormonal work-up for the recently bereaved widower asking for Viagra for his holiday with his new lady-friend next week, yet feels the need to excuse that action because he is talking to an academic.

Isn't science different?

But surely, some will argue, clinical reasoning is different from deciding on the relative prices of soap powder, working out the cottage cheese for a recipe or pricing the stamps for a parcel. Medicine, they would say, is a science and therefore the knowledge that clinicians use needs to be of a higher, scientific order than that of a shopper, a cook or a post-office customer. Isn't it the point of all those years of clinical training to learn to think scientifically and not like ordinary folk?

There are two problems with that argument. The first is that medicine is not just a science; it is also an art requiring judgement and skills that go far beyond pure science. No one would dispute that. So, whatever its scientific core, a clinician's knowledge-in-practice-in-context must extend much more widely into arenas that more properly resemble the decision making of other people involved in complicated everyday situations. Therefore if we wish to help enhance the place of scientific evidence in clinical decisions we are obliged to understand exactly how that works. The second problem is that even the firmest knowledge at the core of medical science cannot be divorced from a wide range of social, organizational, political, economic, ethical, cultural and historical factors that have shaped it. The production of scientific knowledge is also an art (Latour 1987; Chalmers 2003). We will return briefly to this assertion in Chapter 9; here we will explore only the first argument – the relationship between the scientific and practical aspects of clinical knowledge.

There is of course no question that the codified, propositional knowledge of medicine and increasingly the other clinical professions is based on scientific research. People are pleased to think of medicine as being scientific: for the general population the science brings reassurance; for the profession it brings intellectual exclusivity and a welcome emotional detachment; above all for everyone it brings a greater chance of averting the consequences of disease. Yet the scientism has long been seen as a double-edged sword (e.g. Mishler 1981). Most people would want to encourage medical research and expect their clinicians to be fully up to date with the latest scientific developments in their field. Yet, as both the popularity of complementary medicine and the steady stream of critiques of orthodox medicine attest, many people are also dissatisfied with clinicians' reliance on science at the expense of a more holistic approach to their patients. Kathryn Montgomery, for example, alleges that:

> the assumption that medicine is a science – a positivist what-you-see-is-what-is-there representation of the physical world – passes almost unexamined by physicians, patients and society as a whole. The costs are great. It has led to a harsh, often brutal education, unnecessarily impersonal clinical practice, dissatisfied patients and disheartened physicians.
>
> (Montgomery 2006: 6)

Based on her ethnography of a US teaching hospital, the thrust of her argument is that, whereas medicine mis-describes itself as a science, all the evidence points to its reliance on discourses, judgements and decisions (including the contradictory maxims we encountered in the preceding section) that go way beyond the confines of science. The eagerness to make medicine into a science, she insists, distorts and limits practice but fortunately most doctors tend instinctively to realise that. 'Medicine', she maintains, 'is a learned, rational, science-using practice that describes itself as a science even though physicians have the good sense not to practise it that way' (ibid.: 36). Her accusation of misguided scientism may apply to US university hospital physicians and even to some of the academic clinicians that we have worked with in UK universities, but the Lawndale GPs were under no such misapprehension. They were far too pragmatic to describe what they did as scientific. Indeed they were often quite humorously offhand about the contribution of scientific research to their work, even though of course they would if pressed accept (and sometimes quote) the scientific base that, usually tacitly, underpinned their diagnoses and treatments. (See p. 69.)

Of the many reasons why Lawndale GPs might justifiably have no such pretences to medicine as a science, we will highlight just four. In doing so, our intention is not to revisit the old chestnut of whether medicine is an art or a science. We are simply reasserting that it is both, and that there is therefore no justification for claiming that clinical decision making is so strongly scientific that it cannot be subject to the patterns of professional thought and behaviour seen in other arenas described by Schön, Eraut, Lave and others.

First, as we have described, despite the scientific core to their work, there simply are no scientific answers available for many of the problems that clinicians have to deal with – many patients have illnesses too diffuse and indefinable, or complicated by other factors, for the science to be applicable. Many clinical problems at Lawndale and Urbcester fell within the grey or unresearched areas for which one can only interpolate and hope, which is a more common occurrence than most people realize, since the research is often restricted to relatively atypical patients. For example, most of the scientific results that guide treatment are based on clinical trials in adults under the age of sixty-five without concurrent disease, and yet a third of Lawndale's patients are over that age, often with multiple pathology.[19] Second, it is not feasible to undertake a properly scientific approach to choosing the best treatment for a given condition, since that would require at minimum a critical systematic appraisal of all the clinical trials with a detailed account of the caveats, the internal and external validity and statistical confidence intervals and the likely confounding factors. The clinician rarely if ever does this for a given patient, but may be lucky enough to find that someone else has done it for them, for example on the Cochrane or Joanna Briggs database or as part of the preparation for a clinical guideline. Even then, the result is inevitably a set of probabilistic general principles. Yet, and this is the third problem, such general scientific deductions are not logically structured to deal with the vicissitudes of particular individuals in complex circumstances.[20] Put simply, it is of limited help for a GP to know that using treatment X in a certain group of patients has a Y per cent chance of success. After all, when faced with an individual patient the outcome will not be Y per cent: it will be either 100 per cent (he gets better) or 0 per cent (he doesn't). At some point, therefore, the probabilistic scientific generality, however secure it may be (and often it is not), needs to be translated and adapted for a specific case, with all the (non-scientific) judgement that entails. So the GP may, in other words, find herself unscientifically (but clinically very sensibly and logically quite unavoidably) weighing up imponderable factors that may help predict whether this patient is likely to be in the successful Y per cent or not. Fourth, a clinical scientist's ideal is to pare diseases down to their simplest possible linear causes (e.g. the HIV virus causes AIDS) whereas the reality is a web of causes (AIDS is due to not just the HIV virus, but also the host response and the social, sexual, psychological, economic, organizational, commercial, religious and political processes that contribute to the spread, the manifestation and the management of sexual health and the spread of the virus; see, for example, Gill 2006). Based even on just these four examples of the clinical limitations of scientific medicine, we can see that science-based guidelines are going to be of limited value compared with the broader and more adaptable knowledge-in-practice-in-context that clinicians internalize as they become proficient – their mindlines. It is to this process of developing mindlines over the course of a career that we now turn, beginning with their early professional education.

Chapter 3: Summary

We show that mindlines incorporate many of the features of illness scripts, heuristics and rules of thumb that are well described in the literature as the means by which clinicians decide what is wrong with their patients and what to do about it. However mindlines also seem to include a much wider range of considerations. Although founded partly in the 'high ground' of generalized, science-based, codified, textbook knowledge, mindlines share many of the features of 'knowledge-in-practice-in-context' that is needed for the 'swampy lowlands' of specific individual cases, as has also been widely described in the literature about practical knowledge.

4   Growing mindlines

Laying the foundations

This chapter is about the way clinicians acquire the core of their mindlines during their early training.

❖ *Jim was explaining how he still makes use of the science he learnt at medical school thirty-five years ago. Having begun to hear about bisphosphonates, for example, he read 'lots about it here and there, like in the* BMJ*', until he 'got the gist of it', and then went back to basic principles about osteoblasts and osteoclasts and worked out how bisphosphonates might work on the bone and what the consequences might be before he prescribed them. He admitted that in doing this he was unusual compared with many of his colleagues, but he enjoyed that part of his work.*

❖ *This week's rep is a likeable and intelligent young man who clearly knows his stuff, so the assembled group of GPs warm to the debate. The rep talks about osteoblast activity and the role of strontium in mending microfractures. Peter smiles wryly and asks about the costs compared with a generic bisphosphonate before raising a question based on the NNT (numbers needed to treat) and the distinction between the relative roles of strontium and bisphosphonates in increasing bone density to help prevent hip fractures. I reflect that Peter clearly has a lot more scientific knowledge than usually meets the eye.*

Because the Lawndale ethnography could not address early education directly, much of this prologue is based on our field notes of observation of third-year medical students at Doppton Medical School, UK. We join them as they are beginning their two-week psychiatric module.

❖ *The course leader is giving his introductory pep-talk: 'While you're on this attachment you'll need to get the core conditions sorted out in your minds. And you'll need to get confident in taking histories. Those are the most important things [. . .] There are deliberately very few lectures. The main thing is see lots of patients and read the basic texts to get the basic knowledge.'*

❖ *During a class discussion about a patient with hallucinations, the students are being quizzed about the things that they should ask the patient. They are palpably ticking things off the history-taking guide that they were given in the introductory session, which they know they have to memorize. (When started? How often? Content? Does he act on them? Insight? . . .)*

They call them out until the list is exhausted. The tutor looks pleased and moves on to the next 'list': other points to actively ask about. He ends by saying 'Don't forget about risk' (which they had). 'You'll fail if you don't ask about risk.'

❖   *During another case discussion, the tutor is taking the students through the key points of taking a history from a depressed patient. After going through the familiar list of set questions to ask so as to reinforce it in the students' minds (duration, associated symptoms, appetite, sleep, libido, suicidal tendencies . . .) he embarks on a more free-flowing discussion about techniques for negotiating with patients and motivating them to accept treatment. Many of the tips he is giving are formulations of his accumulated tacit knowledge, often about dealing with hypothetical situations (what if the patient were to say this or do that?) for which there would be no clear answers. Several stories of past patients illustrate his points graphically.*

❖   *The students are preparing to make a group presentation as part of a learning exercise designed to change prejudices about mental health. Ostensibly the idea is to make a presenta-tion to persuade others that they should, for example, revise their views about schizophrenic or depressed patients. But I can see that the underlying aim is for the students to confront their own prejudices (an assumption I later confirm with the tutors). As the group that I am following are preparing their presentation about post-partum depression, they begin to share many stories about doctors who have behaved well or badly in respect of depressed patients. Some arguments break out; quite deeply held views are being dealt with. But, by the time they make their presentations, they are all toeing the group's 'party line' about doctors needing to be more sympathetic towards depressed patients. During the final presentation by one of the other groups on schizophrenia, someone asks them what surprised them most in the materials they read while preparing their presentation. 'The fact that 80 per cent of people in a survey said that it's OK to refuse to let a flat to a schizophrenic.' 'And what shocked me most', says another 'is that until yesterday I would have been one of those 80 per cent.'*

❖   *In an exercise to teach students how to administer the Mini Mental State Examination (MMSE) the tutor appears to be doing three things simultaneously: driving home the fact that there is a fixed structure to it that they need to remember; giving very practical tips from her own experience on how to conduct and interpret it (e.g. what to do if a question seems to upset the patient); and guiding the students through reflection and feedback on their attempts to use it.*

❖   *Becky and Hitesh, two very able students, take a history and MMSE from an actor who is simulating a patient according to a brief written by the tutor, a practising psychiatrist. Their 'consultation' with the actor (who they are led to believe is a real patient with obsessive compulsive disorder) goes reasonably well but they occasionally have to hand over to each other as they dry up or forget what they should be asking next. Eventually they get most of the story – albeit in a fairly inchoate manner. But by the time it is presented only a few minutes later to the tutor, it is structured exactly as they have been taught in the history-taking guide, and covers all the key points that were in the actor's brief. Apart from some tips on how to communicate the findings more effectively to colleagues (e.g. how fast to speak) and one or two minor details, the tutor is satisfied. But he notices that Becky had been less confident than Hitesh about asking some key questions. He therefore moves on to the more subtle topic of the manner of taking a history (hard-nosed fact seeking versus easy conversational style) and gives them very practical tips for achieving a workable compromise. ('Well, what I've found works in those circumstances is . . .'). He reassures and advises Becky: 'At the beginning when you're still nervous you'll find you're more task focused – more Jeremy Paxman than Jonathan Ross.[1] But as you go on you'll get more comfortable. It's very difficult to teach. Watch doctors who are good at it and ask yourself how they are doing it. It will come with time.'*

❖ *I am chatting to Hitesh about how much he has come across protocols and guidelines during his clinical attachments. 'Yeah when I was on ICU it was all done by protocols. But then I went straight to GP and it was, like, "Well she's depressed but I don't think I'll give her SSRIs" . . . and yet the week before on ICU it was, like, "If the patient's shocked then you do this and this and this!"' He slaps his thigh at each 'this' to emphasize the contrast.*

Inexpressible knowledge

When we asked Lawndale practitioners what had led them to deal with any given clinical condition or situation in the way that they did they would perhaps, if they could answer at all, tell us a story about an incident that stood out in their memory, or reminisce about someone who taught them a particular aspect of what they had done, or allude to something they may have heard or read. But such answers made sense only if one already had a broad understanding of the underlying principles and theory that their answer had taken for granted. If we pressed them to explain the whole picture, we would be met on the whole with an unusual degree of inarticulacy. Given their generally high levels of both knowledge and fluency when we questioned them about most things concerning their practice, we must assume that their hesitancy was due to the difficulty they found in identifying the precise sources of the whole picture.[2] Or perhaps they were just surprised that we were asking such a naïve question. After all, if you asked experienced clinicians why they diagnosed and treated a certain disease the way they do, it would be worrying if they singled out the exact moment when they learnt all about it, or if they simply pointed to a guideline. One would rather expect them to have acquired a wealth of knowledge and skills over their entire clinical careers and to have the confidence that comes from a lifetime of learning that has gone far beyond any particular instruction.

Equally, it would be questionable whether a clinician who could give only the basic scientific facts was maturely competent to deal with the problem. Experienced clinicians might be expected to mention factors ranging from pharmacology through family circumstance to defective local services. And indeed, as we have seen in Chapters 2 and 3, Lawndale clinicians dealing with even the most routine cases were bringing to bear a very wide range of knowledge that had been blended into mindlines that encompassed far more than the canon of knowledge to be found in books, lectures and guidelines. In this chapter we will explore how clinicians initially acquire the foundations for this lifelong ability to use knowledge-in-practice.

As would-be clinicians grow into fully fledged professionals, each continually constructs a unique combination of all the different elements that blend to form their own fund of 'personal knowledge' (Polanyi 1958)[3] which is updated throughout their clinical careers. This is the basis of the knowledge-in-practice-in-context described in the preceding chapter, and it consists of a potentially infinite set of elements, many of which are incapable of being explicitly expressed. Such range and complexity are of course true not only of professional practice, but of any human activity. Just try and list, for example, all the knowledge and skills needed to do something as straightforward as preparing a meal and eating it with friends. They range from the economics of food shopping, through the selection and (safe) preparation of the food, the application of recipes to the available resources and the ethics, health concerns and idiosyncratic tastes of the diners, through to the fashion and etiquette of the dinner table, the cultural conventions of conversation, the subtleties of tone, expressions and body language, even to the ability to balance peas on a fork. How much more so for clinical practice? It is not surprising therefore that clinicians find it impossible to articulate all that they know – let alone how they came to know it – about managing any given clinical situation. As Michael Polanyi famously put it, 'We can know more than we can tell' (Polanyi 1967: 4).

Digging the foundations

By 2002 our observations at Lawndale had already shown us that the multifaceted mental resource we have called mindlines blended knowledge that had been absorbed from the countless sources to which clinicians are exposed throughout their careers (Figure 4.1). That being so, we next needed to explore two key aspects of mindlines, their substance and their growth. The substance of mindlines consists of the multilayered complexity of deeply ingrained knowledge-in-practice-in-context, which would emerge as we explored further the implications of our fieldwork. But the second line of inquiry – the growth of mindlines, or how they are laid down over time – would need to include not only the clinicians' early training but also the extensive and complicated series of transitions that had taken them from callow student to autonomous senior practitioner. Our original study, though, had been designed before it revealed mindlines to be a key concept, so we were now faced with a methodological challenge: the clinicians were working with mindlines that had already developed long before we met them, so how could we trace their origins? We were able to gain the occasional insight by reflecting on the Lawndale data, especially our discussions with trainee GPs, but one of the features of mindlines is their deep embeddedness – hence the senior clinicians' aforementioned inarticulacy on this topic – so we could not draw robust inferences from what they told us about the knowledge and skills acquired during their training.

To try and probe further into this question we therefore carried out brief supplementary participant observation studies in a US and a UK teaching hospital to watch medical training in those two very different environments. We also reflected on our own clinical training and on what we could glean on this subject from, between us, well over half a century of teaching and organizing training programmes for doctors and nurses at all levels and stages of their student and

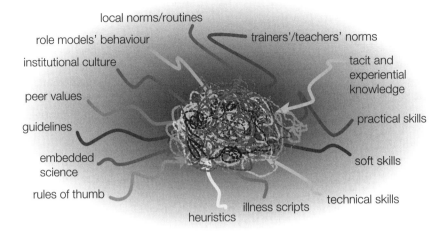

Figure 4.1 A schematic representation of some accumulated contents of mindlines.

professional careers. In order to try and hypothesize how clinical mindlines are developed we also searched the work of educationists and sociologists who have documented how clinical students, trainees and practitioners become proficient in their work and we delved into the wider literature about the acquisition of practical skills through education, apprenticeship and organizational learning. It was never the purpose of this exercise to provide a full description of the education process.[4] Our quest is merely to outline how it may be possible that clinicians develop their mindlines. Given that most of the Lawndale clinicians, doctors and nurses alike, would have begun their training with a large dose of biomedical science (such as anatomy, physiology, biochemistry, pathology, pharmacology, microbiology and epidemiology), we begin that quest with an old debate: just how important are all those basic sciences to a clinician's mindlines?

Biomedical sciences

'As a practising doctor, I have never ever, even for *one nanosecond*, needed to know anything whatsoever about the Krebs Cycle!' one of our eminent professorial colleagues would snarl when arguing for a rebalancing of the medical school curriculum. His irritation highlighted how little of the technical knowledge taught to students – not just that abstruse piece of biochemistry but many other supposedly more relevant pieces of science – eventually seems germane to actual clinical work. The defence has always been that even if the science that underlies the practice ultimately has only indirect, even subliminal, relevance it gives the more direct practical knowledge more rational sense. So, the argument goes, even though few if any practising doctors might be able to recount the complex biochemical interactions of the Krebs Cycle, or the potassium retention mechanisms in the renal tubules, or the role of osteoclasts and osteoblasts that they doubtless expended huge efforts to learn as students, the fact is that much of what they do is based on such science. Therefore there is always the possibility, especially in unexpected situations, that they may require some of that knowledge, however dim and vague the recall, to make sense of things. There are many other arguments around this topic. Those who want to teach more basic biomedical science claim it both reflects and fosters medical progress; critics riposte that it just serves the interests of the academics who teach it, or that it is a way of maintaining the elite status of medicine by unnecessarily mystifying its knowledge base. On the nursing front, similar arguments have raged as to whether the emphasis on the underlying science base serves principally to help the patients or to enhance the nurses' own professional status.

Fortunately we do not need to enter those debates here. Our concern is to try to estimate the degree to which the biomedical sciences taught to students lay at the core of the mindlines that guided, in this instance, the doctors' actions at Lawndale.[5] As we were in no position to quiz the clinicians directly without losing their cooperation (and in any case they were unlikely to be able to give accurate answers about the real influence of the science base), this was not easy to judge. What we can say is that we heard very little reference to scientific detail of any kind. This is not to say, of course, that the clinicians' work was not rooted in scientific principles. The overall basics seemed sound enough and when necessary – for example when teaching or when listening to lectures from local experts or perhaps trying to trip up the pharmaceutical reps whom they often jocularly accused of trying to 'blind us with science' – the GPs' discussions did reveal glimpses of deeply embedded, if dimly recalled, biomedical principles or more recent, scientifically informed reading.[6]

The detailed knowledge might have long since faded, but we cannot know if the GPs would have been capable of, say, diagnosing lobar pneumonia or prescribing antibiotics without some vestige of the biomedical basics. It was of course quite possible for them to get by on the automatic pilot of pattern recognition (Chapter 3) and routine practice without needing to adduce the underlying science, but the science was not so redundant as they might sometimes claim. Where a case followed an unusual path they would have floundered without it. If the problem required more thought, one could see that by having some of that deeper knowledge to fall back on they were much better placed to work out the best course of action. Certainly when reading up about the problem in the medical literature or discussing it with an expert who was well versed in the science, then if it were to make sense to them they needed that background scientific knowledge – as any lay person who has attempted to do the same might attest. And, of course, their patterns of thinking were mainly structured, by now instinctively, on broad-brush scientific principles even if the scientific facts had faded. So our conclusion is that, whilst it may be easy for the clinicians to be dismissive about the need to use the underlying science, mindlines do at some level contain the elements of such knowledge – even if not the full details of the Krebs Cycle, and even if much of it is vague, vestigial and rarely consciously recalled.

There is good evidence to support this view (see Woods 2007 for a recent review), despite the fact that several 'think aloud' studies (e.g. Patel *et al.* 1989; Boshuizen and Schmidt 1992) have suggested that experienced clinicians do not use their biomedical knowledge when dealing with clinical problems because it plays little part in the pattern recognition that is the basis of most diagnoses (Chapter 3). But other work suggests that doctors 'simply do not recognize (and therefore cannot verbalize) how their knowledge of physiology, biochemistry and the other sciences is indeed shaping the way they view, organize and interpret clinical information' (Woods 2007: 1174). Schmidt has proposed an 'encapsulation theory' whereby, as clinicians develop their skills, the biomedical knowledge and clinical facts become integrated, embedded and subsumed ('encapsulated') into the diagnostic categories and patterns (Schmidt and Rikers 2007). The same team also showed (Rikers *et al.* 2004), in a well-designed study of the way biomedical concepts are related to clinical ones, that experienced clinicians were able much more quickly than students not only to diagnose clinical problems but also to link them to the relevant biomedical building blocks. And this was despite the fact that it was, of course, the students and not the older doctors who had most recently been steeped in those biosciences. Other experimental studies suggest that knowing the underlying science helps students to learn and remember disease patterns more easily because it provides an organizing principle that helps them to categorize clinical conditions more coherently. The science, and in particular an understanding of causal mechanisms, acts as the 'glue' that holds clinical features together (Woods *et al.* 2007). It seems that all that early learning does allow clinicians, when they have had practical experience, to develop a coherent knowledge structure that can as a result be more easily accessed even many years later (van de Wiel *et al.* 1999). That being so, we can draw two tentative conclusions: first, biomedical sciences are indeed an important part of the early laying down of mindlines; and, second, they remained an important, if perhaps 'encapsulated' and unrecognized, part of the Lawndale practitioners' mindlines.[7]

Beyond bare bones

It should go without saying that students from all healthcare disciplines acquire from the basic sciences not just facts, but also a wide range of both intellectual and practical skills that are the main focus of the clinical curriculum and take many years to acquire. The intellectual skills include the analytical and problem-solving skills and pattern recognition that we discussed in Chapter 3 and whose development is such an integral part of clinical training and hence of mindlines. The range of practical skills is vast; for example among medical students[8] they range from communication, history taking, blood taking and clinical examination skills, through learning how to read radiographs, ECGs and MRI scans, to avoiding drug interactions and carrying out simple operations (see, for example, Williams *et al.* 2008). The process of imbibing these skills until they become second nature has rarely been better described than in the following passage by Michael Polanyi, who, before he became a physical chemist and eventually such an influential thinker about the nature of knowledge, had trained in medicine.

> Think of a medical student attending a course in the X-ray diagnosis of pulmonary diseases. He watches in a darkened room shadowy traces on a

fluorescent screen . . . and hears the radiologist commenting to his assistants, in technical language, on the significant features of these shadows. At first the student is completely puzzled. For he can see . . . only the shadows of the heart and ribs with a few spidery blotches between them. The experts seem to be romancing about figments of their imagination; he can see nothing that they are talking about. Then as he goes on listening for a few weeks, looking carefully at ever new pictures of different cases, a tentative understanding will begin to dawn on him. He will gradually forget about the ribs and begin to see the lungs. And eventually, if he perseveres intelligently, a rich panorama of significant details will be revealed to him: of physiological variations and pathological changes . . . He has entered a new world. He still sees only a fraction of what the experts can see, but the pictures are definitely making sense now and so do most of the comments made on them. He is about to grasp what he is being taught; it has clicked. Thus, at the very moment when he has learned the language of pulmonary radiology, the student will also have learned to understand pulmonary radiograms. The two can only happen together . . . a joint understanding of words and things.

(Polanyi 1958: 101)

Thus, argues Polanyi in this oft-quoted passage, grasping a new way of seeing or doing things is almost always inextricably linked to learning the associated language. Polanyi continues:

Having changed my profession and moved from Hungary to England, I have forgotten most of the medical terms I learned in Hungary and have acquired no others in place of them; yet I shall never again view – for example – a pulmonary radiogram in such a totally uncomprehending manner as I did before I was trained in radiology. The knowledge of medicine is retained, just as the message of a letter is remembered, even after the text [that] had conveyed either kind of knowledge has passed beyond recall. To speak of this message, or of medical matters, is therefore a performance based on knowledge.

(ibid.: 102)

There is, in other words, an asymmetry: whereas one cannot properly learn the terminology of medicine without also learning to do what doctors do, a trained doctor, he says, instinctively perceives, thinks and acts like a doctor when the detail or even the language has faded. Our Lawndale observations – and indeed our own experience as clinically trained academics who have not practised clinical work for decades – concur with that conclusion for other healthcare professionals too. The basic scientific knowledge may lapse, but what remain indelible are the principles such as the ways of perceiving and interpreting illness and disease, and of thinking through how to deal with them. Just as basic science may be 'encapsulated' within mindlines, so, perhaps, one might argue, it is these principles – the last things to fade – that form the durable skeleton upon which hangs all the detail of the mindlines as they subsequently accumulate.

As students, most of the Lawndale GPs who underwent a traditional medical course would have spent perhaps two or more 'preclinical' years learning the bio-medical sciences before starting to learn their clinical skills. And in the main they would have learnt these skills from observation and experience, in the manner of an apprentice. One has often heard clinical students talking about learning 'by osmosis' or 'sitting by Nellie', or the sardonic 'see one, do one, teach one'. Nurses, in contrast, have long been taught and examined upon their practical skills in a very explicit and structured way, and it is only relatively recently that medical students have been afforded such an approach for fundamental practical skills such as how to measure blood pressure, give a subcutaneous injection or perform cardiac massage. Also more recently, but still not universally, medical undergradu-ate teaching has moved away from the preclinical/clinical model towards much earlier clinical exposure that allows students, as they learn the science, to simulta-neously relate it to the clinical problems they must deal with. This trend towards linking the theory more closely to the practice has partly been in recognition of the finding that professional expertise and skilled decision making are neither the mere application of medical science nor an ineffable art, but go hand in hand with the science and therefore need continual and mutual nurturing right from the start of training. In an increasing number of nursing and medical schools there has additionally been a shift away from rote learning of the syllabus towards problem-based learning that encourages the students to find out for themselves the science relevant to real, or at least realistic, clinical problems (Boshuizen 2009).

Socializing and socialization

Whatever impact these educational transformations have had – and we need not discuss their appropriateness or effectiveness here – at least one thing remains relatively impervious to change as students increasingly learn to think and act like clinicians: they need to rely on each other as well as on their teachers. Students quickly learn that their colleagues are an important touchstone, and it is a habit that stays with them throughout their clinical careers.[9] Whether, as in the old days, working as a group to dissect a cadaver or present a project such as a community profile, or nowadays collaborating in their problem-based (perhaps inter-profes-sional) learning groups, they learn a great deal from their fellows. Sometimes that learning is explicitly about the content of the course – questioning, checking and relying on each other's knowledge, giving each other tips, competing or cooper-ating in preparing for examinations and so on. However, inevitably what they are also learning from each other is how to be a student and ultimately how to be a practitioner who is an accepted member of a peer group. The curriculum, mainly directed at the technical 'core' of knowledge and skills, always carries with it a large penumbra of the professional mindset conveyed by teachers and other established professionals. However, that mindset is also largely mediated by one's peers, a tendency that is apparent from the first days as a student, which is unsurprising since peer-mediated learning is a behaviour pattern laid down from one's preschool days onwards. It is through their colleagues that students become socialized into the cultural environment that impacts on what they learn and how they think and behave.[10]

Such socialization has been well described, for example in the classic study of Kansas medical students in the 1950s carried out by Becker and his colleagues (Becker *et al.* 1976). They also found that, because the curriculum was so over-whelmingly large, students needed right from the very start of their course to be selective about what they learnt. Most chose to learn what they needed to in order to pass their examinations rather than what they thought would matter to them as clinicians.[11] This was partly because at that stage of their careers the students could have no idea what they would actually need to know when they got into practice, partly because passing exams was the imperative without which they would get no further, but partly also because that quite simply was the medical student culture. Becker and colleagues found that the selection of what to learn was profoundly influenced by the peer group, and our observation as teachers suggests that little has changed in that respect among contemporary students. But more importantly there are clear parallels among mature practitioners. Even at the pinnacle of their careers, the GPs at Lawndale were likewise constantly having to be selective about the overload of new information to which they felt subjected, and were very skilled at filtering it in ways that among other things complied with what their colleagues felt was or was not worthy of attention, just as they doubtless had done at medical school.

There is never complete agreement, of course, between what students are being taught, what they are learning and what they actually need to know,[12] but somehow every successful student learns to negotiate a compromise between the three that allows them to become a clinician in respect of not only what they know but also how they think and behave. The way students prioritize and select what to learn is but one example of the way they learn things that are not part of the curriculum, but which will profoundly affect their mindlines. In this and many other ways, learners are also strongly influenced by their peers and by inadvertent experiences that affect the reliance they place on different sources of knowledge and values. As they progress through their training they imbibe much more than the intellectual and practical skills that we have suggested form the skeleton of their mindlines. The groups of student friends that form and develop patterns of working and socializing together – referred to by Becker *et al.* (1976) as 'compan-ionship' – along with the stratification into different types of students with differ-ing approaches to the course and to student life in general, lay the foundations for picking up behavioural and attitudinal norms towards patients and colleagues[13] that will shape their very existence as professionals.

The soft skills within mindlines

Implicit norms are a fundamental component of mindlines, because, as we have repeatedly stressed, treating an illness requires knowing not just about the diagnosis and treatment, but also the manner of relating to the patient, the decision whether or not to consider certain social, organizational and ethical contingencies (and, if so, how) and so on. In the past – and certainly when the Lawndale clinicians were in training – doctors and nurses absorbed these aspects of their mindlines in an ad hoc way from their teachers, colleagues, junior and senior role models and peers. This might happen through observation or through the stories so often used to graphically and memorably convey clinical knowledge (see Chapter 6), but which inevitably also act as a vehicle for transmitting soft skills and values. Now, however, the wide range of 'soft' skills that clinicians must absorb during their training (e.g. Mann *et al.* 2005; Rademakers *et al.* 2007) is increasingly entering formal taught courses as well. It has, for example, become the vogue among some medical schools to promote 'professionalism' as a specified component of the curriculum (Cruess *et al.* 2009). Nurses, in contrast, have been explicitly taught professionalism for much longer (Brown and Libberton 2007). Quite what is covered by this term is varied and sometimes vague – anything from how long your hair and finger nails should be through 'patient access, doctor–patient relationship, demeanour, professional management, personal awareness and motivation' (Jha *et al.* 2006: 1027) through 'subordination of one's self-interests, adherence to high ethical and moral standards, response to societal needs, and demonstration of evincible core humanistic values'(!) (Swick *et al.* 1999: 830). Soft skills also include not only the more obvious broad areas such as ethics and communication skills, but also more specific topics that are now receiving attention from educators, as even the briefest scan of three leading journals in nursing and medical education revealed. They include, for example, how one deals with mistakes (Di Vito-Thomas 2005; Kroll *et al.* 2008), 'cultural competence' such as the ability to handle ethnic varia- tions among patients and colleagues (Seeleman *et al.* 2009), emotional intelligence (Satterfield and Hughes 2007), emotional labour (Smith and Gray 2001; Gray 2009), humour (Chauvet and Hofmeyer 2007) and developing skills for lifelong reflective learning (Albanese 2006).[14]

Whether they are explicitly taught or imbibed through the untaught, peer-ori- ented learning from one's contemporaries and role models that is so fundamental to any professional culture, these soft skills of professionalism will strongly shape a clinician's mindlines. The hidden curriculum of acculturation brings deeply held and long-lasting attitudes, beliefs and values (Ajjawi and Higgs 2008) that include not only such items as how one deals with uncertainty (Fox 2000) or acquires the optimal level of emotional detachment – not to mention the potential for dehumanization (Kleinman 1988) – that are the subject of classic research studies (e.g. Fox 1988), but also what degree of failure is acceptable and why, including the unwritten norms by which one judges the competence and reliability of one's colleagues. Charles Bosk (1979), for example, plainly showed in his ethnography of US teaching hospital surgical teams that the doctors learnt during their train- ing how occasional technical incompetence is less of a sin than moral failings such as lack of diligence or covering up mistakes and failing to learn from them. Such norms and values are at the root of all subsequent mindlines, since they determine the degree of acceptable flexibility around 'textbook practice', the depths of knowledge that one is reasonably expected to acquire, the factors (such as dedication and thoroughness) that might allowably compensate for technical errors made 'in good faith', and the skill to know when and where to call for help.

This acquisition of soft skills is linked to the notion of 'organizational culture', the subject of much study by organizational researchers (Martin 2002), which has been shown to alter the way clinicians practise. ('The social value of [the profession's] work is as much a function of its organization as it is of the knowledge and skill it is said to possess' [Freidson 1988: xi].) One of the most influential accounts of organizational culture is by Schein (1992: 8–10) and in Table 4.1 we have applied his cultural categories to the teaching hospital. Students and trainees are immersed for many years in the culture of such places. The values, rituals, habits of thinking and so on become deeply embedded in their patterns of thought and behaviour and therefore inevitably form part of the substratum of their early mindlines and may persist for life. Indeed, eminent schools have been known explicitly to aim to turn out graduates who bear the distinctive stamp of their

Table 4.1   Organizational culture: examples of categories commonly held to comprise an organization's culture, adapted from Schein (1992) and applied to teaching hospitals

1 Observed behavioural regularities when people interact (e.g. rituals)	How and when people speak on ward rounds, how they dress (suit, white coat, scrubs), whether the doctor in clinic fetches patients from the waiting room or sits behind desk
2 Group norms (implicit standards, values, norms)	Degree of thoroughness required. Do we take audit meetings seriously? Long hours culture or 9–5?
3 Espoused values (public official line)	We value our 'customers', best hospital in the area, 'green hospital' policy
4 Formal philosophy (broad ideological principles)	The clinical method, 'dignity' principles, patient confidentiality
5 Rules of the game	How we do things around here, clinical protocols, how to get on in your career
6 Climate	The feeling conveyed by, e.g., physical layout, formality/ informality (Sir? Mate? Buddy? Granddad? Mr X? Johnny?), art on walls
7 Embedded skills (including professional capital – see Chapter 9)	Special competencies that come from the 'St Swithun's' nurse training scheme
8 Habits of thinking, mental models, and/ or linguistic paradigms	Local jargon, block beds on our ward or move patients on to make space for 'lodgers'? Respect or deride community services?
9 Shared meanings (see also p. 142)	Emergent understandings created by group members as they interact with each other (e.g. diverging clinical policies on adjacent wards)
10 'Root metaphors' or integrating symbols	Ideas, feelings and images implicit in emotional or cognitive responses, or as expressed through layout and artefacts – e.g. one-way mirrors in psychiatric wards, 'evidence trolleys' on ward rounds (Sackett and Straus 1998), alcohol handwash dispensers at ward entrance

particular culture. ('You can tell he's a St Swithun's man' is the kind of thing we still hear said of senior colleagues, although how far the graduates ever imbibed St Swithun's *intended* values and mindset as opposed to those of the hidden curriculum and student subculture is open to debate.)[15]

It should come as no surprise that clinicians incorporate such a wide range of learnt skills, attitudes and values into their day-to-day activity. Their training, after all, spends years immersing them in the entire culture of their profession. The point here is that such acculturation was firmly embedded in the mindlines that the Lawndale clinicians had acquired. When deciding how heavily to lean on a mother who did not want her children to have the MMR vaccine, when weighing up whether to refer someone with a skin lesion to a specialist or simply take a chance on one's own diagnosis and excise it, or when deciding whether or not despite the queue in the waiting room to extend someone's consultation because they look close to tears just as they are about to leave the surgery, the GPs were following a mindline shaped by much more than technical, practical knowledge about managing vaccination, melanoma or depression. Professional values and soft skills were an integral part of the mindlines that determined those actions.

Apprenticeship: learning the ropes together

One key ostensible aim of the long periods of clinical training 'on the wards' is, of course, to learn technical clinical skills in a way that integrates the theoretical knowledge that the students will require as clinicians. This is where the theoretical and scientific knowledge begins to be 'encapsulated' (p. 75) as the clinical and practical work envelops the students.[16] Once they enter the wards, they undergo what is to all intents an apprenticeship, by which we mean learning in the real practical situation not only from (in the original terminology of the craft guilds) the 'master' but also from the old hands. During a clinical apprenticeship, learning consists of much more than individuals filling their heads with the new knowledge and skills. Rather, as Atkinson (1981) showed in his ethnography of a Scottish teaching hospital, they learn the version of medical reality perpetrated by those around them (the textbooks may say that mitral incompetence has a murmur that sounds like that but in fact it usually sounds like this) and they learn the attendant culture that characterizes that environment (yes maybe surgeons do things that way but we physicians do it this way).[17] They are, in other words, acquiring practical, experiential knowledge, much of which is implicit and inexpressible. And, importantly, they are doing so by being involved in a social and organizational world in which their activities, the people they interact with and the entire situation are all playing their part in shaping what they know and how they think and behave (Teunissen *et al.* 2007; Dornan *et al.* 2007). For the trainee GPs, amassing their personal stock of illness scripts, exemplars (p. 57), practical skills and much more besides, this period of apprenticeship is neither an individual activity nor one that is separate from everything else that they are undertaking. It is only by such linking of context and content that the students can proceed to the kind of 'elaborated learning' (Coles 1985) that allows them to go beyond mere rote learning to incorporate the flood of new knowledge into meaningful patterns and schemata that will ultimately be part of their early mindlines. This process involves co-participants (teachers, staff, role models, colleagues, patients) and constant exposure to complex events and activities. Students swap stories avidly, compare notes, compete for practical examples of different kinds of patients and activities, share in-jokes and absorb the tales and habits of the people around them (Atkinson 1981; Hunter 1991). Learning on the wards, like clinical practice itself, is, to use Lave's term, a 'situated activity' (Lave 1996: 4). It not only entails knowledge-in-practice-in-context (p. 65) but also imparts the ability to function when placed in *different* situations, when the learner will need to improvise with 'the social, material and experiential resources at hand' (ibid.: 13). The repertoire that they are acquiring includes not only all those soft skills we have discussed but organizational ones too. Finally, the budding clinician is learning an even more fundamental repertoire: how to present 'face' to patients and colleagues. 'Face' is the term introduced by Erving Goffman in his classic analysis (Goffman 1959) of the way people conduct themselves in dress, manner, appearance, speech and so on to present themselves in ways that maintain their plausibility even in the most difficult of circumstances. Inevitably, therefore, as the students develop their ability to think and act like clinicians, the repertoire deeply rooted in the culture of the wards they are working on and the people they are working with gets built into their mindlines.[18]

How is that achieved?[19] During the apprenticeship period – as students and later as qualified practitioners – clinicians are gradually becoming able to engage in the activities they will eventually need to be able to carry out independently. When Becky struggles to get the 'right' balance between relaxed conversation and incisive inquiry, she is acquiring a skill in history taking that will serve her (and will continue to develop) throughout her career. She starts by watching respected colleagues and being given the opportunity to practise on a simulated patient or real patients in whose treatment she plays no part. But as time goes on she has increasing opportunities to become more closely engaged as part of the team (which was also very evident in Oakville [p. 86]). Lave and Wenger (1991), studying how people learn a wide range of crafts, have called this process 'legitimate peripheral participation'. The term describes the gradual but carefully structured and sanctioned movement of the learner from marginal association to full engagement with the sociocultural practices of the community they are entering. Clinical students don the trappings of the role (white coat, stethoscope, nursing uniform) as a symbol of being allowed to partake in the life of the wards, but are only very gradually empowered to become involved with what is going on there. Having seen the actor-patient, Becky was learning not just about obsessive compulsive behaviour, but also, for example, how to listen to patients, how to structure her findings and conclusions to colleagues, how to deal with her own prejudices and (as we saw explicitly discussed by the tutor) whether she would like to be a psychiatrist.

> From a broadly peripheral perspective, apprentices gradually assemble a general idea of what constitutes the practice of the community. This uneven sketch of the enterprise (available if there is legitimate access) might include

who is involved; what they do; what everyday life is like, how masters talk, walk, work, and generally conduct their lives; how people who are not part of the community of practice[20] interact with it; what other learners are doing; and what learners need to learn in order to become full practitioners. It includes an increasing understanding of how, when and about what old-timers collaborate, collude, and collide, and what they enjoy, dislike, respect, and admire. In particular, it offers exemplars (which are grounds and motivation for learning activity), including masters, finished products, and more advanced apprentices in the process of becoming full practitioners.

(Lave and Wenger 1991: 95)[21]

Bosk's ethnography of trainee surgeons in the USA (Bosk 1979) shows in some detail how they gradually, over five years of post-qualification surgical training, reached the inner circle of elite surgery or found themselves excluded because they failed to meet the exacting and largely social criteria of their legitimacy to do so. The move from periphery to centre owed, in his study, more to a trainee surgeon's demonstrating the right moral fibre than mere technical ability. As Becker *et al.* (1976) also noted, part of acquiring the clinical way of thinking is also learning when and when not to take responsibility – which is also, we would argue, a crucial part of clinical mindlines.

Quintessentially, therefore, this process of apprenticeship is a form of 'action learning' that increasingly engages the student with the practitioners, teachers (both people and written sources) and fellow students (Revans 1998 [1982]; Gabbay 1991), all of whom are helping to formulate the learners' mindlines. Their membership of their eventual professional group evolves as they become more acquainted with how things are done, all of which, alongside the technical knowledge that will be examined, become deeply embedded in their mindlines. For Becky, Hitesh and their colleagues, the early foundations of their mindlines include not only 'the basics of depression' but also how to ask about suicidal thoughts without being embarrassed or offensive, and why it seemed to be fine if GPs sometimes do not follow the guidance on using antidepressants, whereas equivalently non-conformist behaviour would be inimical on an intensive care unit. This is true not only of students but of all 'apprentices' including GP trainees. Jason, although fully trained as a doctor, was introduced only under very controlled conditions to being on call for emergency GP visits at Lawndale until he was thought to be able to handle it alone. Thus Lawndale GP trainees went through a similar process of legitimate peripheral participation until they became accepted and trusted autonomous members of the group. (Or not. Two trainees were eventually employed as partners during our time at Lawndale, but one was unable to make the grade as an accepted member of the group – and indeed ended up not becoming a GP at all.) There were already clear hints on the Oakville ward rounds too as to which students and residents were likely to make it to the top and which were not. But, as we shall see in the next chapter, what stood out on those ward rounds, like a rocky outcrop above the smooth ground, was the almost visible strata of mindlines at different stages of development, from the callow student through the harassed residents to the urbane attending physician, and that the 'situated learning' never stops, no matter what stage clinicians are at in their career.

Chapter 4: Summary

Clinicians find it hard to explain the precise reasoning behind many of their rapid but often complex decisions because the underlying rationales may be deeply embedded in patterns of thinking that have become almost instinctive. Using the educational literature and our observations of early clinical teaching we have explored how those patterns are laid down during their training. Clinical sciences, 'soft skills', attitudes and values drawn from clinical trainees' apprentice-like experience of their entire social environment become embedded in their emergent mindlines. Formal knowledge is thereby inextricably melded with a wide range of experiential and tacit knowledge and behavioural norms.

5 Growing mindlines
Cultivating contextual adroitness

Three facets of mindlines are explored in this chapter: how novices gradually develop them to become experts, how clinicians handle new information that has the potential to change what they do, and how they keep their mindlines up to date or seek guidance. The prologue for the first of these topics comes chiefly from our observations while 'embedded' in an internal medicine team at Oakville Hospital in the USA.

❖ *It is 7 a.m. in the 'conference room' at Oakville Hospital. About twenty doctors and students are sitting at several tables nursing their coffees and doughnuts and writing up their notes from the previous day's admissions ready for their 'attending'[1] rounds. The structure of the presentations on the round is all important, so they are focused on working them up, making sure that everything necessary has been not only done and typed properly into the notes, but built into the brief oral presentations they will make to the attending physician. The key is to have written a succinct summary, the 'thumbnail', that has all the necessary points in the right order on a folded piece of A5 that they use as a 'cheat sheet'. Craig, the resident postgraduate year three ('PGY3'), and his team have been admitting the overnight emergencies. He is briefing Chrissie, one of his PGY1s (postgraduate year one), who has to make slick presentations designed to help the attending's decision making: 'You gotta get those thumbnails right. I just wanna hear the pertinent positives.' Then he turns to the fourth-year medical student, Surinder, who is expected to write a fuller account. 'These are things that are going to stick with you whatever you end up specializing in', says Craig, as he checks what Surinder has written about the patient with aortic stenosis and renal failure and makes some suggestions about both content and format. Craig himself has been on the intranet checking every patient's details, looking up the relevant guidance and papers online, ensuring that every angle is covered before Josh, the attending, arrives.*

Josh walks in; he has been up since 4.30 a.m. and has already quietly checked all the patients online. He has his own clutch of thumbnails. He jokes about it having been 'family therapy night' (i.e. a lot of psychosocial problems) and gives avuncular advice on how to persuade a woman with strong religious beliefs to undertake a procedure that is against her religion. ('Here's what I say to 'em . . .'). But his advice ends more ominously, 'She's sicker than shit, by the way', and he makes it chillingly clear that he expects them to ensure she has had that procedure as soon as possible. As they arrive at the patient's bed, Chrissie spouts the thumbnail so fast that I as an outsider cannot follow it at all. But Josh and Craig look pleased with her. Several levels of conversation follow. There is basic teaching (to Surinder – 'Listen to that swoosh swoosh sound') and a clear explanation of the split first heart sound. For Chrissie there is an explanation of the system for ordering echograms. With Craig there is erudite science and one-upmanship about being up to date with the latest literature about the reason why renal failure patients have raised potassium levels and what to do about it. Josh tells them out of interest what they used to do when he first started twenty years ago and asks – possibly faux naïf, I'm sure he knows – 'What do you guys do now?' Chrissie fluffs the answer and Craig contradicts her as he checks the computer printout and then the screen. She finds herself being grilled about it. But Josh ends by giving them all wise advice about excessive testing and inappropriate hospitalization. Nevertheless Craig talks sternly to her afterwards about having got the wrong tests. There is more than a hint of social control going on here.[2]

At the next patient, Surinder presents the patient. Craig stops him: 'No, that's part of the findings. Right now we're talking about the history.' Surinder is moreover giving far too much detail. They continue to steer him to present the salient facts in the right order: the order their own minds are running in so as to make sense of the case, which he is not following properly. Josh makes that point explicitly. 'Let me tell you why', he says. 'We [physicians] talk to each other all day. That's what we do. We spend all day telling each other stories about patients. And we are used to those stories being in a certain sequence and structure. If it doesn't come that way, it's disconcerting.' Later in response to one of Chrissie's thumbnails Josh, reinforcing this same point, smiles. 'Yeah, now that's an important part of the history. [. . .] but if his father died of an MI at the age of eighty-six, I don't care.' 'Pertinent positives only', Craig adds. 'Yeah, but that was better', says Josh. 'Incremental improvement – that's what we like to see.'

❖ *At 'Morning Report' with a group of residents who are sitting in the conference room discussing recent cases (very much in the form of a tutorial-cum-ward round), the lead resident who is running the session writes up each patient on the whiteboard with all the items required in a thumbnail. Each is a highly structured set of abbreviations and numbers quite unintelligible to anyone not trained in its use but it is the main artefact through which they all communicate. The first line of one such schema, for example, is given in Figure 5.1.*

The discussion consists of a series of reinforcements and modulations of the implications of – and the latest thinking on – each of the most relevant items noted, linked to stories about other relevant patients. I reflect that these structured thumbnails on the whiteboard must act like the skeleton upon which the residents' mindlines are continually being built as they compare experiences, rules of thumb, relevant readings of the literature, techniques, complications, cautionary tales, gossip about how other teams (good and bad) have handled such patients and so forth. For many of the matters discussed, a view emerges of the degree

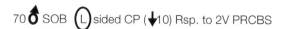

Figure 5.1   First line of a thumbnail.

of acceptable variation in practice, and of what is considered unacceptable. For example, as they discuss a puzzling patient whose tiredness has not been explained, one of the residents ventures: 'Here is my fatigue work-up: TSH, CBC, B12, folate, basic, comp, ESR.' The tutor gently mocks some aspects of it. The resident defends why she checks vitamin B12 levels. They briefly discuss the clinical, economic, organizational and economic merits of doing 'comp' (comprehensive biochemistry) rather than just urea and electrolytes. Others listen to the debate and take note. Someone confirms an element of the debate on their PalmPilot. Someone else quips – 'Wow! If it's written in Up To Date [the online expert system that most of them access through their handheld computers and treat as their bible] it must be real!' They all laugh. They eventually come to an interim consensus on what 'labs' (investigations) would be best in such cases, while another resident is volunteered to check out the literature and report back next time. It dawns on me that this meeting happens every single morning, constantly developing and refining the mindlines for every person present.

❖ *It is 7 a.m. Sita the 'hospitalist' (a grade of senior, fully qualified physician employed by the hospital to manage a caseload of up to thirty inpatients) is engaged in a handover session with a colleague, preparing her day's work. As they talk, she is completing for each patient a highly structured thumbnail that combines all of what Craig would call the 'pertinent positives' about them linked to the relevant tasks required that day. On one set of A5 cards is everything she needs to know, communicate and do about each of twenty-four patients that day.*

❖ *Surinder, Chrissie and I are chatting over a bagel in the middle of their night on 'long take'. Surinder talks about having to get to grips with 'the flowsheets' for each condition. I ask what he means by that. 'Well I get the feelin' that everyone here has some kinda flowsheet in their minds but I don't yet, which bothers me.' I ask if being a student at the moment is about learning all those flowsheets. 'You betcha.' Later on Chrissie is looking very tired, staring at a screen with Mrs Astupile's details on it and saying that the patient should really have an adrenal work-up but she doesn't feel like doing it before tomorrow's round. Anyway the patient doesn't fit the usual picture and may not need it so she will need to look it up later. I ask where she will look. 'Up To Date, I guess – it's where everybody looks. There ain't even any books round here.' (I recall that Craig said he looks everything up online from home before the round, but there are lots of websites that they all visit all the time: online textbooks, guides from other medical schools, experts systems – on one occasion Chrissie, using her cell-phone, even Googled the test she was about to order as we were walking to the emergency room.) I ask if the adrenal work-up is one of those flowcharts Surinder was talking about. She nods and grins. 'Yup! And I haven't done enough endocrine yet to get that flowchart in my head so . . .' She turns back to the screen. When she's finished she tells me the story of a surgeon who derided flowcharts because if we could practise with flowcharts we wouldn't need doctors, and then went on to teach them what to all intents was his flowchart for breast cancer. She laughs at the irony. When I next see her, 3.15 a.m., she's reading about fludrocortisone in hypotension on Up To Date. She needs to be sure she has it all under her belt before the morning round. In fact a great deal of the activity of the rest of the night for both of them is about retyping the notes to ensure they have 'won the game' by getting on top of all the new patients and making sure everything is fully recorded both in the computer and in their own notes (and heads). Everything needs to be in place so that they can begin working on the thumbnails in time for the round at 7 a.m. Surinder even forgoes two very good practical opportunities to see or help with emergencies on the wards so that he can get on with the main business in hand – which is to make sure he has done everything he can to ensure he survives the morning round by having all the right facts and flowcharts ready in his head (supplemented by the odd 'cheat sheet') if he gets 'grilled'.*

❖   *Back in the UK, I meet up with an old friend, Hassim – now a highly successful and wealthy surgeon in Texas. He doesn't know about our research. Enthusiastic, entrepreneurial and ambitious, he explains with due immodesty how he succeeded. When he reads about operative procedures, he says, he is experienced enough to see practical hints that someone less knowledgeable would never spot. He can immediately relate what he reads to a detailed and logical understanding of anatomy and physiology, he says. That gives him the edge when he 'mixes with the big boys', so that when he sees just once how they do something, he can repeat it. 'Like a karate move', he says. 'A novice can see the move a hundred times and still not get it. I get it first time. Who needs formal training when you can do that?'*

❖   *During an interview at Lawndale, Jason says the challenge in hospital was running around making sure that everything that should be done (largely routine) was done and filed in the notes. Coming into general practice as a trainee 'has been a bit more of a diagnostic challenge and a bit more of a meeting patients' expectations challenge – and also I often find myself thinking, "This isn't about medicine at all is it?"' Instead, much of the work, he continues, concerns psychosocial problems that he does not yet feel confident to deal with. He has also noticed there is a lot more multitasking across many different types of task that he has had to learn about.*

During a similar interview Tamsin says how difficult it was when first in general practice not to have had a clear routine of things to carry out for each patient before she referred them to hospital. She found it hard to know where she fitted into the system, for example how far to investigate post-coital bleeding, which she could have easily done as a gynae junior once the patient had got to hospital. The skills she needed back there were relatively simple, and she had had lots of time to see patients, time to ask for advice. By contrast, in general practice it had been 'frightening' to have to deal with the kind of problems that she never had to face in hospital – the variety, the non-specific problems, the social and emotional problems and the different kinds of often tricky decisions that were needed. There were a lot more people and managerial skills involved. 'I'd rather have had an acute MI to deal with any day.' But, she added, the confidence and speed of dealing with things was definitely growing with experience.

❖   *Tamsin spends an hour in tutorial with her trainer, Barry. They are talking through the ways one might deal with various conditions and how she has dealt with patients. What emerges from observing this process is that she is clearly a very competent doctor in terms of her medical training and even, at this relatively early stage of her GP training, her people skills and organizational nous. But on almost every topic there is some aspect of the local situation or system, some piece of tacit knowledge, that she still has to learn, such as what additional factors to take into account, what alternative treatments to consider and why, how to get the system to produce a particular kind of prescription or how to save the patient money and time. Some of this is very specific to Lawndale. But most of it will serve her well wherever she does general practice, even though it is not the kind of knowledge available other than from an expert trainer who sometimes has trouble analysing and explaining it because to him it is just second nature (p. 48).*

❖ *During the resuscitation course for all Lawndale staff the tutor asks them what anaphylaxis is. Ben, the trainee fresh from passing his MRCP, enthusiastically volunteers a complex definition involving antigens, immunoglobulins, chemical levels and all sorts. He is teased and chastened as the tutor smiles and says, 'Well actually all I was looking for was that it's a severe allergic reaction involving the circulatory and/or respiratory systems.'*

❖ *Two of the senior partners challenge Ben over coffee about his tendency to do glucose toler-ance tests (GTTs) strictly according to the guidelines. 'Why do it?' they ask. 'The diabetes just becomes official, scares the patient who now thinks they'll die blind and legless and increases their insurance premium. Why not just regularly keep an eye on their blood sugar?' He stands up for himself, including a nice joke about diabetic men at least being able to get free Viagra. Clive then quotes several studies and statistics at him (about, for example, the changed criteria for diabetes since GTTs were redesigned, and the incidence of diabetes retinopathy in people with marginally high blood sugars) that appear to persuade Ben that maybe doing a GTT is not as logical as he had thought. 'Well', Clive softens, 'it's different in hospital. Clearer. We just can't apply those criteria in general practice. Maybe we should ask the diabetologist along to give us a talk.'*

❖ *During a GP contract meeting, there has been a long discussion about the difficulty of using a simple three-item questionnaire to diagnose dementia before eventually agreeing to have the questionnaire as an easily accessible prompt on the computer. This long argument is puzzling me. It wouldn't be hard to learn the three questions by heart – it would probably take them less time than they have just spent discussing why they can't read them out. What is really going on here? Maybe, once they are fully trained, doctors are averse to rote learning. Certainly a lot of the points they are making as they resist adopting the questionnaire suggest strongly that such things (like guidelines too) have to be individualized to suit both the doctor and the patient. It seems to be the mark of a good professional. Anyone can read out a question but adapting it and thinking about it requires experience and skill. No wonder the one nurse present looks miffed when someone suggests that they and not the doctors should be the ones, if anyone, to read the questions verbatim to patients.*

Developing expertise

It will be clear by now why, in addition to absorbing a vast amount of technical knowledge, by the time they have started to practice, all clinical students have acquired skills,[3] attitudes, practices and values that go far beyond the consciously taught curriculum. 'People do not simply learn *about;* they also learn . . . *to be* . . . Learning, in all, involves acquiring identities that reflect both how a learner sees the world and how the world sees the learner' (Brown and Duguid 2001: 200).[4] We turn now to examine the processes by which all of those components of learning may become embedded as mindlines during the practitioner's development from neophyte to expert. We begin by revisiting Patricia Benner's (1984) classic study of the way practical knowledge becomes embedded in clinical work. Her research, which led to considerable changes in nursing curricula, set out to refocus attention onto the actual roles and competencies that good nursing entails and how they are acquired. Benner made use of what was then the emerging work of the Dreyfus brothers – Hubert, a philosopher, and Stuart, an applied mathematician – who had written a swingeing critique of the 'wishful thinking' that artificial intelligence could ever replicate the way the human mind works (Dreyfus and Dreyfus 1986).[5] They showed that computers could probably never match the subtleties of human thought because expertise entailed such a large degree of 'intuition'. Moreover, they concluded, 'Competent performance is rational; proficiency is transitional; experts act arationally' (*sic*; ibid.: 36). In doing so, the Dreyfus brothers adduced many fields of activity, from learning a language to playing chess to flying aeroplanes, but much of their empirical evidence in fact came from Benner's study of nursing.[6] The key to both the Dreyfus brothers' and Benner's models is that expert knowledge transcends logic, is deeply embedded in practice, and cannot be readily expressed.

Their emergent models suggest that experts acquire this transcendent knowledge-in-practice in five stages: Novice, Advanced Beginner, Competent, Proficient and Expert. Those stages, to which we will add one further one, 'Contextually Adroit', help to give some structure to the chronological growth of a clinician's mindlines, but before we explain them we should state several caveats. First, the stages were never intended to be seen as discrete entities, but are convenient conceptual categories (ideal types) that help analyse how practical learning progresses. Second, as Benner herself showed, a person can simultaneously be at any or all of the stages when engaging in different segments of their professional work. The notion that people develop in their professions by moving sequentially through the five stages, although sometimes misguidedly used as the basis for curriculum design, is a travesty both of Benner's own observations and of common experience. We can all recall times when we were expert in some parts of our jobs and yet novices in others. One learns quickly to become an expert houseman or intern while still being a novice surgeon; a surgeon may be peerless in the operating theatre but barely competent at breaking bad news sensitively; Tamsin, a trainee GP at Lawndale, was an excellent young clinician but initially felt all at sea over many aspects of being a novice general practitioner. Even an expert with all the requisite skills for a new job may well need to learn the ropes either because this place has a different way of doing things or because they have new responsibilities. (A senior hospital surgeon once volunteered to JG that the most frightening time of his career, despite all his skill and experience at that stage, had been his first few months as a consultant.[7]) Third, Benner's model recognizes that even the best people can fail to progress through all the stages in all aspects of their day-to-day work. (That technically peerless but insensitive surgeon may never learn to break bad news . . .)

We would add two further caveats. It seems reasonable to assume that, as the learner goes through the stages from Novice to Expert, what develops is not just the practical learning on which Dreyfus and Benner focused but also the whole range of people skills, organizational and political skills, and ethical and cultural values. They are all accumulating, adjusting and interacting with each other as the learners synthesize their growing professional capabilities (Ajjawi and Higgs 2008) and develop what some would call their professional artistry (Fish and Coles 1998; Titchen 2009). Becker's landmark study of medical students (Becker *et al.* 1976) showed, for example, that they adopted very different cultural 'perspectives' as they progressed from being preclinical novices to hospital interns, and these perspectives profoundly altered their technical and practical learning (p. 78). A significant part of the learning undertaken by the Doppton psychiatry students was designed to change their culturally embedded attitudes towards mental illness and, although this was explicitly led by the teachers, it was also played out and influenced strongly by the peer group (p. 70). Likewise, even as fully fledged experts, the Lawndale GPs and practice nurses were continually subject to the subliminal influences of their peers not only in their clinical roles, but also in the knowledge, attitudes and beliefs that underpinned the entire range of roles that we observed. At every stage, then, not only clinical skills but also cultural and professional norms are being developed and honed. Our final caveat is that Benner and especially the Dreyfus brothers seem to play down the fact that every one of the five stages, even the Novice stage, involves the learner in understanding crucial situational knowledge: 'Who does what and how around here? How and where should I fit in? What do I need to know to get on and how and where will I find it out?' (Box 3.1). This level of skill, although usually additional to the other skills, makes it quite possible to get by in routine work without many of them – as the occasional clinical impostor has demonstrated. It is to stress how important this kind of knowledge is – going well beyond what most people would assume is meant even by expert knowledge – that we have added a sixth 'stage' of Contextually Adroit. To be fair, Benner and the Dreyfus brothers are quite aware of the place of context, but in our view they do not give it enough emphasis. They even suggest that context plays no part in the Novice stage, whereas it clearly does – as the following published reflections of a medical student from a two-week 'shadowing course' clearly illustrate:

> [we] were all obsessed with the seemingly endless and daunting administrative tasks: 'Which bloods go in which bottle?' 'How do I call the porters?' 'What am I actually supposed to write in the notes?' 'Where can I go for a quick cry when the consultant shouts at me on ward round?
>
> (Feest and Forbes 2007: 15)[8]

Context is crucial at every stage and will shape what is being learnt, including the formal knowledge that is being acquired.[9] For example, trainees working where there are no community physiotherapists will develop different mindlines for the management of stroke patients from those of their colleagues in better provided locations.

With those caveats in mind, we can now explore how the different stages contribute to the way in which mindlines are laid down during the clinician's training. The Novice stage consists mainly of acquiring objective facts and 'rules' that are relatively inflexible – eliciting clinical signs and knowing the protocol for what to do next if you find them, for example. This includes the sorts of learning that can be examined in an objective, structured clinical examination, such as how to administer and score the Mini Mental State Examination to detect the degree of dementia. But it cannot help in judging when the dementia warrants social services support or compulsory admission to hospital, and nor can that sort of learning be objectively assessed. The Novices' thinking is necessarily somewhat plodding and linear as they get to grips with all the new information and try to assimilate it. The Novice stage parallels observations (Boshuizen and Schmidt 2000; Boshuizen 2009) that students solving diagnostic problems tended to use logical deductive thinking rather than pattern recognition (pp. 56, 75). By the time they reach the Advanced Beginner stage clinical students are much better at coping with real situations because now that they have some concrete experience behind them they are learning to recognize similar sets of events. They are already beginning to move beyond mere facts, rules and logic. Things often appear strange and overwhelming, and Advanced Beginners need to concentrate very hard to take it all in, but they are learning to discern the key elements of the patterns such as illness scripts and routines that will increasingly help them to work like real clinicians. They also begin to spot much more quickly the aspects of a situation that really matter. In contrast to the more explicit and measurable content of the Novice stage, a good deal of what the Advanced Beginner acquires is tacit or judgement-dependent; they can now cope better with situations that do not follow the norm. The fund of tacit, personal, experiential, practical knowledge that is acquired at this stage and melded with the (increasingly encapsulated) theory learnt as a novice becomes, we would argue, the bedrock of the clinicians' eventual mindlines.

The transition from Advanced Beginner to Competent is an important part of turning a person who knows all the relevant facts into one who can be canny about using them (what many texts describe as the difference between 'know *that*' and 'know *how*'). This progression reminds JG of a particularly stressful period as an overconscientious new house-surgeon (intern) when he was slavishly dealing with one patient after another, taking much longer than the time available to him. To survive, he needed to acquire the skill and confidence to take the necessary short cuts that make the job efficient, and with repeated experience he became more able to quickly get to the nub of each situation and to prioritize and plan the tasks. His survival in the job depended on reaching the Competent stage, character-ized by the ability both to grasp a constellation of events, get to the heart of the matter (as opposed to going through predetermined steps, relevant or not) and deal with any consequences, and also to organize his work more effectively, even when it meant bending the rules. These skills, just as much as the development of illness scripts, the encapsulation of biomedical knowledge and the honing of practical techniques, become embedded into a clinician's way of thinking. Indeed one of the (few) arguments in favour of the stressful jobs that many junior doctors experience is that, by going through that white heat, they are forced to learn to cope resourcefully with the demands of their later careers. Furthermore, since reliance on the skills of others is crucial if a junior doctor is to live to tell the tale (Brown *et al.* 2007), an important part of that process is acquiring the skill of knowing how and when to depend on colleagues,[10] as Tamsin did at Lawndale (p. 128).

The move from Competent to the next stage, Proficient, is a quantum leap, for it is at this stage that thinking ceases to rely mainly on logical progression and becomes more 'intuitive'. Benner's use of the term 'intuitive' does not suggest innate, inspired, irrational or untutored, but refers to the capacity for instantaneous pattern recognition (pp. 56, 75) and the ability to get to the core of a problem, to spot the salient features, without the need for conscious deliberation. Just how these things are done defies logical description or explanation. This ability is related to what Polanyi called 'connoisseurship', something that cannot be taught except 'by a long course of experience under the guidance of a master' (Polanyi 1958: 54; Smith 2008). It applies not only to technical competencies but also to wider skills and considerations that will eventually need to be balanced against each other (Smith *et al.* 2003). For example, when the Doppton psychiatrist, a consummate communicator, was tutoring Becky, who had found it difficult to ask a patient certain questions, he reassured her that even though he could not possibly explain or teach it to her, the knack of finding a comfortable balance between interrogating a patient and conversing with them would come with time, especially if she watched doctors who were good at it and, as he put it, 'try to fathom what they are doing' (p. 71).

At the Proficient stage as Benner described it, a clinician has developed the ability to just sense from the situation as a whole when there is something wrong with a patient and to home in quickly on the necessary steps to rectify the problem. This can come about only with considerable experience and is clearly related to the emergence of pattern recognition discussed in Chapter 3. But, until she becomes expert, the proficient learner still tends also to need mentally to check back with the learnt rules and maxims (as in the Oakville 'flowcharts') and may often need to pause and think the actions through. So, for example, whereas Tamsin after nearly six months of being able to work autonomously as one of the team of GPs still needed to check drug doses in the *British National Formulary* several times a day, the Lawndale partners had to do so relatively rarely. Being mainly at the Proficient stage, she still needed to think through a lot of her decisions and to explicitly discuss a significant proportion of them with a more expert colleague. The contrast with Barry, her trainer, was that he as an Expert no longer needed to rely on analytic principles for the majority of what he did, making it quite laboured for him to explain to her in the tutorial why he would take a certain line with a patient (p. 48). Within their area of real skill, and where things are proceeding normally, an Expert's grasp of the problems and their solutions just happens. Indeed – and the example often quoted is the difference between the way expert radiologists read a radiograph by quickly comprehending the picture it conveys (almost a Gestalt), compared with the way in which students are taught to systematically check every aspect of the film – 'if experts are made to attend to the particulars or to a formal model or rule, their performance actually deteriorates' (Benner 1984: 37). This is why Heather told us (p. 23) that she did her nurse triage the way she did and no longer 'by the book' (Greatbatch *et al.* 2005).

Of course things often do not go normally, and so the Expert is also adept at thinking deliberatively about a problem. But, unlike the merely Competent practitioner, theirs is a different kind of deliberative thinking that rapidly forms whole patterns, quickly taking in a very broad range of matters related to the intended goal, but also cutting straight to the ones that count and cutting out the rest (which Gigerenzer 2007 claims is one of the keys to heuristic thinking). This was doubtless part of the reason for the emphasis on the 'pertinent positives' that were being drilled into the Oakville interns as they struggled to produce the 'thumbnails' that just came naturally to the attending (consultant) physician, who, moreover, was much more able than they were to immediately consider a wide array of factors and focus on the ones that influenced his decisions. So, suggests Benner, when we ask an expert what they would do in a hypothetical situation they are likely to say 'it all depends'. Small wonder then that, in contrast to the interns and residents of Oakville who so frequently checked their 'flowcharts' and other sources of guidance, the attending physician rarely needed to do so. This insight makes it less surprising that we never saw Lawndale clinicians consulting formal guidelines or other normative sources while they were problem solving. When things were going unexceptionally these expert clinicians had no need for the guidance; and when things were out of the ordinary there was no guidance available that would take account of all the variable circumstances that 'it all depends' upon. For guidelines it is Catch-22 again (pp. 5, 30): when it's a routine case, experts don't need the guidance; when the case is out of the ordinary, the guideline doesn't apply.

The description that Benner gives is somewhat idealized. The fact that experts rely on their well-developed intuition does not guarantee that they come up with better answers; they get things wrong and can perpetuate the misguided, even dangerous, eminence-based practice that brought about the need for EBP. The unacceptable variation in GPs' prescribing of antibiotics, for instance, that cannot be explained by case mix clearly implies that expertise cannot always be reliable. As Josh himself pointed out to us, attending physicians do sometimes consult the flowcharts because there is evidence, for instance in the work of Peter Pronovost, that care can be improved when they explicitly follow checklists (Gawande 2007). For these and other reasons Benner's account of the development of expertise has been controversial (see Darbyshire 1994).[11] We suggest, however, that her general picture, bearing in mind our earlier caveats, does go some way towards helping to understand how mindlines are laid down as clinicians progress through the five stages. But it is important to note the additional need to be contextually adroit, as our observations suggest, since skilled clinicians take much more account of the particular circumstances than Benner and the Dreyfus brothers seem to imply. (Imagine an expert Lawndale doctor transposed to Oakville or vice versa.) Echoing Lave and Wenger's (1991: 33) point that 'even so-called general knowledge only has power in specific circumstances' we found that not just general expertise but also knowledge of the immediate context was a key component of an expert's mindlines. That context is of course linked to the roles, goals and networks that we saw played such a part in clinical decisions (Chapter 2). Not only is context a function of the place where one works, but it also alters with time. Some of the expert skills that the Lawndale doctors and nurses were so adeptly using three years ago would no longer serve now because of the ever-changing flow of local contingencies, changing values and technical advances that inevitably continue to suffuse and refashion their expert mindlines.

Spiralling knowledge

The second prologue in this chapter is about the way clinicians process new information.

❖ *During a coffee time conversation about the trustworthiness of different sources, the GPs are saying that it is often difficult to know what to believe, especially when drug companies are putting about different stories and results to try and win market share. In the end it is an accumulation of 'weight of evidence': how many different and relatively trustworthy sources build up one way or the other. The more the journals, opinion leaders, press, central (official) guidance or patients mention something the more likely they are to take it seriously, they tell me. They do not mention critical appraisal, which is left to the more trustworthy sources, who are assumed to be more expert in such techniques.*

❖ *Tony, while referring someone to have their cholesterol level checked, addresses the question of whether it should be done fasting. He always used to insist on a fasting level but a highly respected local professor[12] had said it was not necessary. The speaker had enthusiastically quoted 'a lot of literature' to support that view and Tony had taken note of his advice. That talk had also 'lodged a number of other things in my mind. He really sounded like someone authoritative who knew what he was talking about. And it was relevant to me as a GP.' After chatting with others afterwards, and then with the Lawndale team, he had decided not to do cholesterol levels fasting any more. (This topic kept returning to practice discussions and never quite seemed to be resolved as an agreed protocol.)*

❖ *Jean, meanwhile, has attended a course given by a leading national expert on contraception, the main points from which she later relays to her colleagues at a practice meeting (p. 105). She tells us later in an email: 'Please don't go away with the idea . . . that bland statements are made by consultants which myself and other GPs accept as gospel without knowing if there is evidence to support what's being said . . . Most of us read various journals and whilst a few of these facts are new e.g. ellaone (which I then independently looked up after the course to cross-reference what I'd been told) most of the learning is based on what we already know. Also the time slot for this type of learning is quite short and does not lend itself to in depth discussions about trial data. Most GPs are pragmatists and make up their own minds about information based on the perceived validity of the source coupled with their own pre-existing knowledge.'*

❖   *'Before reading the stuff last night for this meeting I'd have definitely said I'd want warfarin at my age if I had AF but now I'm not so sure', says Tony during a presentation he is making on atrial fibrillation at a practice meeting. Some of the other GPs are surprised at this change of view. To drive the point home, and as now the temporary resident expert on this topic, he quotes a recent patient, not the material he had read up, and then elaborates at some length on 'the subtleties of it'. Only then does he refer them to various sites where they can find more information – and I see that he is quoting from a magazine article in front of him. When I ask him later he admits that he got nearly all his information from a recent issue of* Guidelines Update *which he had seen lying on Nick's desk the previous day and thought 'Oh good – that saves me a lot of hunting around. It's all fairly standard, all in one place, well referenced and everything.'*

❖   *In response to my question as to whether she doubted the authority or validity of the sources that her colleagues were reporting during a clinical meeting (p. 105), and if so why or why not, Shellie writes: 'I know [speaker] is an excellent source of info on contraceptive issues. We all trust our colleagues to feed back to us from teaching sessions in the same way that we would do to them. We all have our own responsibility to make sure we understand and can justify our clinical decision making. I think most of us – if we were going to undertake a major change in the way we practice – tend to try and make sure our information comes from a reliable source, and get secondary evidence to back it up.'*

❖   *Email from Clive: 'Just been to an educational meeting at the health centre – title – depression and its management given by [specialist doctor from hospital elsewhere in the county]. Looked interesting. Reflection – dreadful talk not focused on GPs needs, arranged by drug company. On way back with Jean we were both challenging his assertions as heavily influenced by drug company sponsorship.'*

❖   *At morning coffee it is the 'rep' day. They allow one pharmaceutical representative each week to come, whom they see collectively at 10.45 for fifteen minutes. 'I used to see reps to get info but it wasn't a good use of my time. I'd rather spend that time speaking with colleagues. So we limit it to one coffee break a week', Tony explains. It is the same ritual each time. They banter, give the rep minimal time, and interrupt with questions that vary from mildly challenging (tolerability? cost?) to quite deeply technical to outright (never rude) mocking. It depends on how well they know the rep and how much they really think the new products (or other offers of, for example, helpful equipment or courses) are worth considering. Then usually – as they pick politely at the cakes and fruit the rep has brought them – they settle into an exchange of different views and experiences, as well as half-remembered results of various studies or lectures or consultants' opinions and practices regarding the drugs in question. The rep always leaves a lot of information/promotional material. Some GPs glance at some of it but most of it soon ends up in the bin. ('It's like junk mail at home', laughs Tony. 'You throw it out but only after you make sure there's no cheque in the envelope!') It strikes me as an apt metaphor for how they handle what the rep says, too, except that it takes a lot of examining and discussing to see if there is a 'cheque' worth banking. This morning after the rep has gone some of them get into a debate about the relevance of randomized clinical trials as a source of evidence, quoting examples where the exclusion criteria rendered them unreliable. Other times they swap stories about their experience with the drugs that the rep had been promoting, or things they have heard or read elsewhere. Sometimes the rep targets one sympathetic GP and chats quietly to them afterwards. 'I don't think the reps influence what we do', says Tony, 'although, come to think of it, we did find we were prescribing more PPIs [proton pump inhibitors] after the Wyeth rep kept coming round.' I comment to Peter that reps often seem to stress that the local consultants use their drug. 'Yes — as if we don't know that already!' he smiles. 'But it's their way of saying "Come on you chaps. Get with it. Keep up!" Yes they do quote the consultants a lot, don't they, come to think of it. But, hey I don't care who uses it, I'm not going to prescribe that when it's £1 for four puffs and salbutamol is a penny a puff and works perfectly well!' The rep a week later tells me: 'I completely disagree with the hard sell approach we're told to do. It never works with doctors. They know the drugs they use and the doses. They won't change unless there's good reason.' When I put this to Shellie she suggests that the best time to get GPs to use a new drug is when the old ones are not working and they are desperate for a new alternative.*

❖   *Tony sees a patient with irritable bowel syndrome (IBS), who says he has 'a cupboard full of things like Fybogel, and they haven't worked.' Tony suggests a string of other alternatives until he finds one the patient is not already disillusioned with; it is something that can be bought at the supermarket and is being advertised on television. When asked later, Tony explains he often gets ideas for treatments such as this from the patients themselves, especially what the currently fashionable diets are. But also he gets them 'from things I've read about here and there and from trying things patients tell me, things I've read, and things I've tried. These kind of develop as an accumulation of what I feel is the best way of dealing with it. But I also need to talk to the individual patient to get a view of what they think matters to them, and what their individual triggers and stresses might be.' When you say you read things, what sort of things? 'Oh, not the* BMJ *sort of thing.* Pulse *[a GP magazine]-type things, summaries. For example, I picked up the other day that SSRIs might be useful in IBS. I can't remember where I saw it. One of the magazines like* Pharmacology, *I think. This triggered a memory in me to think about this and go and look it up. Should I perhaps be using an SSRI? It was a flag for me to check whether this might be worth using [. . .] But then', he laughs, 'there's a lot of things I feel I need to come back to and never do. In fact I've now tried to impose a rule on not accumulating journals that I'm not really going to read. If I haven't read it within two or three days I try now just to throw it away. What's the point of having all the journals piling up which I'm really never going to get round to read? Who are you fooling?' He laughs.*

❖   *Interviews with Jean suggested that when developing the practice protocol for heart failure (p. 33) she did so largely by accessing local hospital guidelines produced by a team led by a respected local cardiologist — who, she said, was clearly very knowledgeable and had doubtless 'drawn upon all the evidence'. She supplemented this by reading two published guidelines, and synthesizing this with her own current practice. When she presented the suggested protocol to the practice team, they robustly debated it on the basis of its practicability, the other clinicians' experience of patients in their own practice, the acceptability of variations between their own routines, the ways in which the practice team and computer system could help or hinder the execution and recording of the new protocol, the level at which the new protocols might improve remuneration as well as provide high-quality care, and comparisons with other well-regarded practices (either local or visible via the internet).[13] So, for example, the decision to call all patients with coronary heart disease for an annual check-up, when her proposal had been twice yearly, was, as she said later, 'Arbitrary discussion really. I mean some of which was you know "what are we actually trying to achieve when . . . they come to the nurse?" and I think it was probably felt that [. . .] there was no particularly good logic between, you know, between writing twice a year, so I think it was felt that an annual thing was probably appropriate as a starting point anyway and then we can see.'*

❖   *Peter is being interviewed about his use of guidelines: 'I think there's got to be a certain amount of flexibility in them so yes I think you do [read them] and I think that was actually one of the things that was clear from our meeting the other night that we are interpreting them slightly differently. We are being, I suppose we're being flexible but also we're perhaps asserting our own views, which may well, is it right or wrong, and these are the things that we needed to discuss and refine. [. . .] There are always grey areas and that's I think where we were expanding the other night. In protocols [such as that] . . . there are always examples that, you know, people do remember, you know. "I've got such and such who has been on this medication" and so discussion does come about that way. I suppose you've each got to have done a little bit of homework on it otherwise you can't have a really fruitful discussion, you can have people so entrenched in their own views they're not prepared to change. [. . .] But I suppose things I've found most useful have been the open discussions to see what people's views are and then if you can back those discussions up with some hard evidence you know actually come away with something concrete from the meeting.'*

To complete our review on the way in which mindlines grow, we must now turn to the way in which clinicians, even expert ones, 'learn the ropes' of a particular context and continue to do so as the ropes constantly change. Linked to this, therefore, is the question of how new ideas are spread among health professionals. In the world of evidence-based practice, the implicit underlying model of the spread of innovation – new ideas, new knowledge, new practices – is founded in Everett Rogers's classic *Diffusion of Innovations* (Rogers 2003 [1995]). Bringing together research findings from a wide range of disciplines, he forged a highly influential model for the way in which innovations are generated and spread. He posited a five-stage model of the process by which people decide to adopt and use an innovation. Their prior behaviour and attitudes towards the problem in question and towards new ideas in general (e.g. 'early adopters' and 'laggards' were his terms), their own socioeconomic characteristics, personality variables and communication behaviour (e.g. their networks), as well as the relative advantage, compatibility, complexity, trialability and observability of the innovation, all played key roles in whether they pick up on it. If they do, they tend to seek more information, try it out, decide whether it is useful or not and then maybe spread the word depending on their own communication channels (e.g. whether they are opinion leaders or change agents or not) and the way in which their organization aided or inhibited innovation. But, complicated as his wonderfully clear book of over 500 pages made it sound, the spread of ideas is nothing like so simple! For example, the seminal study by Andrew Van de Ven and colleagues (1999) revealed that the process of organizational innovation was much more haphazard and much less linear than Rogers's model of diffusion might suggest. Although there may be common patterns such as a number of (non-linear) phases in the advance or demise of an innovation, each is subject to unpredictable contingencies so that, 'whatever route is taken, the innovation journey is highly ambiguous, is often uncontrollable, and involves a good deal of luck' (Van de Ven *et al.* 1999: 65). It is not surprising, therefore, that the attempts at disseminating evidence-based practice that assume the more linear (though still complex) progress envisaged by Rogers have usually foundered. The spread of new ideas in health services is anything but a linear process (Fitzgerald *et al.* 1999; French 1999; Dopson and Fitzgerald 2005).

Our focus here, however, is not on organizational innovation per se, but on how clinicians acquire and process new research evidence. We will, like most who discuss the way in which knowledge is developed and shared in an organizational context, begin with the seminal work of two Japanese academics, Ikujiro Nonaka and Hirotaka Takeuchi, who set out to understand how some extraordinarily successful Japanese companies created new knowledge (Nonaka and Takeuchi 1995). This is a rather different question from ours, since we are interested not, as they were, in the way organizations manage the invention and growth of new knowledge, but in how clinicians in an organizational context manage the acquisition and adoption of new knowledge. Nonetheless there is sufficient overlap to provide useful insights. The key point is that, '[a]lthough ideas are formed in the minds of individuals, interaction between individuals typically plays a critical role in developing these ideas. That is to say, "communities of interaction" contribute to the amplification and development of new knowledge' (Nonaka 1994: 15). Nonaka and Takeuchi's observations led them to set great store by tacit knowledge, which they subdivided into two components, both of which we have discussed already in this and the preceding chapters. One is tacit technical knowledge, the 'know-how' of informal craft-based skill that cannot be formally pinned down (exactly how to place the cannula when setting up a drip; the 'nose' that instantly told Clive that the lady describing 'ice in my chest' was seriously ill). The other, largely unconscious, component – echoing both mindlines and the illness scripts within them – is 'the schemata, mental models, beliefs and perceptions so ingrained that we take them for granted' (ibid.: 8).[14] Nonaka and Takeuchi found that these two forms of tacit knowledge, technical know-how and unconscious schemata, represented the driving force of success, which far outweighed the explicit, formal, codified knowledge that the companies could write down, count or include in their information systems.[15] This led Nonaka and Takeuchi to explore the growth of that tacit knowledge in organizations, which they suggested took the form of what they called a 'knowledge spiral' (often called 'SECI' because of the four major stages of Socialization, Externalization, Combination and Internalization). Drawing usually on this work, 'knowledge management' gurus now stride across the commercial and public sector amid a cacophony of catchphrases and management speak, intent on making fortunes by mining the untapped wealth of organizational tacit knowledge.[16] We, however, intend to be more prosaic; we will simply use the SECI spiral (Figure 5.2) as a tool to help reveal how clinicians in healthcare organizations develop and share their mindlines. In doing so, we – like those knowledge managers and their gurus[17] – will shamelessly adapt and mould the original SECI spiral to help in our analysis. So, although it is helpful to distinguish the phases of knowledge development at Lawndale, we should note that we did not see the clear sequence implied by the SECI spiral. The stages that we outline here are – like those of the Benner/Dreyfus model of the growth of individual expertise – no more than convenient categories, ideal types that, while often simultaneous and intermingled, could be identified among the observations we made.

The first stage, *socialization*, involves people transferring tacit knowledge to each other, without necessarily making it explicit.[18] It is learning 'how we do things here', typically gleaned by observation of, interaction with, and feedback from colleagues who show you the ropes. A good deal of what goes on in the 'sitting by Nellie' aspect of the apprentice-like training, or the chat in hospital dining rooms, or the general gossip in the bar at conferences and courses[19] lays the groundwork for this way of learning. At Lawndale it was evident for example in the coffee room, as when Adam gradually had his overzealous investigative approach mellowed by his colleagues' jocular 'role sending' (p. 36). It was also ever present as an undercurrent of the more formal meetings and, of course, in trainee supervisions. Patients also played their part in 'role sending'[20] and in helping clinicians develop specific and local tacit knowledge – either individually during consultations or through the 'Friends of Lawndale' meetings.

At the second stage, *externalization*, people's tacit knowledge is made more

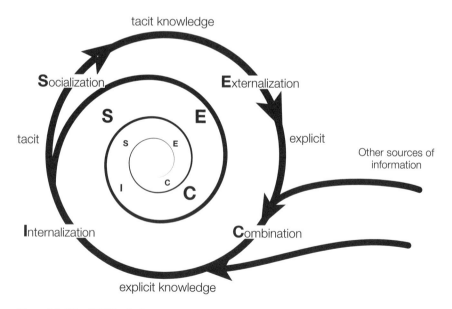

Figure 5.2 The SECI spiral.

explicit, mainly through informal interaction as they talk to each other and become better at expressing it in words and images.[21] Metaphors, analogies (Douglas 1987: 45–53), jokes and above all stories (Chapter 6) are the key to this process as people try to make collective sense of their own and others' tacit knowledge.[22] The result is the formulation of explicit knowledge in a form that is understandable by all participants, perhaps even captured in practice policies. Usually, however, that crystallization into policy involves also the third stage of *combination*, when other sources of knowledge – and this might include new knowledge from research – are brought to bear and amalgamated with the explicit formulations of the originally tacit knowledge, which may as a result be substantiated, perhaps strengthened, perhaps attenuated, before being made available for others to access. Thus, when Barry produced a practice policy on the management of kidney disease after several group discussions had strongly shaped the policy (p. 153), he ensured that he had also checked it against a number of written sources of evidence. The result in this instance was a local policy, but the combination stage may in other circumstances result in lectures, textbooks, editorial reviews or guidelines in which clinicians codify their collective wisdom in a form that is accessible much more widely. Fourth, and back once again at the level of the individual, there comes the final stage of the SECI spiral, *internalization*, when practitioners transform the combined knowledge into something that makes sense to them in the light of their own existing knowledge and experience. As a result they may or may not incorporate the new knowledge into their mindlines and hence into their daily practice. It is here that new and old knowledge compete, as it were, for a place in the internalized knowledge-in-practice-in-context, which, once in place, can then be further shared and modified as the spiral continues indefinitely.

This knowledge spiral has important implications for evidence-based practice, to which we will return in Chapters 7 and 8. Many types of evidence are involved, and all undergo some kind of transformation. When there is a new piece of evidence, say from recent research, that practitioners need to absorb, it does not merely fill a knowledge gap or simply supplant the incorrect knowledge held in the individual's mind. Rather, it enters the mêlée of the SECI spiral, to be integrated with existing knowledge or perhaps examined and discarded.[23] The knowledge provided by researchers, systematic reviewers and guideline writers is generally context free, but needs to be used in a specific context and combined with 'colloquial knowledge' that will include a very wide range of material regarded by the practitioner as 'evidence' (le May 1999; Rycroft-Malone *et al.* 2003; CHSRF 2005a,b; May 2006). Indeed the very essence of clinicians' practical skill is embodied in their collectively honed ability to apply context-free knowledge to specific situations taking account of a very wide range of clinical and non-clinical considerations (Chapter 2).

The 'evidence' advocated by the EBP movement may be vitally important, but for clinicians it is just one source of additional information among many others that they need to take into account as they contextualize it, both within their well-developed existing mindlines and in terms of the individual case they are dealing with. Over time, contextualizing and combining all those sources of evidence usually occurs not as a decision taken by one individual once and for all, but as part of the social process of continuing discussion among colleagues. Put more simply, before new knowledge can lead to a behavioural change, clinicians will actively relate it to what they and their trusted colleagues already, possibly implicitly and tacitly, know or believe. They will assess its relevance, benefits and disbenefits, and in effect 'negotiate' a final position in which they may or may not be persuaded to incorporate the new evidence into what they do. In short, for research evidence to inform practice, it must be subjected to a social process that continually and repeatedly transforms it from the explicit knowledge that emerges from the research world into something suitable for internalization as part of the mindline, the knowledge-in-practice-in-context that is used in the clinical world. Research knowledge is thus inevitably altered before it is used.

Indeed, most commentators on knowledge management (e.g. Davenport and Prusak 1998; Ahmed *et al.* 2002) would not consider evidence from the research world or any other outside source as meriting the term 'knowledge'. They prefer to define 'knowledge' as 'information used in a context'. So, whereas researchers or the Department of Health may like to think of some new piece of evidence as 'knowledge', such commentators would define it merely as 'information' when it is first introduced into the clinical world (Figure 5.3). It becomes 'knowledge' only when the practitioners have collectively and/or individually combined it with their own experience, skills, 'intuition', ideas, judgements, motivations and inter-pretations (Ahmed *et al.* 2002). Timmermans and Berg (2003: 203) also concluded

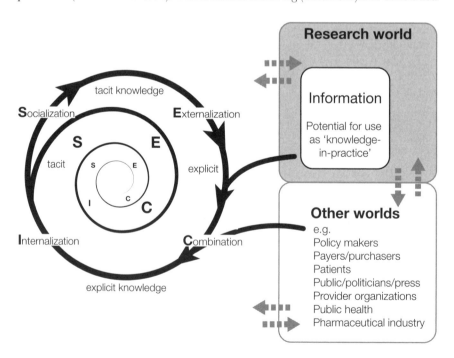

Figure 5.3 How information enters the SECI spiral and is transformed into knowledge-in-practice-in-context.

from their seminal studies of the way clinicians use the standardizing tools of evidence-based healthcare that 'physicians more often than not see guidelines as just another piece of information'. In this way the practitioners transform the evidence so that it fits into their context in ways that enable them to practise it.[24] This may even happen when the GPs appear superficially to be ignoring the research-based evidence. As May and his colleagues conclude in their study of the reasons why GPs appear to ignore the evidence on brief interventions for alcohol abuse:

> our argument is that to see our [GP] respondents' perspectives as evidence of a 'gap' between clinical evidence and everyday practice is to miss the point. For something *like* brief interventions has been normalized into their work and is evident in their accounts even when they rejected, or did not recognize, the particular label of brief interventions for this work. By normalisation we mean that a set of practices that seem to accord to the broad principles of brief interventions are routinely accounted for as being embedded, locally, in clinical practice, and that they are interpreted and adapted flexibly according to the contingent requirements of specific settings.
>
> (May *et al.* 2006b: 396, their emphasis)

Our contention here is that the evidence in question had been transformed by the SECI spiral until it was no longer visible either to themselves or to those lamenting their 'failure' to follow the evidence, which, as May and his colleagues found, in many hidden ways they actually often *were* following in the only ways that were feasible in the circumstances.

Our own previous research (Gabbay *et al.* 2003) found that new information introduced to groups of people attempting to formulate local policies for healthcare was batted about until it was unrecognizable (see Figure 7.1) but that the groups' deliberations nevertheless adopted the evidence sufficiently to anticipate national 'evidence-based' policy (see also Chapters 7 and 8). Much of the content of the practice meetings found Lawndale clinicians similarly discussing and 'processing' new information that they had gleaned from reading, from reps, from lectures and from colleagues so that it could be combined with other sources and with their existing knowledge before (perhaps) being absorbed. The result was inevitably to transform the new information before it was included in a practice protocol or internalized as a change in practitioners' mindlines.

Keeping experts up to date

We turn now to examine the way in which experienced clinicians used new information to keep up to date.

❖ *When Lawndale, in response to a new item in the GP contract, is developing a new practice protocol for identifying and managing patients with possible early kidney disease,[25] the task immediately generates a host of unanswered questions about workload, relevance to local needs, potential distress to patients, and conflicting priorities for care. 'To what extent would we be (dangerously) over-investigating patients who are already being checked regularly for other related conditions? What impact would this have on our nurses' and the hospital laboratory's workload? How much distress would be caused to patients with marginally low test results by being suddenly labelled as having kidney failure?' As part of their strategy for answering these and many other questions, Lawndale arranges a local lunchtime educational session on this topic, attended also by twenty or so GPs and nurses from other local practices. It turns out to be a commanding presentation from a local nephrologist with many data-filled slides and much clinical advice on the topic. Yet, invited precisely because the GPs need her to answer the questions that are troubling them, the speaker is simply not able to do so satisfactorily despite all the information she is giving them. The audience reaction, which ranges from unmoved to sceptical to hostile, reveals that GPs from other practices have very similar concerns to those at Lawndale. The nephrologist handles some searching questions authoritatively, but makes little headway in combating the underlying scepticism in her audience. They maintain that much of her expert nephrological guidance is simply not feasible in the primary care setting. When she states, for example, that 'it takes just five seconds to test someone's urine' some of the attendees exploded: 'What about the time it takes to call the patient, arrange for the MSU [mid-stream urine] to be taken, process the forms, review them, call them back . . . ?' In short, the medical-scientific mindset that underpins her talk goes nowhere near dealing with the managerial, health promotion and other considerations that concern the GPs about conforming with the new requirements when dealing with their patients. Indeed the specialized hospital context within which she practises and which informs her whole way of thinking means that even the clinical information she is giving them is of little use. At their next practice meeting the Lawndale GPs, reassured that they are generally not out of line with GP colleagues elsewhere or with the essentials covered by the nephrologist, cheerily declare themselves 'none the wiser' as they set about resolving the practical details of managing chronic kidney disease (CKD). (See p. 152.)*

❖   *At another of the same series of lunchtime educational sessions, this time presented by the local diabetology professor,[26] I notice that before the lecture he is deep in conversation with Tony and it sounds to me almost like a mini-tutorial as he answers some queries Tony has about diabetes. When Tony introduces him to the audience he lauds the speaker, saying 'I find he always gives the latest scientific evidence, but also makes it useful for clinicians'. The speaker further establishes his credentials by immediately reminding the audience that he speaks at least thirty times a year like this to GPs 'so don't worry it's not promotional'. He gives three clear practical messages about when not to prescribe a particular class of drug – glitazones – based on recent science, which he displays in impressive graphic form, but not so as to allow the audience really to absorb the detail. The slides strike me as mainly having the effect of lending authority to the very clear, pragmatic 'take-home message' as he calls it. He also conveys how he is on the inside track of 'Big Science' in diabetes ('as I said only last week to the editor of the Lancet . . .'). He repeatedly stresses how things have changed in diabetes (using several times the locution: 'Now, in 2007, I wouldn't do XYZ any more, but I would do ABC' or 'In 2007 the science tells us we should be doing . . . PQR'). The audience lap it up because, it seems to me, he is indeed both very practical and simple about where their practice needs to change, and also clearly an 'expert' they can trust (and is anything but promotional). When they ask questions he gives practical, pragmatic* answers often along the lines of 'Well, this is what I would do in those sorts of cases . . .' Unlike the renal session, the answers are in tune with whatever the GPs have been concerned about. After the session the pharmaceutical rep who had funded the lunch greets a local GP on his way out: 'The Prof is very good isn't he?' She laughs nervously. 'I hope he hasn't put you off [prescribing their brand of glitazones].' 'Oh no not at all', he answers politely if untruthfully. I catch Nick winking at Barry; he says 'I can see a change in our practice policy coming on.' Barry smiles, nods and points to the voluminous notes he has taken.

❖ Tony had told me on another occasion that he had attended a lecture by the same diabetologist and had been meaning to summarize his notes. Why? For yourself or for your colleagues? 'Both. I've always thought it would be very useful for us to do that for each other, but we don't tend to do it because we don't always have the time. If I've been to something really good, and I think it may or may not benefit my colleagues, it seems only sensible to pass a note around which might then stimulate some discussion or trigger some further thinking about it. And for my own purposes, having written notes would do the same. I should put them on my Palmtop. It'll act as a good trigger for later.' Tony had then gone on to recount the key points from that earlier talk as a sort of mental checklist which he had clearly internalized, even though he hadn't yet written it up on his Palmtop. I had commented at the time that he did seem to have it all already fairly well rehearsed, and asked whether he had talked to colleagues about it, rather than writing them a note. 'Well it all sounds so obvious really when you just say it. I think a note stimulates discussion. You can put it in your CPD file, it's an opportunity to start talking about things. Perhaps we should use email more to do that sort of thing. It could act as a trigger. For example, Jean has just sent me some information about a patient through an email. I will use that as a trigger to respond to her later with much more information about that patient in case she needs to know it.'

❖ I am invited to the first of a series of clinical meetings, attended by most of the Lawndale GPs, that – as Tony suggested above – take the form of presentations from partners who have recently attended courses, so that they can pass on any key points they have learnt. The first presentation is on contraception. Jean has already circulated some notes about the course she had attended, which had been given by an eminent emeritus professor of gynaecology, consisting of a summary of the key points (i.e. matters where there might have been doubt or unacceptably varied practice). As she begins elaborating on the notes in some detail, several heads begin nodding vigorously – especially the three women GPs who do a lot of the family planning work in the surgery. Very soon they are chipping in with their own confirmation of many of the points, or slightly varied suggestions. Nick tells a brief story about a patient, which is picked up on by some of the others and used to elaborate one of the points in the talk. Clive queries how often a particular condition is likely to occur. More practical questions are opened up by others. Answers and suggestions start flying, always brought back firmly by Jean to the main points that were made in the original talk, but often also reinforced, elaborated and explained, especially by the three women who seem to know a lot about family planning. I notice a few 'Aha's' and 'Oh I see's', including from the women, and some brief notes being taken as a result. Some scepticism is voiced by a couple of the partners about the costs of some of the suggestions, but these are batted away by the enthusiasts, who argue that it's actually more likely to result in overall savings.

Their (unsubstantiated but plausible) argument seems to be accepted. Increasingly, there are questions exposing gaps in knowledge that Jean or the other women partners willingly fill in where they can. An extraordinary amount of information is exchanged in the mere eighteen minutes that this section of the meeting lasts. But no one ever once queries the authority of the original talk, or the evidence on which its points were based. As this is the first such meeting they have had, I send a brief email questionnaire to check the above perceptions of what they have learnt, which are amply confirmed. They respond (see also p. 96) that they trusted the original speaker and their colleagues and assumed that as none of those who know about these topics doubted the proposed suggestions they were valid (and they were probably aware that Jean would have checked anything dubious – as indeed she had). They each list a different range of ways that they will amend their practice following the discussion, and the response is similar about the second presentation that day, which had been on rheumatology. Peter adds: 'The thing with this sort of discussion is that it is very easy to relate it to your own experience (i.e. recent patients) and you get instant feedback/answers to those extra questions that pop into your head (or someone else's head for that matter!)' Tony comments: 'This form of knowledge sharing is excellent and allows for discussion amongst colleagues and a chance to get a "feel" for how other colleagues apply this knowledge in their own day to day work [. . .] I also reviewed which medications can induce liver enzymes and have included these [in my CPD reflections].'

❖ *A group of GPs at a reunion are in the bar discussing what one learns from GP courses. Sue is frustrated. 'I don't think we do enough to keep up in our practice. I go on courses and get lots of new ideas that I bring home but my partners always find a reason to reject them. Sometimes they are justified but often it's just ingrained habits and defensiveness.' Jim is surprised that she is so positive about the courses. 'I find they are usually a waste of time – you usually know everything they are telling you and they rarely pitch it right.' 'Oh it's worse than that', says Phil – a GP in a large industrial city, who has a reputation for being a strong-minded and outspoken individual but a good clinician – and he launches into a story. He and all his colleagues had been required by their primary care trust to attend a mandatory lecture on antibiotic prescribing, which, as Phil put it, was 'given by a pharmacist or somesuch . . . When he'd finished I was livid. I stood up and told him it was a load of bollocks. I told him, "You have no bloody idea how we work. What's the first thing to think about when deciding whether to prescribe an antibiotic?" He stands there dumbstruck, of course, so I tell him. "The patient's postcode! There are parts of our practice where we know they have no local support, not even easy access to phones. And then there are the articulate middle-class areas where it's much easier for the family to phone for the right help if things deteriorate. It's easy enough not to prescribe the antibiotic with the second lot but with the first lot you're actually putting them at risk" [. . .] So then I ask him, "What's the second thing to think about?"' Phil's dramatic pause is broken by Jim: 'The day of the week?' he suggests. 'Exactly!' Phil shouts triumphantly. 'We wouldn't prescribe on a Monday but definitely would on a Friday. And that's what I told that pillock from the PCT. "So why don't you take your f***ing guidelines", I told him, "and f*** off coz you've just no bloody idea how we work!"' Phil's point, which was immediately obvious to his GP pals but apparently lost on the pharmaceutical lecturer, was that patients could come back to him if they got worse during the week, but that, because over the weekend they would be at the* *mercy of out-of-hours services who didn't know the patient or the history, he would err on the side of caution and prescribe antibiotics.*

Formal educational courses were obviously a potential source from which research evidence could find its way into practice. There is a large literature on the place of formal lectures as a way of educating practitioners, and much of it suggests that they are very limited as a method of influencing practice (Forsetlund *et al.* 2009). All too often the lectures that we observed failed to 'hit the spot'. The contrast between Tony's diabetologist, who seemed to press all the right buttons, and the beleaguered nephrologist, who did not, was very telling. The difference was the skill of the lecturer in recognizing and appreciating the different needs of day-to-day practice, and in adapting his message to the real concerns of the practitioners. The diabetologist showed that, despite the difficulties that the nephrologist personified, it was possible – if relatively rare – for experts to escape their own context and enter that of their audience, so that they engage with the hands-on, multifaceted aspects of primary care practice.[27] Unfortunately that was unusual. A great deal of formal educational material, like most research-based knowledge, deals almost exclusively with clinical matters, whereas – as we saw in Chapter 2 – clinical decisions are rarely purely technical but instead are a balance between tensions that such sources rarely touch upon. One reason why Phil had been so abusive about the PCT pharmacist's lecture on antibiotics was the speaker's ignorance of the non-clinical, organizational aspects of the GPs' many complex roles, goals and networks that are crucial to their work. (Another reason, of course, might also have been his need to mount an aggressive-defensive claim of the tribal superiority of frontline GPs over the PCT managers and pharmacists but that is another, not unrelated, story.)

Good professionals keep up to date and are continually learning their craft (Davis 2009); the Lawndale GPs were no exception. They were genuinely enthusiastic about continuing professional development, and embraced keenly the RCGP's move away from achieving a set number of hours of educational meetings per year to a more varied, self-directed form of learning. They set up regular small group meetings to discuss clinical topics, review critical incidents (such as 'near misses') and the results of audits and, where appropriate, discuss them further with the wider practice team. The ethos that the GPs espoused went beyond simply taking part in learning events to ensure that the lessons, once properly and (usually) collectively reflected upon, had an impact on their practice. This process involved ascertaining current best practice and identifying areas where they needed to improve, learn new skills or otherwise develop themselves as clinicians. Having each year set themselves personal development goals and selected the means by which they would achieve them (e.g. by attending courses and lectures or through well-focused reading) they would each have to show their appraiser that they had done so. They would then discuss this with their colleagues at the practice meetings so that it fed into the overall learning plan for the practice.

In keeping with these requirements for annual appraisal, Clive, for example, each year produced an exemplary annual CPD portfolio that filled an A4 ring binder some 3 cm thick, full of reflections, notes, audits and feedback data covering the clinical, managerial and interpersonal aspects of his practice. The folder, which aimed to record what he was learning, for example from educational courses (both live and online), from articles and guidance consulted or received, and from insights gained by reflecting on day-to-day activities and meetings, showed that he took seriously the need to reflect on his practice and maintain his learning. In a formal document such as this, which is required of all practitioners in order for them to continue to be 'of good standing', what better way for Clive to prove to his appraiser that he was keeping up to date than by emphasizing the place of authoritative articles and guidelines that he had referred to as key sources of new knowledge? Yet, although these did indeed sometimes appear, apart from a few notable exceptions his reflective notes suggested they had had only a limited effect on his thinking or practice. The majority of his CPD portfolio, even in this formal record of evidence of learning, suggested that it was *practical* sources such as audits, critical events, unusual patients, meetings and discussions that had provided the most potent sources of new knowledge and changed practice. But he 'admitted' when we interviewed him about this that he needed to read more learned journals, and that others, such as Jean, were much more diligent about doing so. However, the sources that different GPs used would depend very much on their individual learning styles, be it a preference for abstract thinking, actively trying things out, or reflecting on their own and others' experience (Kolb 1984), and Clive's was clearly very different from Jean's. Whatever their preferred mix of styles, the fact is that they were all continually learning new things that amended their mindlines.[28]

Like most clinicians, the Lawndale clinicians had developed their favourite 'information-seeking heuristics' (Box 5.1), but, whatever the source, its contribution to their CPD could always be seen to be deeply embedded in the SECI spiral. Written sources were approached in two main ways: either browsing, usually in an idle moment, or specifically searching out some item to help with a particular question. They browsed many sources, including some of the 'highbrow' medical journals, but more usually perused the popular doctors' magazines, colloquially called the 'GP comics', that are mailed free of charge to practices in the UK, or material that happened to come across their desks such as the many sources of guidance from the NHS or commercial information about new products. Such reading – or rather skimming – was anything but systematic and many such sources were regarded with some scepticism as likely to be in their different ways unhelpful or misleading. Before being put into practice, items gleaned from those sources needed to be checked out – sometimes by further reading, but almost always by discussing them with trusted colleagues to check out not only their credibility but also their feasibility in the local context – all of which contributed not just to their shared expertise but to their shared contextual adroitness.

When there was a need to search for specific information to deal with a specific point, each had their own natural propensities and preferences. When asked, for example, where he might learn about a particular group of drugs, Tony quickly mentioned a list of main sources including the National Prescribing Centre's *MeReC Bulletin*, the *Drug and Therapeutics Bulletin* and several sources of useful

Box 5.1 Information-seeking heuristics

Sources and types of information/evidence that practitioners have volunteered as informing their practice (distilled from a decade of ACLM's interactive EBP lectures with qualified nurses).

Types

- experiential
- research
- theoretical
- policy
- custom and practice
- trial and error

Sources

- peers (within and outwith own professional group)
- experts
- patients
- opinion leaders
- own experience
- reflection on own practice
- stories and case studies
- audit (including complaints reviews)
- national/local policy
- local protocols
- national/local guidelines
- integrated care plans/integrated care pathways
- benchmarks
- education (study days, teaching and mentoring)
- newsletters/cascades
- networks
- professional meetings
- conferences/workshops
- journals
- systematic reviews
- websites
- textbooks
- representatives from drug/devices companies

reviews, and even lamented that they were not yet available in an electronic form to use quickly during surgery. When Barry had to develop a practice protocol for chronic kidney disease (CKD), he – a relatively young partner – went online to consult local and national guidelines and the National Service Framework, did some simple Google searches and looked up reliable websites aimed at GPs, some of which were recommended by email discussion groups or magazine articles that colleagues had passed on to him. In contrast, when Jean was asked to draft a practice protocol for heart failure, she turned to the local (printed) hospital guidelines produced by a team led by a respected local cardiologist, who, she assumed, had 'drawn upon all the evidence'. (She had recently attended a course run by him on this topic.) These guidelines 'reinforced' her existing practice, but she supplemented them by reading two other sets of published guidelines, she told us, just to be sure. She also carried out an audit of Lawndale's current practice, which they knew needed overhauling. All of these were synthesized into the policy she brought to the meeting.[29] On the occasion that she had attended the course by the eminent gynaecologist, she was happy to accept the expert's views because they accorded with what she already knew or what she was hearing from other sources, and where she had doubts over some of his new suggestions she had looked them up and discussed them at a later meeting with her partners.

Written and oral information from many sources went into the mix that was eventually combined and codified into written policies or internalized into individual practice. The clinicians had learnt, rightly or wrongly, to treat the different sources with different degrees of respect and to some extent this too was a social process. The doctors were openly dismissive about what they were told by representatives of the pharmaceutical industry. When listening to presentations (which were always kept very short) from reps, the GPs would often vie with each other to make subtle, sometimes coded remarks that undermined what the rep was saying with a degree of humour perceptible only to their colleagues. (The more experienced reps would spot this and engage in banter that they turned to their advantage if possible. By colluding with the humour they might gain more trust.) But, despite the GPs' open cynicism, the reps were not necessarily without influence, especially those whom the GPs had got to know over the years. To a lesser extent advice or guidance from the Department of Health and its local PCT representatives was also regarded with suspicion – perhaps because they believed, like the GP commenting on commissioners (p. 22), that PCTs had a naïve view of the place of guidelines and protocols in practice, or perhaps because they suspected (probably unfairly) that the PCT's motives might be unduly biased towards cost-saving. Whichever it was, the practitioners had developed what they felt was an instinct about which sources to take note of and which to ignore. The PCT pharmaceutical adviser, for example, had earned the respect of the practitioners and was a particularly welcome and well-trusted source. Above all, however, the most trusted sources were colleagues who were known to be expert in a given clinical area – be that local hospital specialists or colleagues within the practice.

There are three main observations to be made here. First, practitioners had their own hierarchy of evidence that differed from that usually promulgated by the EBP movement (see, for example, le May and Gabbay 2010). Second, and relatedly, the ethos for finding out about new developments was not one of deep and scholarly immersion in the literature. What mattered was the ability to know which sources to trust so that one could efficiently find reliable short cuts to keeping up with new developments – information-seeking heuristics? (p. 57) – and more often than not that meant knowing who was 'in the know' and nurturing the capacity to pick their brains. The third lesson is that, whether the clinicians were actively seeking some new piece of information (e.g. to help prepare a practice treatment plan) or whether they had happened across some new idea that needed to be considered (e.g. the suggestion that there may be untoward side effects with a drug they commonly used), the new information was almost always processed by some discussion with trusted colleagues, and consequently adapted and transformed before being internalized and put (or not) into practice (Chapters 7 and 8). Another important feature of this process was that if some item of new information were being found in several different sources – suddenly turning up in many of the written sources and/or being talked about by more and more people – it was much more likely to enter the discussions that would lead to its being taken seriously and combined as appropriate with existing knowledge.

The crucial point, in summary, is that the GPs were constantly grazing a wide range of written and oral sources that conveyed new evidence and information with the potential to be incorporated into their mindlines. Anything of interest would be checked out while being fed into the transformations of the SECI spiral where it was shared, combined and then tacitly personalized as knowledge-in-practice-in-context (Figure 5.3). Whatever the sources of such information, and whether it was eventually internalized or rejected, there was inevitably some way in which it was combined with the knowledge and beliefs that the clinicians already held in their mindlines. And the key to integrating that new information into people's mindlines seemed to rely a great deal on informal interactions among colleagues, when the new ideas were blended with experiential evidence. Much of that process entailed telling each other stories – or what Tony once told us were 'anecdotes with a purpose'. Our next step was therefore to explore storytelling.

Chapter 5: Summary

We have explored how mindlines develop as a clinician moves from being a novice to becoming a 'contextually adroit expert'. Our analysis, which relies on our own ethnographic observations as well as a critique of the existing literature, points to the crucial relevance of 'knowledge-in-practice-in-context'. In any given context, new information, whether tacit or explicit, becomes transformed by the complex social processes described in the SECI spiral (Socialization, Externalization, Combination, Internalization) that enable clinicians to amalgamate it with other relevant knowledge before using it. Information from research, education or other formal sources becomes practical knowledge only after that social process.

6   The place of storytelling in knowledge sharing

Our examples of the place of storytelling in the exchange of knowledge begin among the Lawndale clinicians.

❖   *The QPA requires that ten emergency hospital admissions from the practice be appraised and reported, detailing what happened and the lessons learnt. At a QPA meeting Jean opens with an anecdote about a recent emergency that makes them all laugh. (She had sent the patient to Marge for a blood test, during which the patient developed chest pain. Marge sent the patient to Rose, the triage nurse, who referred her back to Jean, who sent her to hospital.) Over the next fifteen minutes, six more stories follow, in which the main events surrounding the admission and the lessons are recounted, often with black humour at the storyteller's own expense, and clinical lessons (was this 'acute coronary syndrome' as the hospital said or angina or pericarditis?) and critical comments about the local services (positive and negative) are quickly shared. The lessons conveyed by the stories are never challenged or critically commented on.*

    The next item is about the quality of the premises and whether to change the front doors to automatic. Those in favour (receptionists) tell several brief stories of patients having trouble with the heavy front doors. They are unconvinced by Janet's explanation that the doors' resistance/weight has been tested and approved in a formal disability inspection. But when Clive tells them about another practice that paid £13,000 for automatic doors and ended up being sued by a patient who got caught in them, the argument is over. Lawndale keeps its doors as they are.

    There follows an item on repeat prescriptions. More brief anecdotes about the way different doctors approach it lead to a proposal to audit and change the system. A little later in the same meeting Clive asks the district nurses not to use a certain type of urine dipstick because there are too many false positives. He briefly mentions some of the accepted criteria for screening (which sound to me like the standard WHO criteria [Wilson and Jungner 1968], though that source is never mentioned), but the message is not clear to the nurses who use the test. Then he tells the story of a thirty-year-old man who was recently unnecessarily sent to the hospital for cystoscopy because of a false positive urine test. Now they understand.

❖   *In a taped interview, Tamsin comments on what is good about Lawndale: 'I think there is definitely a feeling of teamwork. Actually the fact that not many practices would have everyone sit having coffee together, just even just to chat. Just to sort of catch up with things and the fact that everyone is . . . always available to talk to . . . They may be busy; they may be stressed or something but they're always willing to help. And encouraging.'*

❖ *Five doctors and the practice manager come in to get coffee within a few minutes of each other. It is a typical coffee break; usual banter. Among other things they tell me the flu epidemic is subsiding. Shellie asks Janet about coding flu vaccines. Janet tells them how people have been doing the coding and the vaccinations have been panning out. Rachel quotes the code by heart; someone questions it and then they agree that is the one. Two anecdotes follow about using the computer system to record vaccinations and one about how they are maintaining the current stocks of vaccine. They talk about the busy surgeries, which leads within a few minutes to the exchange of four brief anecdotes about a variety of personal experiences (about their own childcare compared with others, about their own illnesses, about the idiosyncrasies of colleagues, about the behaviour of a doctor they once worked with, three about current patients, how they had dealt with them and what other specialists had said about them, and one about a patient years ago). Almost all of the stories contain some kind of useful information that could potentially impact on the way the others might react to similar events in future. These include a useful contact at the local hospital, varieties of flavours in paediatric medicines, how to deal with moderately controlled epileptics who think they don't need help, hints on how to present an audit successfully, the best drug to use in post-prandial somnolence, and much else.*

❖ *Another coffee break. Rachel has just reeled off en passant what she does whenever she has a man with suspected prostate disease. She quips that before it comes to doing a rectal examination she makes sure he comes back to see a male doctor. Several others share stories – more or less risqué – about cross-gender and same-gender vaginal and rectal examinations, during which it emerges that there is a spectrum of views about the advisability of women choosing female doctors and men male ones, and everyone – amidst the laughter – has the opportunity of reconsidering this question, which some visibly seem to do and maybe had not done previously. Then Clive changes tack and relates a story of how he was teaching a registrar about migraine when he suddenly thought, 'This boy has just done his MRCP. He knows much more than I do – who should be teaching who here?' 'Yes', says Peter, 'but they [neurologists] don't see the same kind of migraine that we do.' Several anecdotes follow about how the statistical and qualitative differences between hospital and primary care populations have led to errors, poor guidance and poor hospital services. Adam uses the opportunity to talk about a case of diarrhoea that didn't follow any pattern he had learnt in hospital when doing his MRCP. The others are able to help him decide how to deal with it.*

❖ *Six GPs are talking at coffee about measles. They talk about their own families. They move to the problem of persuading parents that the MMR vaccine scare is unwarranted. They share several striking statistics that they have tried (e.g. UK 1200 annual hospital cases of mumps down to 800 cases in total, now up to 8000 after MMR scare, and so on). 'I just tell the mums that I looked after two kids with measles who died. That usually does the trick', says Clive with a wicked grin. 'Yes', says Adam, 'I've tried talking about a third of children being carried away with measles in an African village, but the mum just said "If the child dies of measles that's God's will; if she gets autism, that's my fault."' There is a quick cascade of further stories about patients' beliefs. Chickenpox is mentioned. Ben, who recently did hospital paediatrics, tells a story about a child who had thrombosis – a rare complication that Rachel, Clive and Shellie clearly had not heard about, judging from their reaction. Then follows a quick stream of story-capping about TB and tropical diseases surprisingly seen locally, leading to another exchange of four or five quick accounts (about themselves and their families, about things seen, told or read) of the side effects of antima-larials and how they are best dealt with. Then some racy, funny stories about local sexually transmitted diseases lead to a serious exchange of tips for tracing contacts and concerns about the administrative problems and a further discussion comparing the STD services of neighbouring towns and the relative helpfulness of their websites and how to judge them. They have been talking for just under twenty minutes when Peter starts to leave to go and see some patients. Clive is beginning a story about the side effects of Cox2 inhibitors. Peter stops at the doorway. 'This is one I've taken', he grins, making as if to lean back into the room, ear cupped, to listen to the end of the story.*

❖ *Jim admits 'When I was a houseman I rarely went to the doctors' dining room because it seemed to me to be elitist. Then I realized that I was missing out on the chance to learn about the things that really mattered. In amongst all the bravura, bitching and banter a great deal of precious know-how was flying around.'*

❖ *Audrey quickly realizes that a thirty-five-year-old woman, recently moved to Woodsea, who has come about her acne has really come because she is depressed. She writes a 'prescrip-tion' to go to the local gym. She spends several minutes explaining why it might help her depressed feelings and if it doesn't to come back in two weeks, when antidepressants might be worth trying. 'Poor thing, she's homesick but doesn't realize it', says Audrey to me, rather maternally, once she has gone. I ask why the gym. 'We know that exercise helps – probably biochemically – but also I find that in cases like this just going out and meeting people at the gym also helps. We can always go on to the pills if it doesn't – it's worth a try.'*

❖ *At their (tetchy) lunchtime meeting the Urbcester doctors discuss how they could use the intranet to alert each other to useful bits of knowledge. 'I saw a brilliant article in* Pulse *the other day, for example, on ophthalmic emergencies. We ought to be able to share things like that quickly on the net.' (Someone asks her where the article was and makes a note.) They quickly agree that the intranet system as it stands is far too clunky and restrictive for such things, and begin swapping a lot of frustrated stories that highlight their doubts and difficulties, for all sorts of reasons, in using it. They start laughing at someone's anecdote about a child in the surgery who switched their computer off at the mains, but someone else caps the story. 'I had a child try and blow its nose on my shirt the other day. That just about summed up that consultation!' The tension is finally released in an explosion of laughter. As it dies down, Frances says 'Why not shift all that crap out of Jane's old office? I don't know why we can't have a doctors' room with a kettle, tea and coffee there where we can discuss patients and talk to each other. It's crazy that we don't.' 'Or what about Craig's little cubby hole room?' asks another GP. Someone adds: 'If necessary I'd give up my consulting room and we could put a fridge in there too.' Others excitedly chip into the reverie with more ideas until the chair brings them back to the main discussion about improving the intranet expert system. The mood drops again. After the meeting I interview Ramesh, who comments to me how good it is that they now have a meeting like this every week as there is no other opportunity for them all to talk. 'Six months ago even that meeting would only have lasted ten minutes', he tells me, 'because there was no proper leader to chair it. But it's so important to share information and it's not been happening until now.' Ironically, Ramesh is the person charged with developing communication via the intranet, which would diminish the need for the very kinds of meetings he is praising.*

Stories and the sharing of practical knowledge

Storytelling, or swapping anecdotes,[1] formed a large part of the Lawndale team's informal clinical discussions about practice; they were always telling each other stories and learning from them. Yet anecdotes are often frowned upon by healthcare professionals as unscientific. And rightly so; anecdotal evidence can be perilously misleading. An anecdote about an unusual case – or more likely a series of similar anecdotes – may sometimes lead to a useful hypothesis that can then be tested scientifically. But in terms of developing clinical science that is its limit. Any clinician whose knowledge relied on something so unrepresentative and idiosyncratic would be dangerous. Yet still we find that clinicians incessantly tell each other stories as a way of sharing knowledge (Hunter 1991: chapter 4; MacNaughton 1998). Why? The answer is not only revealed by a moment's reflection on one's own intellectual development, but also amply confirmed by the psychological literature. As Jerome Bruner, one of the most influential cognitive psychologists of the twentieth century, formulated it, there are

> two modes of thought, each providing distinctive ways of ordering experience, of constructing reality. The two (though complementary) are irreducible to one another. Efforts to reduce one at the expense of the other inevitably fail to capture the rich diversity of thought.
>
> (Bruner 1986: 11)

The first, which he calls the logico-scientific mode, is typical of formal clinical knowledge. The second is the narrative mode typical of the kinds of knowledge exchanged in the prologue to this chapter. Throughout our lives, much of what we find out about the world is through the narrative mode, through stories of one type or another (Schank and Abelson 1995). It is a fundamental part of how we understand the world and cannot simply be dismissed. Thus it is that when people chat about things, and this includes their work, they tend to do so in the form of stories and in this chapter we explore the many reasons why that is such an effective way to share knowledge and why – as many have observed (p. 101) – storytelling is such an essential part of how knowledge is shared, integrated and internalized (Brown *et al.* 2005).

We cannot escape the fact that stories and anecdotes are a very powerful way to communicate ideas, increase our knowledge (Benner *et al.* 1996: chapter 8) and even trigger action. This may be one reason why clinicians use them as ways to help their colleagues to readjust their practice (MacNaughton 1998; Cox 2001), or in our terms to modify their existing mindlines. They seem instinctively to know that by using the power of a story they are more likely to affect their colleagues' behaviour. 'We are more persuasive when we tell stories' is one conclusion that Schank draws in his extensive review of the psychological role of stories (Schank and Abelson 1995: 7). As psychologists from Dewey onwards have recognized, and as William Osler, Florence Nightingale and all good clinical teachers and reformers have always instinctively known, stories about concrete events are an excellent way to make people take note (Osler 1905; Nightingale 1860). We saw in passing in Chapter 4 that clinical teachers often use stories to help embed scientific and clinical ideas in their students' minds. During the process of acquiring their basic, scientifically based mindlines, stories – from teachers and from their own and fellow students' experience – are a powerful aid to learning (Cox 2001). Moreover, this learning reinforces the place of stories. Being such an easily recalled aspect of the training that one has received from respected teachers and role models – for it is the teachers' stories that so often stand out in the memory – anecdotes become legitimized as a powerful way of transmitting and sharing clinical knowledge.

Perhaps storytelling is *too* effective since, by being so deeply ingrained in our mental processes, stories are much harder to forget than other forms of information. The 'stickiness' of stories and the ease with which they can lead us to think or do something different is therefore a double-edged sword: they are a very good way to spread information, but also to spread misinformation. A misleading story is more likely to be remembered – and hence to corrupt one's mindline – than an isolated misleading fact. One can understand, therefore, why anecdotes are heavily discouraged as a blight on scientific, evidence-based practice. Yet there is a danger of throwing the baby out because the bathwater looks dirty. If stories are such a key currency for information sharing, the evidence-based practice movement shuns them at its peril.

Not only are stories a memorable way to convey information, but they are also an important means by which clinicians make sense of the complexities of day-to-day practice, especially when their mindlines are challenged by something that doesn't quite fit the pattern they have learned. Simply by formulating a narrative, a practitioner can begin the process of comprehending, say, a patient who doesn't fit the norm, or of resolving conflicting evidence about best practice. That formulation can involve piecemeal 'bricolage' (Levi-Strauss 1966; Weick 2001: 62–63; Gobbi 2005) by which they try to resolve anomalies by exploiting fragments from varied sources such as empirical experience, the written word or other stories they have heard. Once clinicians have developed their mindlines (Chapters 4 and 5), the daily informal exchange of information structured through the formulation of such narratives allows clinicians to help each other cope with challenges to their existing mindlines and adjust them. Sharing and hearing such stories therefore allows a continual checking and upgrading of their practice.

In this regard, the clinicians are no different from people who work in other sectors that have been studied. Brown and Duguid (2000), drawing largely on their work on knowledge management at Xerox – and in particular Julian Orr's seminal study of the way that photocopier technicians learn on the job (Orr 1997) – have stressed the role of stories in what they call 'the social life of information'. In the organizations they were researching, they found that instruction manuals, top-down directives, protocols and other formal sources were of relatively little actual use. Instead, people found it more helpful to learn from others who were doing similar work; a great deal of the knowledge they picked up was from each other's (and their own) experience. The photocopier engineers, for example, shared knowledge informally through the innumerable opportunities that they created for themselves to simply chat about their work. And such chat, Brown and Duguid report, largely took the form of 'constant storytelling' (ibid.: 106). The tales they told each other – whether, say, over coffee, in the locker room or while actually working together on a difficult job – were a good way to put things into some sort of coherent sequence and hence to make sense of why things happened and what might be the next step. Stories also helped them to compare notes, to pass on useful tips and to help integrate people's knowledge and experiences. Stories, it turned out, were a key way for those professionals to share *practical* knowledge that went beyond the canon of formal knowledge that their organization expected of them (Brown and Duguid 1991), and there is no good reason to assume that clinicians are any different.

Theoretical knowledge (an understanding of the renin–angiotensin cycle and its effect on renal potassium retention; the role of sodium/potassium balance in cardiac arrhythmias), gobbets of abstract information (ACE inhibitors can cause high potassium levels) or isolated rules of thumb (be careful about prescribing potassium supplements to someone on ACE inhibitors) are better retained and recalled when they are linked to a narrative (Mrs Jones had a worrying arrhythmia when she was on that ACE inhibitor because she forgot to stop her potassium supplements). The same information is much less forgettable when it is anchored in specific experiences in the form of stories.[2] This is all the more so if the story is oral rather than written, because the listener can actively engage, challenge, check, reinforce and more (Connell *et al.* 2004). That is why Tamsin stressed how important the coffee room was for Lawndale when compared with other practices where she had worked, and why the Urbcester doctors were right to want one.[3]

In summary, anecdotes and the story-form are the natural currency of a great deal of informal talk. There is ample evidence that 'conversation' is a crucial part of the way organizations – including healthcare – adapt and evolve (Boden 1994; Czarniawska 1997; Jordan *et al.* 2009). It would be surprising if clinicians did not use something that helps information to stick, makes it easier to share practical *nous*, is an efficient shorthand way to convey information. Moreover, because stories often contain elements of metaphor, analogy and other expressive imagery, they are highly effective in conveying tacit knowledge that is otherwise difficult to articulate (Nonaka 1994: 20). It is therefore unrealistic to insist that anecdotes be removed from day-to-day clinical discussion. Before condemning them, it is important to be quite clear about the difference between the story or anecdote as valid and generalizable knowledge (which it is not), or as adequate grounds for persuading someone to alter their practice (which it may or may not be – depending on the validity of the knowledge it conveys), or as a graphic way to convey information (which it inevitably is).

What's the story?

It therefore behoves us to explore further the many features of stories and story-telling that make them such a fundamental part of the way clinicians develop their knowledge and their mindlines, beginning by clarifying what, for present purposes, we mean by a 'story'.[4] We will not delve into this too deeply as it is the subject of fierce debate among literary academics (see, for example, Loewe *et al.* 1998; Eggly 2002), but most stories comprise the following components:

- some *main characters* (e.g. the patient, the people, circumstances, events or objects linked to the illness);
- some *coherent actions and events* (who did what and when to cause, exacerbate or ameliorate the illness);
- some discernable *plot* (how the illness developed, was treated and eventually turned out) with perhaps some *forces of good and evil* (bacteria, drugs, drug companies, carers, scientific advances, lack of resources, the government);
- a *complication* or conflict that needs resolving (the guidelines said do this but she wanted me to do that);
- a *moral* (don't use that treatment in those circumstances).

A story with such elements can also be constructed as an internalized narrative (told, as it were, to oneself). That helps the clinician make sense of all the complex and often disjointed components of the case. Audrey (p. 114) sees an unhappy woman with acne (main character) and quickly constructs in her own mind the story that she is homesick and in danger of becoming frankly depressed (plot). Previous similar stories have had a happy ending because exercise raises serotonin levels (forces of good and evil) and patients who join a gym meet new friends, which cheers them up (coherent actions and events), develops their social capital, and helps avoid the need to take antidepressants (conflict). As she then tells this story to the patient (and perhaps in future to colleagues if her approach works) it conveys the moral that you can avoid medical depression with sensible lifestyle changes.

If she were to tell that story to colleagues it would probably be only a couple of brief sentences. (I had a lady in the other week who looked depressed. One of those exercise prescriptions and two weeks later she was right as rain!) When stories are told in that way, one can detect that many of the implicit elements are unspoken but understood by both the speaker and the listener, with the result that only a terse, truncated version need be told (Connell *et al.* 2004). The listener, after all, not only already knows the story up to this latest episode but also shares the core aspects of the collective mindline on depression, serotonin and local knowledge about the background of the woman with acne. The listener may also feel gently chided for often moving too quickly to prescribing a possibly unnecessary antidepressant and may or may not take that on board. As this last point suggests, for a listener whose mindlines share many of the same elements the story usually connotes the practitioner's conflicting roles and goals (Chapter 2). The *clinical* role's narrative is that it is sometimes worth trying the gym before the pills; *preventively*, this approach might help other patients avoid depression; *managerially*, it helps reduce the drug spend; *professionally*, telling this story represents informal peer review (the listeners may contribute other evidence for or against) that may promote some reflection and change of practice, as well as maybe promoting the speaker's image as a good clinician.

The brief telling of this story therefore will be likely in some small way to influence the mindlines and hence the future actions of both the person who related it and the listener. We know from a range of organizations (Denning 2005) that people who need to decide how to act may be more likely to respond to a relevant story rather than to a theoretical or statistical fact or indeed, when they have any choice in the matter, to being told what to do (especially, we might add from our own observations, when being told by a remote and unknown authority at the Department of Health or a royal college).

Relating stories; stories relating

One reason why stories are more likely than abstract discourse to lead to action is that narratives are 'related' not just in the sense of 'being told', but also in at least two other senses of that word: *connecting* (relating ideas and people to each other) and *empathizing* ('I can relate to that'). As each story is told, it can remind the listener of another from their own repertoire so that, as the conversation develops, each tale is being mapped onto the listeners' relevant stories (Schank and Abelson 1995). They may or may not begin to empathize from their own experience. This in turn has the effect of inducing listeners to review what they have experienced or heard about the topic in question. The conversation therefore allows each person to amend their view of that topic, be it to confirm, question or revise their existing views – or in this case their mindlines.

The process of empathizing with a story also has the effect of altering the narrative as heard, especially where it is being directly linked to the listener's own concerns. When the listener is using the story to further their own thinking, what they hear may be different from what others might be hearing or even from what the storyteller intended. With stories more than with other types of information, people live and feel the ideas being conveyed. While listening, they imagine how they would react in those circumstances, or plan what they might do as a result of hearing this. Many conversations consist of little more than connecting, comparing, complementing, combining, competing, contradicting or capping each others' stories. The reason is that the participants are concurrently relating the stories to their own experience and situation. In fact psychological studies suggest that it is this process of triggering the listener's own internalized narratives, rather than the simple process of hearing the other person's story, that tends to change one's views or stimulate action (Schank and Abelson 1995: 26). Storytelling therefore also involves 'relating' in the sense of 'interacting'. While listening to a story the 'little voice in the head' is already planning how to respond, either in the conversation or by subsequent actions (Denning 2005: 114). That aspect of the storytelling, the active listening and internal response, is what leads the listener to action.

We have seen (Chapter 5) that stories are one of the main means within the SECI spiral by which experiential and tacit knowledge, which are otherwise difficult to convey to others, are brought to the surface in a form that can be shared. By telling each other about concrete, practical experiences clinicians expose the unspoken assumptions that underlie their way of doing things. In other words, the stories imply inherent knowledge that is intrinsic to the events and actions being recounted. As a new young casualty officer, JG told a fellow novice how he had referred a patient with a relatively minor abdominal stab wound to the resident surgical officer, who had immediately and pointedly asked 'How many units of blood have you cross-matched?' He hadn't. And in relating this story to his colleague he didn't have to say any more – the raised eyebrows did the rest. Both had quickly learnt through that short story that in this situation and this team the threshold for cross-matching blood rather than just requesting a blood grouping was much lower than they had previously understood. That brief story not only confirmed their implicit knowledge (the threshold they both had in their mindlines) but conveyed how that internalized knowledge now needed to change in this new environment. By sharing the story as new junior doctors they were, as Hunter (1991: 81) has put it, engaging in both 'instruction and social bonding'. Without the need to laboriously itemize their implicit clinical pathways, they both now knew what to do next time. Through a story just a couple of sentences long, they had rapidly and collectively exposed and adjusted the mindlines that guided their management of abdominal stab wound patients in that hospital.[5]

Narratives in healthcare: the place of stories as boundary objects

As we saw with Audrey, stories also play a part when used with patients.

❖ *Peter's patient has a chronic urinary tract disease. The two of them pore over charts and algorithms, discuss urodynamics and pros and cons of various antibiotics – it sounds to me just like a clinical case conference. Unlike the next patient, with whom suddenly Peter is using very simple language and still having trouble getting the message across about how to treat duodenal ulcers. Then Peter tells the story of the scientist proving the link between ulcers and* Helicobacter *by drinking down the 'bugs', which the patient immediately remembers seeing on TV.[6] Then he understands, and Peter can talk him though his laminated algorithm for managing ulcers (p. 21) – one of the very few times we saw a guideline referred to with a patient present (p. 25).*

❖ *A man whose wife is in hospital is in the urgent surgery because he fainted after having abdominal pain yesterday. He had been sent to casualty, where investigations revealed no explanation and they referred him back, still perplexed, to his GP. Clive explains how you can get vasovagal attacks when you stand up, especially when you're stressed and aren't eating properly because your wife's in hospital. 'The blood wasn't able to get up to your brain, that's all, so you went pale and then flushed up again, which is why the hospital thought you were very red.' Then while checking the man's blood pressure, Clive goes on to explain that the pulse was also slowed down because of the propranolol he's taking. 'If it happens again, sit down or, better still, lie down. And be careful driving . . .' and so he continues, piecing different aspects of the story together as he also explains vasodilation in a hot bath and the fall in blood pressure when having a pee. The man smiles, visibly relieved. The whole story now makes sense.*

❖   *One of us (ACLM) while writing this book develops a strange rash (must be the new shower gel) shortly after experiencing some hot flushes (must be that time of life). Later that day she gets some severe pains down her legs (must be the long walk to work). The story, disjointed as it is, more or less makes sense and life carries on as normal. Then she begins to feel ill enough to go and see her GP. 'Yes', says the GP, 'it could be a coincidence. But there is another way of putting all this together, you know, that we really shouldn't ignore.' A few hours later the hospital confirms the diagnosis of viral meningitis. The story told thereafter becomes one about not ignoring unusual presentations of meningitis, and not being tempted by benign interpretations of apparently unrelated symptoms.*

It is clear that stories are a way of making sense of unstructured, complex events and interpreting them in their context. There can be several concurrent narratives: in primary care there is not only the story of this illness episode but also the stories of the person's life to date, of their family, of the place that they live, and of the biopsychosocial disease processes that might be involved. All of these interwoven narratives that are inter-related within the internalized story may have a bearing on how the practitioner comprehends the illness and deals with it. Over the past two decades the importance of this phenomenon, under the rubric of 'narrative medicine', has been increasingly acknowledged not only for the features that we have described, but also as a counterweight to other recent more reductionist trends, in that it stresses the importance of an empathic and holistic approach to patients (Box 6.1; Greenhalgh and Hurwitz 1998; Greenhalgh 1999; Launer 2002, 2003, 2006; Hurwitz *et al.* 2004). Rita Charon for example defines it as 'medicine practised with the narrative skills of recognizing, absorbing, interpreting, and being moved by the stories of illness' (Charon 2006: 4). But it has also been claimed to be an effective way of improving quality of care (Greenhalgh *et al.* 2005a) and has led in the UK to excellent patient support initiatives such as www.healthtalkonline.org (Herxheimer and Ziebland 2000), which have made illness narratives widely accessible to patients and clinicians.

The concept of narrative medicine leads us to the important relationship between the patients' stories and the practitioners' stories (Clark and Mishler 1992). After all, patients usually tell their clinicians what ails them in the form of a narrative, and indeed the clinician will then usually explore it further by 'taking a history' (i.e. developing more of the narrative). We will return to this crucial interaction (p. 182). Here we wish only to stress that, because patients also make sense of their illness in narrative form, the clinician finds it easier to relate (in the

---

Box 6.1 The value of narrative medicine as summarized by Hurwitz and Greenhalgh (1999: 49)

- In the diagnostic encounter, narratives:
  - Are the phenomenal form in which patients experience ill health
  - Encourage empathy and promote understanding between clinician and patient
  - Allow for the construction of meaning
  - May supply useful analytical clues and categories
- In the therapeutic process, narratives:
  - Encourage a holistic approach to management
  - Are intrinsically therapeutic or palliative
  - May suggest or precipitate additional therapeutic options
- In the education of patients and health professionals, narratives:
  - Are often memorable
  - Are grounded in experience
  - Encourage reflection
- In research, narratives:
  - Help to set a patient centred agenda
  - May challenge received wisdom
  - May generate new hypotheses

Reproduced with the permission of BMJ Publications.

'telling' and 'connecting' senses of that word) what is happening to the patient as a narrative. In other words, not only does a narrative format help clinicians to formulate something coherent for themselves, but it makes it easier for them to communicate that story to their patients and engage with them. One of the important features of storytelling, after all, is that one can adapt the story to suit the audience – colleagues, examiners, students, patients, family – as one is going along (Hunter 1991). One can also use that device to help 'translate' the story between those different audiences, for example by recasting the patient's story in different terms to persuade the mother to take action or the local consultant to see them quickly. When the clinician and the patient communicate through telling each other their versions of the illness/disease, each is using the story as a 'boundary object',[7] something accessible to the separate worlds of both the patient and the doctor. Each sees the event differently, but at least each can try to construct narratives that they think will make sense to the other while still doing justice to their own view of what is happening. The narrative form is therefore their common currency, which will make it much easier for the doctor to relate to the patient about the illness (Launer 2002; Eggly 2002). Abstract and statistical facts about the incidence of depression, lifestyle, biochemical changes and the pros and cons of antidepressant tablets will cut little ice with Audrey's woman with acne.

But, by making such scientific facts individualized and concrete, the recasting of the story also humanizes them (bad brain chemicals are reduced by exercise; mad scientists swallowed bacteria to show they cause ulcers; blood rushed away from the brain and needed to be coaxed back; your rash, leg pain and flushes have a common cause), which helps explain the situation to the patient and enables the clinician to apply an individual solution.[8] We are not suggesting, of course, that stories always improve communication. Far from it (Sharf 1990; Clark and Mishler 1992). It is perfectly possible for the clinician to 'rewrite' the patient's story in a way that alienates them from each other (Hunter 1991: chapter 7), and we saw instances in all our observation sites when this was clearly happening.

An example of the way in which stories can become the common currency between people with different backgrounds and responsibilities occurred when we were working over several months with multi-sectoral groups of people from various local authority, health and voluntary organizations, and service users to develop local services for elderly people (Gabbay *et al.* 2003; le May 2009a). Our role was both to help them develop local policies on, for example, convalescent services for people discharged from hospital and also, while providing the groups with research-based information, to observe how they used it. (For brief details of the methods see p. 137.) We quickly found that, whatever the topic or the type of information being provided, the participants tended to swap stories, some of which, although usually short and spontaneous, became the key shared currency upon which the groups built their policies. Although we deliberately made research results and other relevant (mainly abstract and statistical) data available to the groups, they almost never introduced these into their discussions: they preferred anecdotes about their experiences. That was the most common form in which the groups shared their knowledge. The lay and voluntary-sector members seemed to find that the easiest way to make their points, while the professionals tended instinctively to use stories to relate their accumulated knowledge and experience about the subject and about the local organizations and the people who ran them. Even when participants were asked to summarize research papers or formal documents for the group, they usually focused on one small aspect of the research that they wanted to emphasize by lapsing rapidly into a story relating to their own similar experiences that confirmed or refuted the research. This might then elicit similar stories from those who empathized with that experience, or occasionally counter-examples from those who didn't. The acceptability of the stories was partly based on the credibility and authority of the contributor (le May 2009a). Our conclusion in those studies was that new knowledge was being internalized by linking it to people's own experiences, and that the telling and the hearing of stories were an important vehicle by which that was happening. Whether a story from a doctor or a service manager carried more weight than one from a patient or vice versa depended partly on group dynamics and partly on how well the story chimed with the individual and group views. But stories were the medium that made the knowledge accessible to all the participants, whatever their background, and however hard we tried to get them to use more formal knowledge sources.

Stories can not only act as boundary objects to bridge the differing worlds of

people with different training and backgrounds; they can also help health practitioners link the often disparate sectors within their own worlds. For example,
the clinician qua scientist inhabits a world of generalized knowledge that often
fits ill with the less certain world of individual patient care that they also inhabit.
One of the essential tensions but also one of the essential skills of the clinician is
marrying general scientific theory to particular, complex and often idiosyncratic
instances (pp. 30, 68). Individual clinical stories, once one has learned how to
construct them appropriately, become a key way to relate the general to the specific. One can coherently – as with Audrey's depressed patient with acne – weave
oneself a single narrative comprising such diverse elements as brain biochemistry;
the statistical likelihood, based on trials, of the relative benefit of exercise and
antidepressants; the psychology of health belief models; the sociology of social
capital; the woman's family background; and her beliefs about depression and/
or exercise. Once having constructed the narrative, one can see more clearly what
the next episode might be, in this case a referral to the gym. It also is perhaps
in this way that – as Karl Weick suggests (Weick 1995: 120, 127–131) – stories
help to perpetuate paradigmatic beliefs even when the evidence for them may be
equivocal. (To what extent can one really scientifically justify the concatenation
of elements in that story about exercise, social capital and serotonin levels? Yet,
however tentative the causal links between them, the story makes them sound
plausible, and so they persist.)

Never-ending stories

Relating each individual story to the appropriate mindline helps the clinician to
see how a specific case fits the pattern not only of the illness script but all the other
elements of the story, including experience of actions taken (e.g. treatments tried,
colleagues contacted and explanations given) in the past.[9] And conversely the
accretion of such stories (one's own and those of others), accumulated over many
years of practice, is what helps mindlines evolve. This may be one way in which
mindlines become complex and flexible guides to action. Founded on broad and
detailed scientific knowledge, they are capable of being continually reinterpreted,
applied and readjusted with each particular and more or less unique narrative
instance of that broad knowledge. By the way they transmit knowledge and relate
experience to existing knowledge, stories are therefore intimately linked to the
continual reshaping of a clinician's mindlines.

Stories also play a number of other important roles. For example storytelling
makes it easier to discuss the many patients that do not easily fit the norm. Not
only does the construction of a coherent narrative help make sense of the anomalous case, but it exposes legitimate queries about the boundaries of the norm.
So a story about an unusual event is useful not only to check out whether others
have had the same experience, but also, as the fund of stories on this topic grows,
to help to collectively test out the boundaries of 'acceptable' deviation from the
usual pattern of events or actions in a given condition. Such information sharing
can sometimes also be important for furthering medical knowledge. Without the

capacity to share informal anecdotes, the coincidences are less likely to be spotted. Such brief stories can in this way strengthen the clinician's capacity to question the norm and hence not only to adjust their own mindline, but sometimes also to alter the received view. As Hunter has put it, the anecdote 'serves the skepticism that is essential to scientific medicine' (Hunter 1991: 82). As two or three anecdotes are shared and start to become a 'case series', so begin the first steps towards a more fundamental shift in collective knowledge. Sometimes this can even lead to new discoveries. The informal sharing of anecdotes about isolated instances of a very unusual tumour, Kaposi's sarcoma, was one of the key events that led to the recognition of AIDS as a new disease.

An associated feature of the anecdote is the chance that it gives to colleagues to comment on a niggling problem that one wants to air informally. This occurs particularly when a less experienced clinician describes events to senior colleagues without wishing to make it sound like a formal consultation. 'Yes I've had several like that and they've all spontaneously recovered' is a very reassuring response to a tale told by someone worried about an unusual case. More experienced clinicians may act as 'witnesses' to confirm their junior colleagues' experience or knowledge, but may also use the opportunity to adjust their practice ('Actually, in that situation I have found X works better') – and more often than not that is precisely what the storyteller was seeking. Shared narratives about patients are a crucial vehicle by which colleagues both confirm their mindlines but also apprise a colleague of a need to change their practice towards the local collective mindline. Such stories can include cautionary tales. More formal case presentations can of course also have a similar function at, say, audit or critical event meetings; but these also take the form of story swapping, the key difference being the amount of detail that the format allows. 'Anecdotes with a purpose' therefore play a role in introducing discussions that help the speakers test out ideas or seek help for problems that might range from a worrying patient to a query about a new research finding or guideline to a report in the press. The subsequent exchange opens up a channel for informal collegial help that plays an important part in supplementing or amending the speaker's mindline – and indeed that of others who are engaged in the conversation.

Stories are an extremely efficient way to make a point, not least because they so often assume a similar pattern and are almost always embedded in a set of common assumptions such as shared or collective mindlines. Much of the content can therefore go unsaid (as in the two-sentence story about blood grouping for abdominal stab wounds), allowing many implicit elements to be relayed 'silently' because they are taken for granted. This also has an excluding/including effect, in that anyone who does not share those assumptions, background information or similar mindlines will find the narrative incomprehensible. Only those already in the know would have learnt anything from hearing most of the stories that we heard being told about clinical matters. And, as Bosk (1979: 109) suggests in his ethnography of elite US surgical teams, 'story telling is the anteing-up of clinical credentials . . . Having a ready stock of stories serves notice that one has been around and knows what is going on.' His junior surgeons' stories were often couched as 'horror stories' (cautionary tales) told sometimes against themselves. They were a form of social control as well as collegial bonding, of norm reinforcement as well as tension relief, of role demarcation as well as pomposity pricking. Moreover, as we shall see in Chapter 8, stories are a way to justify one's actions by fitting them into a narrative that gives them meaning that is acceptable to people, real or imaginary, who might judge them. In these and other ways, stories are a way to reinforce one's identity as belonging to a status group and to gain the respect of colleagues in that group (Orr 1997: 174).

In short, stories have both knowledge transmission (or transformation) roles and social roles. Not only did the clinicians reformulate and regenerate a great deal of knowledge when swapping stories, but in doing so they also collectively reinforced their professional roles and relationships. The fact that stories, one of the chief methods of communication, carry both cognitive and social functions when people learn practical knowledge from their peers may not be surprising as we uncover how knowledge and social interaction are inseparable aspects of communities of practice.

Chapter 6: Summary

Whatever the dangers of anecdotal evidence, clinicians – like all of us – transmit a great deal of information in the form of stories. Using illustrations from our work, we review the important properties of the narrative form that have been shown to make stories a fundamental part of knowledge sharing, including their memorability, their role in helping to make sense of disparate events, and the way they ease communication and action. Sharing stories also helps clinicians maintain their collective sense of identity. Stories help practitioners combine new information with other relevant knowledge and make it easier to communicate with their patients.

7   A community of clinical practice?

The focus in this chapter is the way that practitioners rely on each other to help improve their knowledge-in-practice-in-context.

❖ *A fifty-five-year-old woman asks Tony if she should have a cervical smear every three years or every five. As they talk about it he decides on three-yearly. Later I ask why he didn't opt for five. 'Ignorance really', he says. 'We tend to go for three-yearly here up to a certain age but I don't know the exact cut off, so I played safe. Jean is the one who knows about smears; she'll tell me what the guidelines suggest and I'll be happy to agree because I don't have the knowledge. But if I had good evidence for moving, say, to five-yearly then I'd take her on.' At that moment, Nick appears at the door and joins our conversation. He says (as I recall) that their protocol is to do it five-yearly except in women aged twenty to forty because of the higher incidence of cervical cancer in the younger women. He personally can't see any point in doing them at all over fifty-five but the practice tends to do it five-yearly anyway, so he would have tried to persuade her to wait. But when Tony explains how anxious she was about it, Nick concurs that he might in that case have relented this once, even though the lab service can barely cope with the volume of samples from five-yearly intervals for that age group. Then Nick says he had come to ask Tony about another patient with an unusual connective tissue disease; he shows Tony the ECG and takes his advice.*

❖ *Clive pops down to the treatment room and asks Rose, one of the nurses, for advice about a patient with a split heel. She runs through the options and says what she would do. As we walk back to Clive's surgery he tells me that he is pleased that nothing she said suggested he was on the wrong track. Later in the same surgery he and Angela, the lead practice nurse, discuss a leg ulcer, and he accedes to her suggestions. The previous day, Heather had asked Nick to help sort out a very complicated problem in a diabetic lady whose leg ulcer she was dressing and the two, together with the patient and her husband, had arrived at a solution that none alone would have come to.*

❖ *Tamsin says in her taped interview: 'As I've seen repeated things I'll know what to do now but with new things I'll ask another GP. They all practise differently. You know that if you ask the same questions to different GPs they'll all come back with slightly different management plans. . . . Say someone comes with a one-week history of a productive cough. Some people will think it's viral and be really mean and not give antibiotics. Others will be maybe less, you know maybe it's been going on a week maybe there's a bacterial bit and maybe it is viral but maybe we should give them some antibiotics. Also some would take a [skin] lesion off and others would refer. Some use one class of antihypertensive, some another.' Are there limits on the differences? '[Yes for] regular things. But when none of us know we send round an email' (or discuss it, for example the thyroid problem she had raised at coffee that morning). 'So we do use each other as knowledge' (and she says she uses people that she knows have specific lead expertise within Lawndale). 'But sometimes it's just whoever's door is open' (when she usually tells them what she would do and then, she says, listens to how they would do it and adjusts her approach if necessary). The other trainee, Jason, on the other hand, says he usually tries to look things up before asking colleagues.*

❖ *Nick opens a clinical meeting by stressing that the aim is to share and verify information 'because sometimes what you're told isn't true'. Each person presents something they have recently read or heard and the others debate it. Ben opens with a paper he has read that suggests that patients with irritable bowel benefit from metronidazole (antibacterial) and a low-fibre diet. 'Low fibre?!' splutters Peter – 'like burger and chips?' They laugh. 'What's the evidence?' asks Barry, equally sceptical of such a revolutionary notion (IBS has traditionally called for high-fibre diets). Adam, keen as ever, has done his homework and gives details of the trial. Peter says that yes he has heard the idea of 'friendly bacteria' being useful. 'Yes, they're called Bifidobacteria somethingorother' adds Adam. 'Friendly bacteria', though, is the term they all start using. I can't help thinking that they have picked it up from television adverts for yogurt, not from learned journals, but the term sticks. They decide that probiotic yogurt with 'friendly bacteria' is less likely to have side effects than a prescription of metronidazole. There follows a discussion in which they appear to share their mindlines and bits of things they have read about when to use antibiotics in treating IBS, even though – as Jean characteristically reminds them – this is not in the guidelines. Some realize that there are differences in the length of time they prescribe metronidazole for, say, diverticulitis. (Four or five days? Seven days?) Embarrassed laughter suggests that some mindlines are being hastily revised. Add cephalosporins? Or just a 'bog standard' antibiotic seems to work, says Jean. 'Won't that wipe out the friendly bacteria?' No, says Jean and quotes a recent discussion about a patient with a respected local consultant to support her case. Ben agrees with her, based on what he learnt during his recent hospital training.*

The conversation continues in this vein as they posit and question their different antibiotic regimes for various tricky conditions including sinusitis. There are some anecdotes of things seen or experienced, some references to things they have read. Some nodding; some perplexed looks. A couple of the GPs are writing occasional notes. Others appear to be making occasional mental notes ('aha' moments of raised heads, eyebrows and forefingers). The medical student hardly stops writing throughout. From subsequent one-to-one conversations it seems that some of the GPs checked some of the ideas later (through discussion or looking things up), dismissed some of the new ideas they heard, and tentatively incorporated others.

The rest of the fifty-minute meeting includes a description of a local pulmonary rehabilitation service that Tony visited 'because we prescribe it without knowing what it really entails'. The partners' ears seem to prick up when Tony mentions that the rehab team can refer patients straight on to Westchurch Hospital. Is this a potentially useful short cut for their respiratory referrals to the hospital? They swap stories about such patients who could be eligible and agree to do an audit.

❖ *Peter (taped interview): 'unless I'm going over them [guidelines and protocols] frequently then bits may disappear so it needs to be ingrained I think on my brain to be a good protocol and I suppose what these [QPA] meetings are doing is reinforcing the good practice. So although we're not actually going line by line through the protocols we're going over the things that we really think are important and that actually forms the basis of the protocol [. . .] So the ones that we develop within the practice I think you're much more likely to use not necessarily by taking the piece of paper off the shelf but because you've been involved in developing it, so it will be ingrained in your brain better.'*

❖ *Amid the usual gossip, banter and laughter at coffee, Clive mentions that the lab results seem to be consistently showing low potassium levels, which several of the other partners have also noted. They think it is an artefact. The conversation moves to the vexed question of how patients are told about 'abnormal' results. Clive suggests an implicit pragmatic classification that he tends to use for abnormal results (e.g. 'abnormal but don't worry', 'abnormal and urgent') and posits how he deals with them. Rachel (a younger, salaried, part-time GP) reels off the way that she tends to deal with near-normal potassium results. This makes Clive revise his three-point classification to a four-point one. The others are obviously listening and seem to be mentally noting what has been said, nodding, but saying nothing further about it. They go on to discuss the possible causes of low potassium, which someone suggests includes extra-cellular leakage of potassium ions when blood specimens are left hanging around. Later Adam (the bright young new GP registrar) rushes in for a quick coffee; Clive asks his view, as someone who has recently been working in hospital medicine and is likely to know about such things. (Clive had earlier commented how much they learn from the young registrars, but had jokingly told me not to write that down). There is much laughter as Adam explains how cellular leakage would actually increase the serum potassium level. But they are no further in explaining the spurious results so Nick says he will ask the lab and bring the answer back to a (formal) practice meeting.*

Two years later when chatting to Tamsin (who had replaced Adam as the trainee) I notice that when asked for an example of something she has picked up from the others in the practice she chooses to mention the fact that one need not be concerned about the occasional low serum potassium.

❖ *Clive is talking about our emerging findings about mindlines and the use of evidence. He says our analysis is 'spot on'. He comments how he notices that he and his colleagues 'glean' (his word) what is thought to be best practice from things written by consultants, from snippets of reading, and from each other in the practice. Each of the partners, he says, has recognized areas of expertise, and they tend to keep each other up to date in that way.*

Meanwhile in Urbcester . . .

❖ *Ben – reputedly the keenest user of Urbcester's intranet expert system – is wondering which antibiotic to use for a patient on warfarin. He looks in his well-thumbed* British National Formulary. *Still not sure. He phones a colleague to ask and then writes his prescription. What a shame, I think, that they haven't got that coffee room yet (p. 114).*

Trusted sources

The clinicians' mindlines did not exist in each individual's island of personal knowledge. They were being implicitly shared and checked, refined and continually developed through interactions between colleagues (Figure 7.1). Whilst each practitioner would carry in their own mind what they regarded as the most appropriate way to manage a given situation, they also built up a fairly good idea about each other's ways of dealing with similar problems. Through their discussions they were able not only to ascertain what others thought was regarded as appropriate practice but also to learn from the ways in which they might subtly modulate that ideal depending on the exact circumstances of a particular patient. Both the theoretical 'best practice' and the nature and applicability of the modulations were continually subject to this subliminal process of reassessment and adjustment, which might sometimes also involve reference to trusted sources such as books, review articles, websites etc. (pp. 20, 109) or formal educational sessions. But the sources that provided the GPs with the most relied-upon and efficient short cuts to the up-to-date practice were their professional networks. They found it most helpful to hear – often in narrative form (Chapter 6) – what trusted colleagues thought about, say, a new suggestion for managing a clinical condition: what they had heard about it, whether they had come across reliable evidence for or against it, whether they had tried it and with what results, and so on.

Local experts from the hospital provided one useful source of such information and this occurred by several means. One was simply to learn from their example. The fact that GPs shared the care of many patients with local experts at the hospital gave them many opportunities to see what hospital specialists considered to be appropriate practice and where necessary to recognize when their own practice was out of line. It is of course a source of frustration at many hospital trusts that GPs often fail to pick up or even deliberately ignore such cues from the specialists, but this resource of expertise was generally an opportunity that GPs at Lawndale were keen to grasp, as were many other GPs we have talked to. 'If I see that the local [hospital] consultant has started using a new drug I might well look it up and start checking out whether it's something I should be thinking about', as Jim succinctly put it. And this is also of course why we often heard the pharmaceutical reps telling the GPs that this or that new drug was favoured by a respected local consultant. If the people in the know use it then surely you should too, was the transparent message – which backfired if they mentioned consultants that, unbeknown to them, the GPs did not respect. The reps were instinctively exploiting what has long been known about the important role of opinion leaders and of doctors' networks generally in influencing their uptake of new ideas (Coleman *et al.* 1966; Rogers 2003 [1985]; West *et al.* 1999; Locock *et al.* 2001; Doumit *et al.* 2007; Lomas 2007; Adler *et al.* 2008).

Not only were the formal interactions with hospital consultants to whom Lawndale GPs referred their patients a useful source but the GPs and consultants also deliberately fostered close informal relations. GPs were often able to telephone a hospital colleague for advice about a patient without making a formal referral – something that is now being encouraged in a more systematic way by the NHS since it not only makes shared care more efficient but also provides a helpful source of specialist expertise. But the Lawndale GPs went even further in forging closer links with hospital experts. They occasionally invited them to spend a day at the surgery, which gave them an opportunity both to pick the experts' brains and in turn to show them what it was like dealing with patients in general practice, so that the specialist might in future be more sensitive to the constraints (and, we would add, multiple roles) of primary care when responding to the GPs' queries. Such visits usually entailed an informal and interactive discussion in the manner of a masterclass about common conditions in that particular speciality, which was a particularly powerful source of expertise about those borderline patients who were out of the ordinary but not quite complicated enough to be referred to hospital. What was particularly notable was the kind of information based on tacit knowledge that was also exchanged (e.g., when the visiting ophthalmologist was explaining the protocol for using certain eye drops, he gave out a lot of his hitherto tacit knowledge about how long they could be stored, how to make the most of the small volumes available, when things can safely be left to opticians) as well as the degree of mutual respect that emerged from the contact, and the evident desire to find ways to communicate more often and more effectively.

Local experts would also be invited to speak at formal educational sessions, such as lunchtime meetings organized by local networks of GPs or perhaps at

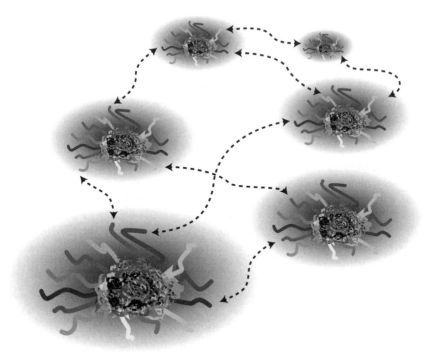

Figure 7.1 A community of mindlines.

more formal courses laid on by various authorities. (See also p. 104 for examples of how these sessions did – and didn't – function as a means of transmitting new knowledge.) The education at such CPD meetings was not confined to the didactic lecture and the plenary discussions. Where the GPs had good relations with the experts, the private informal chat before or afterwards (p. 104) could provide rich and concentrated guidance (often focused around a particular shared patient) on the latest thinking and also the inside knowledge about local services and their foibles. Such informal exchange was also the purpose of many social events such as regular informal dinners for the local medical community, which facilitated exactly that kind of discussion. At these gatherings, the chat around the dinner tables was largely anecdote swapping, gossip, pointed jocularity, cautionary tales, 'war stories', but at the same time they provided a potent source of useful informa-tion about appropriate practice and the boundaries of acceptable care. It was also a chance to find out more about, for example, the strengths and weaknesses of the local hospital and community facilities, and the relative merits of one's colleagues.

Inevitably such exchanges alerted participants to aspects of their own practice that they might wish to attend to. Thus, for example, when Clive had missed a diagnosis on a patient he had referred to outpatients, the local hospital physi-cian had been able to rectify the problem, order the relevant test, and write a brief summary in his formal outpatient letter back to Lawndale. This had alerted Clive to the omission and prompted him to reduce his threshold for ordering that biochemical investigation in future. One evening at a subsequent local doctors' informal dinner, though, the consultant while telling a story about a similar patient also gently and humorously ribbed Clive about his case and elaborated on the lessons learnt. Several other GPs at the table were listening, and none of them was left in any doubt about when it might be appropriate to carry out that lab investi-gation in future. In that short dinner conversation – typical of dozens that evening – Clive's mindline for that condition had been further reinforced and other GPs at that table had also taken the first steps of refining their own mindlines. Moreover there was also an exchange of useful clues about the people involved: everyone privileged to be part of that 'insiders'' conversation saw that the physician was sharp but good humoured and approachable; Clive – a senior and respected GP – had been happy to learn from him; there was clear mutual respect between them; and no one need feel threatened or ashamed – all of which were important lessons about their network and its ethos. By many such small exchanges, each participant was, over time, building up and embedding their store of contextualized, practical knowledge about everything from technical matters and local systems to the reli-ability of the wide range of people with whom they needed to deal (Tables 2.1 and 3.1). And they were doing so in consort with each other.

Important as such wider networking might be as a knowledge resource, most such exchanges at Lawndale in fact occurred within the surgery itself, where everyone was known for the areas in which they were relatively expert. At both formal and informal meetings within the practice, the exchange of knowledge – not just clinical information but the full range of practical knowledge such as that illustrated in Box 3.1 and the kind of insider intelligence network that we just recounted – was never far away. For the Lawndale clinicians, nurses as well as doctors, it was discussions and interactions, often based around stories (Chapter 6) drawn from either each other's experience or that gleaned from trusted colleagues, that led to new departures in practice being raised and then gradually reinforced or rejected.

Communities of general practice

We saw many examples of mutual consultation between colleagues, each drawing on various sources of knowledge that illustrated how important was the level of trust that each was able to place in those sources. The constant networking was vital in providing a continual opportunity to weigh up the strengths and weaknesses of colleagues and of other sources of information so that they could assess which to rely on and when. A great deal of the social interaction and professional to-ing and fro-ing between doctors/nurses and other practice staff – and beyond – provided the means to check out who or what were the most authoritative and trustworthy places to find things out (both interpersonal but also written or online), and whose advice should be ignored. However, once they had established someone or somewhere as reliable, the clinicians rarely questioned how – or even whether – the information from that source was backed by research evidence. This was simply assumed, because those sources are supposed to be the ones 'in the know'. Barry was quite capable of single-handedly searching and appraising the online literature about contraceptives and the risk of thrombosis for his wheelchair-bound patient (p. 51) but (a) he was implicitly assuming that a trusted textbook whose content had been interpreted by a trusted colleague and corroborated by a (less trusted) pharmaceutical rep was a sufficiently reliable final arbiter to give the best answer – in a few minutes – without having to review the research literature at length in the manner that the advocates of evidence-based practice might have preferred and (b) he knew that this exact problem was in any case unlikely to be covered in the literature.

The type of knowledge exchange that all the examples in the prologue illustrate is typical of what has come in recent years to be known as 'communities of practice', which are groups of people who share similar concerns, problems or passions about a topic – not necessarily work related – and who learn from each other through their formal and informal interactions. They may or may not work in the same organization but, as in Orr's Xerox engineers' locker room (p. 117) and the Lawndale coffee room:

> they meet because they find value in their interactions. As they spend time together they typically share information, insight, and advice. They help each other solve problems. They discuss their situations, their aspirations, and their needs. They ponder common issues, explore ideas, and act as sounding boards. They may create tools, standards, generic designs, manuals, and other documents – or they may simply develop a tacit understanding that they share. However, they accumulate knowledge, they become informally

bound by the value that they find in learning together. This value is not merely instrumental for their work. It also accrues in the personal satisfaction of knowing colleagues who understand each other's perspectives and of belonging to an interesting group of people. Over time, they develop a unique perspective on their topic as well as a body of common knowledge, practices, and approaches. They also develop personal relationships and established ways of interacting. They may even develop a common sense of identity. They become a community of practice.

(Wenger *et al.* 2002: 4)

The concept was originally introduced by Lave and Wenger (1991) in the context of the way people learn, and we certainly found that the Lawndale practitioners were doing a great deal of their learning – improving their knowledge-in-practice-in-context – through their interactions with their colleagues.[1]

As Etienne Wenger (1998), whose name is most closely associated with the term, has argued, communities of practice rely on three essential components that link an individual's practice with that of his or her colleagues. Put simply, members of the community must:

1   be trying to solve similar problems, such as the tasks of looking after the patients or managing a practice and dealing with the external environment that puts pressures upon them ('joint enterprise');
2   interact easily and constructively with each other, which includes of course not only professional formal interactions but also – and perhaps more importantly – informal interactions in the coffee room, at the meal table or socially ('mutual engagement');
3   have in common a wide range of routines, vocabularies, assumed knowledge, concepts, words and gestures that the group uses to carry out its tasks ('shared repertoire').

Wenger (1998: 41) suggests that, 'whoever we are, understanding in practice is the art of choosing what to know and what to ignore in order to proceed with our lives'. That entails not only having access to the right information and skills, but, for example, knowing where one fits into the picture, how far one has the right to be dealing with the problem, what the relevant norms and rules of social relationships are, and how to work with the social structure in which one is operating – right down to handling the dynamics of everyday existence such as how and with whom to hold a sensible conversation. This process tends mainly to involve other people who are also learning or refining these arts. The important point is that the act of learning is as much about social relations – indeed about working out one's very identity as a professional – as it is about acquiring specific knowledge and skills. His analysis leads inevitably to profound questions about how practitioners negotiate a workable relationship between what they know and what they do, how and where they learn to do it, and what their place is in the scheme of things – themes that we will explore further below and in Chapter 8. For now, however, we will simply outline some of the features of the communities of practice that we encountered at Lawndale and elsewhere, and how they led to the shared development of clinical mindlines.

Discussions such as the typical one in the coffee room about potassium levels relied on the relaxed, often humorous informality of the discussions as well as their clearly practical focus and their foundation in relevant experience. The chatting between the GPs around the Lawndale library coffee table was rife with anecdotes about experiences with patients and snippets of things they had heard or come across – at meetings, in the press, on websites, on the radio, from the pharmaceutical representatives, from patients who had heard about a new treatment and so on. Helped by the relaxed atmosphere of gossip, ribbing and inside jokes, each would chip in with what they had read, heard and understood about the topic, or maybe their own or other people's reported experience. They might accept, reaffirm, add, reject, question or challenge new bits of information, often with much mirth and mutual debunking. They might reveal their own current practice, often by telling brief stories about recent patients, occasionally scoring good-natured points over each other, sometimes with admonishments – maybe sharp, humorous or elliptical, maybe logically explained. The occasional cautionary tale would be used to remind each other of the limits – and limitations – of good practice. Good group dynamics characterized by trust and mutual respect helped them to deal constructively with differing or even conflicting views, to expose problems and deficiencies, agree on practical solutions and review them, checking sources only when that was deemed necessary because of lingering collective doubts (as in Nick's offer to ask the lab about unexpected low potassium readings).

The community of practice that we have been describing – the 'coffee room GPs' at the practice – was not monolithic.[2] There were three ways in which this Lawndale community of practice among GPs overlapped with, and was supplemented by, others. First, within the practice, there were several 'specialist' subgroups, both formal and informal, where they would go into more depth over certain topics, and those groups might include other members such as the practice nurses, the practice manager and the phlebotomist. Some, such as a group focusing on diabetes, were set up formally but increasingly functioned as communities of practice. The 'clinical meetings' (e.g. clinical audit or critical incident meetings) attended only by the doctors and practice manager were a particularly potent focus for more formalized community of practice interchange. Other groups, such as the nurses' treatment room, where there was frequent discussion between the nurses and phlebotomist about work, evolved more casually in that direction.

Second, outwith Lawndale, each clinician – and this applied especially to the doctors – also had their own networks of local clinicians, committees, old colleagues, and so on, whom they trusted as sources of information. We have already seen the example of the regular social gathering of local doctors over dinner, but there were many other groups and networks that acted as communities of practice, and which Lawndale could tap into. Clive, with his finger in so many political and administrative pies around the region, was a resource for ensuring that Lawndale was aware of all the latest debates and proposals about, say, contractual or educational changes. Janet, who actively linked up with a network of fellow practice managers, could where necessary contribute a different angle on such questions, and triangulate Clive's GP perspective. Nick belonged to national and regional groups dealing with IT and was able to use those other communities of practice to explore new ideas or problems regarding the practice computer system. Angela used her links with the community nurses to keep Lawndale abreast of developments in that arena, and so on. By being members of many different networks and communities of practice, the clinicians were able to bring the expertise of those other communities to bear on the problems being solved by this one and vice versa – a phenomenon that greatly adds to the potency of communities of practice in spreading knowledge.[3]

Finally, Lawndale's formal practice meetings also evolved into a wider multidisciplinary community of practice that began as a regular practice meeting in 2002 to prepare Lawndale for the Royal College of GPs Quality Practice Award (QPA). It included most of the GPs, the practice manager and the nurses, phlebotomist and receptionists. Indeed there were occasions when almost all the staff at the practice appeared to belong to it until we realized that there were also quite a few of the reception and administrative and secretarial staff and even one or two part-time GPs and attached staff who chose not to take part and whom we as researchers hardly ever came into contact with.[4] But for those who did attend, just as for those who sat in the coffee room or nurses' treatment room, it eventually became very clear to us that the discussions were playing a potent part in shaping their mindlines, both individual and collective, and it therefore is to the nature of such discussions that we now turn.

Information flows in communities of practice

The discussions at those Lawndale practice meetings had all Wenger's core features of 'joint enterprise' (e.g. to improve the quality of care), 'mutual engagement' (which spanned all of the disciplines involved in care) and a 'shared repertoire' of practice (p. 142). Once they had achieved the QPA it was hardly surprising that when Lawndale moved on to the next big task of developing the practice to meet the GP contract the group continued to evolve its role of sharing knowledge and driving practice forward. Yet it is worth emphasizing that – perhaps because our early ethnographic focus had been on the day-to-day utilization of knowledge in the surgery, on the multiple roles and on our emerging notion of mindlines – we were, in retrospect, surprisingly slow to recognize the way this group was functioning as a community of practice, and to see just how crucial it and the other Lawndale communities of practice were to the development of clinicians' knowledge. Despite the fact the questions driving this ethnography had arisen from a research study of communities of practice that we had recently completed elsewhere, it was nearly a year before the penny dropped. Perhaps this was because we were trying hard not to impose the assumptions from that prior research onto what we were observing – or perhaps we had simply not noticed the slow evolution of a project group, clustered around the QPA exercise, into a versatile community of practice.

It is pertinent to give some brief details of that earlier study, since we will now draw on data from there as well as from Lawndale. That earlier work, whose reliance on stories we briefly mentioned at p. 123, had involved four communities of practice, two of which were at 'Haymarket', our pseudonym for a well-heeled area in the Home Counties where our task had been to set up, facilitate and ethnographically observe two multi-sectoral communities of practice aiming to improve local health and social services for the elderly (Gabbay *et al.* 2003). The other two were also artificially constructed, having been set up to redesign outpatient services including ear, nose and throat (ENT) and dermatology (Lathlean and le May 2002; le May 2009a; Lathlean and Myall 2009). Our aim in all four of those projects had been to elucidate how communities of practice (each consisting of up to twenty-five people drawn from primary care, community services, hospitals, social services, the private sector, voluntary organizations and local citizens) processed and applied evidence in formulating their views. To help the groups at Haymarket design improvements to their respective services we explicitly encouraged the use of the best available evidence by providing them both with the bespoke services of a librarian to find any relevant publications, and with expert facilitation to assist them in their deliberations. Data collection for the studies included observing and tape-recording and transcribing the group meetings, interviewing participants and reviewing documents they generated and used.

The Haymarket data showed us particularly clearly that the members of those communities of practice did not handle new evidence as a basis for their policy recommendations in anything remotely like the orderly, linear, rational manner envisaged by the proponents of evidence-based practice (Figure 1.1). On the contrary, their deliberations resembled the apparent chaos of Figure 7.2 in which information brought to the group reached its eventual fate via complex and haphazard interactions. This finding disappointed our funders, who were intent on using communities of practice to spread the rational use of research evidence. But they should not have been surprised at our finding, since anyone who has worked in policy-making groups will recognize the picture and moreover there is an established literature on group decision making that repeatedly describes decision making going through similar processes, variously called, for example, 'muddling through' (Lindblom 1959) or the 'garbage-can model' of organizational decision making (Cohen *et al.* 1972).

Our analysis of the Haymarket communities of practice revealed five main themes that helped explain why the participants treated new evidence in these ways.

- First, they were more likely to accept certain categories of evidence in preference to others. In particular, personal experiences or the views of locally respected authorities, often relayed as stories and anecdotes, became the groups' *lingua franca* (see also p. 119). The acceptability of that information had much less to do with scientific validity than with perceived immediate credibility and relevance. Adoption of any new information required lots of different pieces of knowledge to be transformed and linked to others so that the members could reformulate them in ways that made sense to them. Personalized stories seemed easier to interpret and incorporate into their thinking than abstract concepts or research results.

- Second, we found that much of what went on in the meetings when the group members were processing new information was reminiscent of the organizational processes described in the SECI spiral (p. 100). The participants needed both to surface and communicate their existing implicit (tacit) knowledge, and also to combine and internalize (or discard) the new explicit information that they were getting from external sources or from each other. Judging new evidence for its relevance and its likely fit with local practices required each item of information to be subjected to one or more of a wide range of activities such as weaving it into the participants' personal experience and interests, linking it or building it into a story that helped make sense of it, or finding persuasive ways to discredit it.

- Third, the emergence of a shared view of elderly services and what needs to be done about them was reminiscent of the 'negotiated social order' suggested by Anselm Strauss and colleagues (Strauss 1978; Strauss *et al.* 1985), whose work suggested that people organize their social environment through negotiation, whether explicit or tacit. So, for example, people alter the social structures in which they exist through sharing ideas, exchanging views, bargaining, colluding, arguing or compromising, even though they may not consciously be engaged in what they might recognize as negotiation or even be aware of the results of that process. The original example was a group of psychiatric wards where the staff and patients 'negotiated' their roles and functions; although we also saw that happening at Haymarket and at Lawndale, we are here more concerned not so much with the negotiated construction of roles and functions but with that of concepts, meanings and mindlines.

- Fourth – and it is a feature of that 'negotiation' – the destiny of any item of information was contingent partly upon happenstance. Its fate would depend on such things as who happened to be at the meeting, how easy it was to make the item understandable and plausible to those present, or who commanded the greatest respect, credibility, and even sheer forcefulness, which would vary from discussion to discussion.

- Fifth, the outcome of the negotiation about the desirability and feasibility of putting any new information into action depended on the (often shifting) roles, agendas, power relationships and credibility of the people involved in the discussion (which were themselves being negotiated). This in turn had differential effects on the way the groups collectively made sense of the information available to them. In other words, the way in which the groups reacted to available information – including whether or not they accepted it as valid and useful knowledge – depended partly on the way its members negotiated more or less power and influence for themselves as the group evolved.

This last point in fact had a particular bearing in the case of the community of practice charged with reorganizing outpatient ENT services. Unlike the Haymarket groups, this one was very careful to seek out and review evidence such as national service frameworks, relevant research studies, a recent health technology assessment on audiology services, the available NICE guidance on hearing aids, the existing NHS policy directives and other evidence garnered by consulting colleagues and experts. This ENT group took such sources very seriously; they even on one occasion undertook a formal critical appraisal. This was the only one of the four groups that was acting approximately in the way that the evidence-based practice movement would wish them to. And why was that? The answer, it appeared, was that the two most influential clinicians in the group were meticulous adherents of such an approach, and their way of doing things held sway. Those who didn't like it gradually withdrew from the discussions or even from the group as a whole. This was perhaps why the group ended up somewhat smaller than the others and why, therefore, although much more 'evidence-based', it was rather less representative than the other three of the multi-sectoral views that the groups had been expected to include in their policy making. In contrast, the Haymarket communities of practice charged with improving the care of the elderly remained broadly multi-sectoral and strongly influenced by a pragmatic ethos that was sceptical of the 'dogma' of evidence-based practice. Yet the conclusions of their apparently chaotic knowledge management (Figure 7.2) almost exactly presaged two major national initiatives that recommended, just as the Haymarket groups did, an increase in intermediate care facilities and patient-held records. So one might conclude that however haphazard the processes appeared to be, the Haymarket groups' policy conclusions were not too far off the evidence-based mark.[5]

Many Lawndale discussions had exactly the same feel of the pragmatic, negotiated processes that we had seen in the Haymarket communities of practice meetings. This was certainly true of Lawndale's monthly evening (QPA, subsequently GP contract) practice meetings, but there were crucial differences: the Lawndale

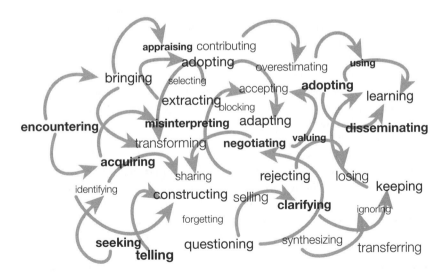

Figure 7.2   What the multi-sectoral, multidisciplinary communities of practice were doing with new evidence. Adapted from Gabbay *et al.* (2003) with permission from Sage Publications.

meetings consisted of people from a single organization, all of whom were health professionals or support staff, most of whom worked together day to day, who had an established (negotiated) hierarchy of expertise across different kinds of topics, and who already enjoyed relaxed relationships that eased efficient communication. Discussions were therefore more focused, better directed and crisper, more able to cover a lot of ground quickly, and hence more productive than at Haymarket. When the partners established these evening meetings, and (unusually for most primary care teams) opened them to all staff including nurses and receptionists, the medical partners, practice manager and more experienced nurses tended at first to dominate. Over the five years that we observed the meetings, though, the ethos of the doctors' coffee break discussions became established in the practice meetings and excellent, inclusive group dynamics emerged. One marker was the rapid and elliptical nature of much of the discussion; another was the increasingly easy humour at each other's expense, regardless of 'rank'; and a third was the growing participation of the non-clinicians. As a result, the meetings became a very effective forum for doctors, nurses, phlebotomist, receptionists and others, chaired usually by the practice manager, to all engage actively in discussions about the practice that were often swift even though they might be complex. Thus, for example, in the summer of 2006, the first discussion on the contractual require-ments about chronic kidney disease, with contributions from six of the seven GPs present, took less than half an hour, but already foreshadowed, in some detail, almost all of the concerns and conflicts that ran through the later debates on this topic, which were very wide-ranging, as we shall see in Chapter 8.

In exchanging and developing ideas on clinical policy most of the participants – especially the GPs and to a lesser extent the practice nurses – were continually exposing and filling gaps in their knowledge, usually by comparing, refining and readjusting not only the way they did their clinical work, but also the underlying logistics such as clinic arrangements and computer coding. Much of this relied on their individual mindlines. But they would also conduct 'reality checks' against actual case records on screen or against each other's clinical or logistical experi-ence. Sometimes too – though much less often, during the meetings at least – they would turn to copies of the literature or guidelines; more usually, though, they would rely on what they remembered of them as long as there was not too much dissent about the content. If there was, someone would usually volunteer to check it out before the next meeting.

At such meetings we were able to see how each participant both contributed the knowledge he or she already had about the subject under discussion and also drew from that of others (often externalized and surfaced through concrete patient-based examples, anecdotes and stories), to amend their own mindlines. They also brought varied skills and resources to the meeting. Each partner had the lead in a number of areas and would prepare for the meeting by checking up on best practice or contractual requirements (not always seen to coincide!) and on current Lawndale activity in that area as recorded in the computer system. The nurses (who all had their own 'lead areas'), phlebotomist and receptionists brought a wealth of knowledge about the locality and individual patients, as well as detailed knowledge of organizational processes including the variations in the ways that the GPs each practised and the administrative consequences. The participants brought other resources to the meetings too. Clive, for example, being on a number of local and national committees and hence epitomizing the value of 'cross boundary flow' between communities of practice, was the main source of knowledge about changing NHS requirements and resources. He tended often to have his laptop on with reference material (usually about the GP contract and QOF) to hand should it be needed, which was quite rarely, since someone there was usually thoroughly briefed about the QOF requirements. Jean would sometimes bring in the local hospital guidelines to help with the discussion and occasionally used them to back up a point she was making. She once won an argument about whether to use urinary dipsticks by saying she had looked it up earlier that day. The explosion of laughter and teasing that instantly defused the dispute conveyed how rarely the meeting referred explicitly to written sources. No one questioned the source, which we later learnt had been a set of hospital guidelines she had found on the internet. Yet, despite such examples of explicit reference to written guidance being very rare, as far as anyone could tell all the GPs seemed abreast of the main points of current best practice and were familiar enough with any guidelines under discussion to criticize them in some detail.

When Jean, for example, brought her draft protocol for heart failure (p. 33) to an early QPA meeting, no one questioned its scientific basis; rather they took its soundness for granted, confident, because they knew she was conscientious, that she had consulted trusted sources (the main one of which, the local hospital guideline, she had brought to the meeting to refer to if necessary). But they robustly debated her suggested protocol, a discussion that again betrayed the many conflicting roles that GPs play. They discussed – in a little over fifteen minutes – its practicability, the ways in which the practice team and computer system could assist or hinder the execution and recording of the new protocol, the acceptability of variations between it and their own varied routines, their own experience of patients, and the level at which the new protocol might improve remuneration as well as provide high-quality care.[6] None of these, of course, were matters that one could consult in the guidelines or literature, but they could be interpolated by sharing views, making comparisons with other well-regarded practices (either local or on the internet) that they had found out about and adding a range of other pieces of information from various other sources. Similarly when Barry – who unlike Jean had primarily used the internet rather than printed guidance to gather the information he needed for this exercise – presented his draft protocol for kidney disease at a later GP contract meeting (p. 153) his colleagues unquestioningly trusted him to have looked in detail in all the right places and summarized the key points appropriately in his draft practice policy, even though he had no special expertise in the topic. However, during the discussion of the kidney disease policy, whenever they felt he might be overzealous in espousing aspects of guidelines that they doubted (and they mostly gave the impression of being quite familiar with what his internet-based sources advocated) they quickly disabused him. He usually accepted any strongly asserted consensual view that a given proposal might be unrealistic. The resulting protocol that was being negotiated into existence was later very well adhered to (p. 156).

The features of the community of practice

In the next chapter we will delve into the depth and complexity that underpinned the negotiation of that apparently straightforward protocol for early renal failure. But since we shall be arguing that the way communities of practice construct collective knowledge in practice has important implications not only for evidence-based practice but for the nature of clinical knowledge, it behoves us first to explore the extent to which this group was actually functioning as a community of practice. There was no doubt that the group showed many of the features high-lighted by Wenger in his original discussion of communities of practice (Wenger 1998). The work of the Lawndale meetings was, as we have already noted, a social activity in which learning occurred as a result of what he calls 'mutual engage-ment' among the practice staff, who shared a clear understanding of the nature of their 'joint enterprise' with all its multiple conflicting complexities (be it the care of a patient, the smoothing of practice administration or the achievement of the QPA). The participants possessed a wide range of what Wenger would term 'shared repertoires' (their vocabulary, their clinical training, their computer rou-tines, their knowledge of the patients and the local services and so on). The group also demonstrated other features emphasized by Wenger: there was rapid and easy flow of information, often through stories. Through their interactions the partici-pants negotiated new shared meanings for the problems they were dealing with, which could entail what Wenger claims is the 'reification' of practice routines. This refers to the way in which artefacts not only arise from, but in some concrete way also actually represent, the things the group talks about. A tangible example might be pop-up computer screens (SOPHIEs) that remind the staff about the agreed protocols and the correct codes to enter into the system (Figure 2.2), but other examples included new staffing arrangements, new investigation routines or audits, practice guidance (Appendix 1) or simply changed thresholds for action. Such new entities, all of which came about as a result of the discussions, arguably formed concrete (reified) links between the discussions and actual practice. This may be why, as the examples in Figure 2.2 and Appendix 1 show, reifications such as practice guidelines and SOPHIEs tended to be much more practical and context-specific than any general guidelines that are available.

As befits the fact that the activities and discourse of communities of practice were first described in a book about the way people learn practical knowledge (Lave and Wenger 1991), we saw a great deal of learning happening during the discussions among the Lawndale practitioners. We also saw new members going through the stage of 'legitimate peripheral participation' that Lave and Wenger describe in that book, as they gradually adopted a more central role in the group. This applied to trainee clinicians (p. 83) but also to other participants such as receptionists and the phlebotomist, who over time became more involved with, and respected by, the clinicians. Like the others who took part in the discussions, they found themselves constantly learning and increasingly contributing what they could to the learning of others, developing their knowledge-in-practice-in-context, and adapting it to the challenges posed by the inexorable evolution of science, best practice, NHS organization and local circumstances, all of which meant that the mindlines required constant updating.

Learning, the *sine qua non* of communities of practice, was clearly happening at Lawndale. Is that enough, though, to allow us to say that the practitioners were functioning as a community of practice rather than simply as a management team or action learning group? Wenger, particularly in his later work, links the learning very closely to other functions of communities of practice, especially their role in helping participants establish *meaning* in what they do, and also their own *identity* in doing it (Wenger 1998). Did we see this in the Lawndale meetings? Indeed we did. As for *meaning*, the participants frequently found themselves having to negotiate what something meant in terms of their work at all levels. How should they interpret an unusual set of symptoms in a patient, the advice of a consultant, a controversial new piece of guidance, a newly reported side effect, or the place of a new drug, dressing or device? The discussions made it easier for them to understand in practice how to interpret such things and who should do what, when and how. As they swapped stories, experiences and information, through what Wenger calls their 'shared histories of learning', problems lost their initial opaqueness as solutions emerged. This unremitting need to clarify components of all aspects of their practice, deeply interlinked with their continuing need to evolve in order to remain competent, up-to-date clinicians, was a key feature of the discussions within their community of practice.

Under the rubric of *identity*, Wenger sets great store by the way in which communities of practice help their members to develop and reinforce a sense of who they are as individuals and how they fit into the context that they are learning about, and also help establish a clearer identity for the group as a whole. Certainly the group discussions, we observed, were helping the participants situate themselves and their work as competent practitioners in several ways (p. 165). When a doctor or nurse contributed to the work of the group, not only were they demonstrating their value to the enterprise (such as helping to ensure that the practice met its contractual requirement) but also they were reinforcing their roles as members of the organization and hence consolidating or improving their own professional positions. Their particular areas of expertise were confirmed (or challenged); their depth of knowledge was revealed and respected (or exposed and repaired); the degree of mutual trust and respect was renegotiated. It was notable, for example, that the salaried GPs who almost never made any contribution to the community of practice were later unsuccessful when applying for a partnership, whereas others who grew in stature through their sound contributions to the discussions and their obvious willingness and capacity to learn later became partners. Other participants such as the phlebotomist and one of the receptionists, both of whom often made incisive comments, grew in stature among the clinicians. Whether this was cause or effect (did they more readily join because they commanded respect or was that respect, and self-respect, growing as a result of their ability to contribute?) it was not possible to say. Probably both. Moreover, by helping to ensure that Lawndale maintained its reputation as one of the very best practices in the area, the active members of the community of practice also raised their personal professional standing among patients, health service managers, and colleagues beyond Lawndale – another aspect of their identity. Finally, at another level still, it was discussions among the community of practice that helped fortify and justify the clinicians' views about their right to decide for themselves how they will deal with patients, rather than be dictated to by the Department of Health or other outside influences. All of these outcomes from the discussions suggest that the participants' learning was indeed linked to the shaping of their identity.

We can be reasonably confident that Lawndale did, therefore, demonstrate the key general functions that Wenger has posited for learning, meaning and identity in communities of practice. But in addition to his rather philosophical considerations he and his later colleagues have also suggested some practical features, most of which it will by now be clear were also features of the Lawndale discussions (Box 7.1).

Le May's criteria for communities of practice in healthcare (Box 7.1), which draw on Wenger and on her own research (Lathlean and le May 2002; Gabbay *et al.* 2003; Gabbay and le May 2004, 2009) were also met. The *membership* criterion was demonstrated in the way that the nurses, phlebotomist, receptionists and less forceful GPs gradually came to contribute more and more of their different expertises as they became involved in achieving the group's goals of improving the general quality of clinical practice and achieving the RCGP awards, contractual rewards and attendant kudos. Lawndale's was what Klein *et al.* (2005) would classify as an egalitarian knowledge-nurturing community of practice, rather than a stratified (hierarchical) or explicitly knowledge-sharing one.[7] Growing *commitment* is especially effective when the members' aims are consonant with the pressures from outside the community, as was the case at Lawndale, where they shared a desire not only to fulfil but to surpass the RCGP's and the primary care trust's requirements. It goes without saying that communities of practice in Lawndale – be they the GPs, the broader group or the focused subgroups – all met the criterion of *relevance,* in this case to the needs of the groups' members, of the Lawndale practice as a whole and of its patients. The discussions were almost always very closely focused on the practical needs of the participants and/or the practice and patients, which – unlike, say, external educational meetings – might include the whole range of concerns stemming from their complex and multiple roles. The *enthusiasm* was clear from the increasing participation, energy and learning that we witnessed in the main meetings as well as the dynamism of most of the informal gatherings (which, incidentally, contrasted sharply with the cagey, uneasy silences that used to characterize the infrequent meetings of a somewhat dysfunctional practice that JG used to work in as a young GP locum). The necessary *infrastructure* was there, for example in terms of ease of access to knowledge or evidence such as library resources and information technology, particular experts and opinion leaders, or information brought from other groups to which the members belonged. Crucially, the community of practice also provided a ready source of relatively reliable opinion about the trustworthiness and relative value of those sources. Being so well networked was one of the many clinical, managerial and interpersonal *skills* of the participants, as were their specific skills in accessing and judging the relevant evidence to inform their discussions. Finally, the discussions we have

---

Box 7.1 **Features of a successful community of practice**

a (Wenger *et al.* 2002)
- Shared domain of knowledge
- A group that get on well, with clear roles and expertises
- A shared enterprise that uses the knowledge to progress in their domain – something they all care about, depend on and value (which makes it more than just a network)
- Different (and appropriate) levels of engagement with the group by different participants
- Interactions both within and (in subgroups or one-to-one discussions) outwith the full meetings of the group
- Evolving membership and task
- Bringing in ideas and new perspectives from outside the group
- A chance to air new and exciting ideas about practice and also to 'tame' and enliven the routine business of, for example, meeting the criteria of the RCGP and the GP contract
- A regularity and rhythm that helps to sustain it

b (le May 2009b)
- Attention to having the right kind of membership, which adapts as the group develops
- Growing commitment to the group's aims
- Relevance to local communities and existing services and groups
- Personal, professional and service enthusiasm
- The right infrastructure to support the work of the community of practice
- The right skills to work as a community of practice
- The right resources to achieve the changes resolved upon

---

described would also have most likely faltered if there had not been ready access to *resources* that enabled the practice to implement their decisions. The fact that the senior partners with Janet's unerringly efficient management could usually press quickly ahead with the organizational changes that arose from the discussions was a great motivator. Again this contrasts sharply with community of practices that we have studied or been a part of (including Haymarket) that have fallen apart because of their frustration and disillusionment with their own organizational impotence.

It should be clear by now that the interactions we observed at Lawndale were strongly suggestive of a fully functioning community of practice that achieved a great deal (Box 7.2). We can therefore now turn our attention to the next question: exactly how does a community of practice impact upon the way that clinical knowledge and, in particular, mindlines develop?

Box 7.2 General outcomes resulting from Lawndale's work following the introduction of the GP contract

1 Positioning of Lawndale as a practice achieving high quality and success
2 Reflection and analysis of practices resulting from the need to examine performance in terms of hitting agreed targets in the contract
3 Increased sharing of individual mindlines so that there was:
    • debate about clinical, administrative and managerial practice as a result of exposing individual mindlines
    • challenging of contract directives when there was a mismatch between the contract details and individual mindlines
    • betterment of the minimum standards laid down by the contract
    • multidisciplinary involvement and debate
4 Collective negotiation of 'practice mindlines' resulting in greater standardization of care within the practice through the exposure, debate and incorporation of individual mindlines (acknowledged as best practice)
5 Making 'collective mindlines' explicit through the alteration of systems for formally transferring knowledge, e.g. practice protocols (sometimes referred to as crib sheets on macros in the IT system) and SOPHIEs (new and existing) within the IT system
6 Alterations in the ways that the IT system was used – e.g. more use by nurses. Greater attention being given to some aspects of care than previously through centrally targeted practice (e.g. smoking cessation)

Chapter 7: Summary

Among the many sources of helpful information that clinicians rely on, trusted colleagues were paramount. Practitioners' personal networks of reliable experts were vital in helping them evaluate new information or situations that challenge their existing mindlines. Central to the way this occurred is the notion of 'communities of practice', groups of practitioners who share similar concerns, problems or passions about a topic and who learn from each other through their formal and informal interactions. Using data from several of our studies, we demonstrate how important this concept is in understanding the social processes by which knowledge is shared and used.

8   Co-constructing collective mindlines

How do clinicians collectively make sense of complex matters and agree collective mindlines? This chapter tries to make sense of that process.

❖   *Extract from interview with Jean: When developing your practice policy on coronary heart disease, did you have any 'official' guidelines? 'Right, probably no, probably not until really the NSF [national service framework] came out I would think, yeah I don't think we had any specific guidelines I mean I suppose probably what many of us have undoubtedly based things on has been following on from what the consultants do. I mean obviously we all read as well but I think in practical terms you tend to learn from what people come out of hospital on and what the local consultants are doing, I mean for instance although we're largely still being told that diabetics you know we should still be using charts and looking at them as primary prevention, I mean the local consultants particularly at [Westchurch] I don't think agree with that. So they generally are treating you know cholesterols that are above five in all of their Type 2s. So personally I think that's probably more what I'm doing to be honest.'*[1] *So in the absence of any official guidelines how did you as a GP and as a team of GPs agree on standard practice? 'Right I mean I would say as an individual first of all that I read the BMJ, RCGP journal and so on, which obviously has actually had various editorials and published the major papers to do with coronary heart disease prevention, so I was obviously aware of it in that respect, but again as I say actually seeing what the hospitals do with the patients that I see, so for me it's both of those things that would really give me guidelines as to what I should be doing, if you see what I mean. As a partnership I suppose that has been a little bit more muddled until the NSF came out, though our nurses have certainly been involved with following up, you know, patients with heart attacks afterwards and we'd agreed to do that. Now I couldn't tell you really where the guideline came from for that [. . .] We also have to, had to do audits for that and certainly coronary heart disease formed quite a large proportion of the audits that we did for that, so that probably, I suppose actually that [audits for coronary heart disease] probably is partly what sparked quite a lot of the practice change to be honest, yes it probably is. Sorry, as I say it's sometimes quite difficult when things evolve to remember what order and I expect if you talk to somebody else they'd say something completely different.'*

❖ *At a taped clinical meeting to review policy on heart disease the Lawndale clinicians are trying to agree on an improvement in their health promotion:*

Clive: So, would you be suggesting that when they come for a well person check that they have all the normal bits done and then we use the Sheffield tables to estimate their risk and decide?

Jean: That's basically what we do.

Clive: But you don't do cholesterols, do you?

Jean: Sometimes. And I think that's what we ought to coordinate into a policy.

Nick: Exactly. But when do you choose to do it?

Jean: If there are two risk factors?

Nick: But you should actually be looking at percentage risk.

Jean: Yes, but if you look at the tables it is actually fairly clear that most men do not need a particularly high cholesterol over the age of about fifty to put them into a high-risk category. So you could actually decide an arbitrary age cut-off for most men.

Nick: But then you should go further and we should then be explaining to them and saying 'do you want it done?'

Jean: Absolutely.

Nick: Because if you have it done, A, B and C may follow, and if they don't want B or C then I don't think we should be doing cholesterols.

Jean: Of course it should be explained to them.

Angela: But the majority of people you are talking about are asking to have it done anyway.

Nick: Yes, but those are the ones who don't need it.

Peter: Yes, and the intervention may not be a statin. It may be dietary. I know which I would choose.

Jean: Interesting, because I would choose a statin if I was in that . . .

Nick: But that just goes to show the dichotomy.

❖ *At a GP contract meeting, this time about congestive heart failure (CHF), the debate is drawing upon what they know about best treatments. The doctors are chipping in about the ways they treat CHF, giving some justification that draws on preferred expert opinion and practices with the addition of 'evidence' sources (mostly local consultants' views, which differ) to back the figures. There is reference to some (disputed) guidelines and to a 'useful' BMJ Learning Module. They begin to worry that they may be differing in their actual practice so they agree to audit their treatment of heart failure. (This subsequently showed they were performing well according to their agreed policy.)*

❖ *Verbatim (edited) field note extract from GP contract meeting: [Time] = 7:28. Janet [Practice manager:] 'We talked last time about identifying pathology from [hospital] letters and entering it [into the computer system]. Are we doing it?' Her smile shows that she clearly knows they are not and the doctors sheepishly admit that, well, perhaps they are not being very systematic. They are using humour and good-natured mutual prodding to get each other to conform. Peter admits he – like the others – has been slow to record some things and tries to explain it away. He ends up laughingly saying 'I'd better stop digging [myself into a hole] hadn't I?' He's teased for it and joins in the fun, as if contributing to the process of prodding himself to do something that has so far not been part of his routine. Nick smiles and says 'It's up to the lead in that specialty to check and kick shins.' For example if there has been a hysterectomy for cancer, they must ensure it's recorded as 'Ca. uterus', not 'Hysterectomy' or else the SOPHIEs for cancer care won't come up on screen when the patient is next seen. Angela, the practice nurse who mainly deals with cervical smears, says it would help a lot from the point of view of taking smears if the patients were correctly recorded on the system. Nick explains that this can be done using a 'filter', and Tony agrees, adding that it would simplify things if she did use one. 'Perhaps, Tony,' says Janet pointedly, 'you should show Angela how!' They all laugh and the discussion moves on. [Time] = 7.35. It seems that a clear learning need has been identified here but no one appears to follow up or teach. Why not? [End of field note extract.]*

In fact this last question noted by the researcher was misplaced. At the meeting the following month, Angela was knowledgeably engaged in a discussion about whether to use the 'filter' before or after letters are printed. Tony – or someone – presumably had heeded Janet's suggestion.

❖ *Clive is reflecting to us that he tends to be at 'the liberal end' of antibiotic prescribing among the partners. They are all aware of each other's propensities. He tells a story (based on a published study of tonsillitis treatment) of a practice where the partners all made a concerted effort to try and conform more, and for a while their prescribing habits did converge. However, a year later an audit, he says, showed 'they had all reverted to type'. (An interesting contrast with Urbcester where the GPs did seem much more forcefully to restrict their antibiotic prescribing.)*

❖ *Clive tells me they have developed good enough relationships for him, as the current practice lead on diabetes, to have noticed that [one of the partners] had done some odd things with one or two diabetic patients and he had gone to chat to him to find out why he had done that. After a discussion of all the ramifications, the partner had been completely accepting of Clive's concerns and had changed the prescription as a result.*

❖ *During a QPA discussion about the need for spirometry to confirm chronic obstructive airways disease a great deal of knowledge sharing and educating goes on as doctors explain the process to receptionists, nurses point out difficulties, the practice manager laments the way computer pop-up reminders are not working, receptionists point out difficulties in using patients' birthdays to call them in for checks. Everyone has some frustrations, something to learn and something to add. 'It takes time! You need to make sure that spirometry appointments are half an hour apart', says Rose, 'and the receptionists don't know that.' 'Then the doctor should instruct the receptionist', chorus Janet and Clive. 'But the trouble is that the doctors don't know that either!' quips Jean and the meeting dissolves into gales of laughter. At the next review, the system for spirometry has, they agree, been much improved.*

Collective mindlines

Much of the discussion that took place about work appeared to contribute to 'collective mindlines' against which the clinicians could check their own individual mindlines – the collective and the individual mindlines reciprocally influencing each other. In that sense at least, the communities of practice were palpably shaping the knowledge used by the clinicians. Not only the explicit correctives about diabetes management or cancer coding, but also the debates about the best management plan for patients with congestive heart failure, the stories told over coffee about recent patients or past near misses, the questioning of an unexpected piece of guidance – all such discussions allowed the communities of practice both to nurture each other's knowledge and to corroborate their views on the best way to practice. This entailed checking and revising individual mindlines when they were out of line and also, if there appeared to be agreement on a sensible modification, altering the collective mindline. As long as the practitioners then kept within the evolving consensual boundaries of that collective view (which sometimes, as with Clive and the off-beam diabetic care, they had not) they could vary in the way they interpreted their own mindlines and implement them flexibly with different patients. Collective mindlines were therefore being implicitly discussed and jointly understood by the whole group, which could result in the norms of appropriate practice being reinforced or, as we shall show below, modified. Thus although collective mindlines were only virtual (and indeed, as we shall ultimately argue, not entities but *processes*) they could manifest themselves through tangible entities that guided practice, for example computerized prompts (SOPHIEs), instructions to staff, set procedures such as investigation routines, and of course alterations in individual clinical practice and its outcomes.[2]

Like individual mindlines, collective mindlines are complex, flexible, context-specific ways of guiding practice that are formed from a mixture of sources melded by time and experience and which are not (and probably could never be, p. 169) made explicit in the form of a comprehensive written guideline. Indeed only certain aspects of the collective mindline are ever discussed. The rest, which are uncontroversial and/or deeply ingrained in each individual's mindline, appear to be taken as read. (There is no need to discuss whether to check blood pressure regularly in a hypertensive patient, but there may be discussion about how often the check should be made and by whom and how to ensure that the record is entered correctly in the computer system, and what departures from the norm are within acceptable limits.) What gets discussed depends on what arises as a concern. For example, the small adjustment to the entering of pathology reports that Janet was reinforcing in the collective mindline that Peter was having trouble with was not a matter of clinical care, but a simple administrative task that, if it became part of how they handled cancer patients, had the potential to improve the quality of care, trigger tertiary prevention of cancer, increase practice income and reduce the unnecessary workload for colleagues. Similarly, in the subsequent discussions on heart disease, the focus was not only on when to do cholesterol tests, but also on how best to fill in the forms, what code to enter and why, and how that leads to different administration with benefits, or not, to the patient and the practice. All of this and more (related to the clinicians' many roles and goals, p. 38) was part of the collective mindline being embedded and reinforced.[3]

One function of both collective mindlines and the processes that go towards their production and maintenance is to act as a repository to call upon when one needs help in recalling aspects of one's own mindline. Memory relies on external as well as internal acts of remembering, and, although these include prompts and formal sources both written and electronic, one's colleagues are also a key repository of useful knowledge. As Engeström and colleagues suggest, 'what would be more natural than to ask your nearest co-worker when you do not remember something?' In modern forms of remembering, they point out, inanimate objects seem to have gained the central mediating role, but other human beings are still there as a special kind of 'external memory aid' (Engeström *et al.* 1990: 144). Moreover, as we have shown, a colleague who understands the complexities of your knowledge-in-practice-in-context is much more likely to provide a more helpful (if not necessarily more scientifically accurate) answer than formal sources. The accuracy is increased if you are calling not just on another individual's mindline, but on a communal resource that acts as what Orr has called a 'collective memory' (Orr 1997). Thus, among the Xerox technicians that he studied, he found that, apart from instances of personal animosity or deliberate exclusion, 'there appears to be every incentive to share information and none to keep it private' (ibid.: 174). We saw in Chapter 6 that the main currency for such information sharing – among Orr's technicians as among the Lawndale clinicians – was storytelling, one of whose functions was to reinforce their identity as members of the group that shares the collective knowledge (p. 143). As Orr concludes, 'their stories celebrate this identity to themselves and to others, while creating another part of the identity: member of the community, contributor to the community memory' (ibid.: 187). By sharing their detailed practical knowledge, they were also building and reinforcing the way they and others saw them as a particular kind of practitioner.

Telling stories and comparing notes allowed the practitioners to develop and share their collective mindlines because the process also, to use the vocabulary of the SECI spiral, helped them to externalize their tacit and implicit knowledge (Chapter 5). Through chatting with each other about their work, they exposed their knowledge-in-practice-in-context and their views about what they had gleaned from their reading and other sources. These glimpses of each other's mindlines could then be combined with what they already knew and with all the other relevant sources of knowledge. Thus their individual mindlines both contributed to the collective mindline and were modified by it when they internalized the new consensus. This collective mindline was also an agreement to try and conform; it placed boundaries around what the community of practice considered to be acceptable practice. Naturally each clinician tended to vary it a little, to revert at least partly to his or her individual mindline and also to implement it flexibly depending on the circumstances. Plasticity within boundaries is, after all, a key feature of mindlines that always leaves room for the individual to use 'common sense'. Yet the very commonality of that sense – the overlapping and mutual moulding of the individual and collective mindlines – is incessantly being checked and validated by the social processes and reciprocal learning that we have described.

The challenge of chronic kidney disease: QOF vs quality?

The learning process was often triggered by challenges to an individual's mindlines from an unexpected experience. This might entail, say, a case that didn't fit the norm, hearing or reading about new developments in practice such as new drugs or devices, or realizing as one heard the others discussing cases that one was out of line with the collective mindline – as in the prologue examples. The outcome of such discussions, via the processes of the SECI spiral, might be a 'negotiated' modification of individual mindlines or collective mindlines or both. Sometimes, though, the challenge was directly to the collective mindline because it came not from the differences between the ways individual colleagues were practising, but from an external source that forced *all* of them to rethink a mindline. One particular example, which we will explore in some detail here since it provides a useful base from which to explore the features of collective mindlines,[4] was a set of requirements about the management of early chronic kidney disease that the Department of Health unexpectedly and controversially introduced into the GP contract and hence to the Quality and Outcomes Framework Indicator Set in 2005 (Box 8.1).

The Department of Health's stated rationales for adding CKD were first its high prevalence – claimed to be up to 10 per cent of the population – and second the recent elaboration of a pragmatically useful way of describing five stages of increasingly severe renal failure based on an eGFR (estimated glomerular filtration rate), which may be calculated from the serum creatinine (Department of Health 2006). The new GP contract documentation supported both of these rationales

---

Box 8.1 Quality and Outcomes Framework for chronic kidney disease

To obtain the maximum points and hence full remuneration for managing CKD the QOF required practices to show that:

1 they could produce a register of all their adult patients with Stages 3–5 of CKD (i.e. with an estimated glomerular filtration rate [eGFR] of $< 60\text{ml}/\text{min}/1.73\text{m}^2$): this was worth 6 points;

2 > 90 per cent of the patients on that register had a record of their blood pressure in the preceding fifteen months (6 points);

3 for > 70 per cent of those patients, their last recorded blood pressure was 140/85 or less (11 points);

4 80 per cent of patients who were on the CKD register and also had hypertension were being treated with either an ACE inhibitor or an angiotensin receptor blocker, or there was a record of a good reason why not (4 points).

Source: Department of Health (2006).

with key references from the American literature (Coresh *et al.* 2005; John *et al.* 2004) but also referred to the NHS National Service Framework for Renal Services, which the Department of Health had published in February 2005 (Department of Health 2005) and which in turn referred to the then still unpublished guidelines from the UK's Renal Association and Royal College of Physicians Joint Specialty Committee on Renal Disease (Joint Specialty Committee 2006). These sources all stressed that, although chronic kidney disease is important in its own right, it both shares and contributes to the risk factors of other QOF domains in the new contract, notably hypertension, diabetes and cardiovascular disease, to which it is closely related.

During the first practice meeting at Lawndale where CKD was discussed, the doctors revealed, amid sheepish laughter, enough gaps in the detail of their collective knowledge (ranging from 'What exactly is the cut-off point for Stage 3 CKD, and why?' to 'What's the likely local prevalence?' to 'Why can't I carry on using the GFR formula that I already use?') to realize that they would not be well placed to make any changes to policy without updating their knowledge, so they agreed that Barry should take the 'CKD lead' by drafting a protocol for next time. At the next meeting the results of his search of local and national guidelines, the NSF, simple web searches and reliable websites aimed at GPs, some of which were recommended by email discussion groups or magazine articles that colleagues had passed on to him, generated considerable discussion (see also p. 141).

His colleagues criticized much of the guidance because they perceived it to be failing to relate to 'the real world'. This perception seemed to link to the lack of practical know-how betrayed in guidance. As we have seen in Chapters 5–7 the most common currency during the exchanges of information at this meeting was geared towards telling or showing each other hands-on knowledge of practices or contexts, for example stories of how they have dealt with problems, demonstrations of how they find and code events on the computer system (and improve data accuracy in so doing) or a review of their methods for ensuring that patients are dealt with by the right person at the right time. The GP contract, like clinical guidelines and educational events, dealt almost exclusively with the GPs' *clinical* role, plus small allusions to the public health and (usually implicit) cost-effectiveness roles: it therefore did not fit easily with their normal discourse that continually blended all their roles (Chapter 2). Not only was most of the content already familiar (or, as we have seen in Chapter 5 and 7, capable of being quickly checked and refreshed) but such sources gave almost no guidance about the concerns actually troubling the GPs. For example (see also p. 104), what adverse impact would the recommended investigations have on the workload of the local specialist services? How much distress would be caused to patients with marginally low eGFRs by being suddenly labelled as having kidney failure? And anyway, just how relevant was a US-derived eGFR formula to a local elderly population? (See Clase 2006.)

Following the first CKD-related GP contract meeting, a local educational session with a nephrologist revealed that GPs from other practices had similar concerns (and not just locally, see, for example, Spence 2006). But, as we described on p. 104, the beleaguered nephrologist was incapable of answering them, largely because she had been unable to take sufficient account of the conflicting roles the GPs must play in order to run a primary care service. If the knowledge she was conveying to them was to be useful, it needed literally to be fit for practice: to fit with their own experiences, needs and practical day-to-day concerns. Clearly it was not.

In contrast, the discussions between the Lawndale practitioners, which slipped seamlessly between the many domains, roles and goals of their work, were part of the continual networking, exchange and refinement of their knowledge-in-practice-in-context. This enabled their multiple roles to shape the very content of the clinical knowledge they were discussing. Take the vexed question of deciding when to label someone as having a level of CKD 3 and hence in need of being clinically followed up and managed. Table 8.1 illustrates how statements drawing on the assumptions underlying different roles affected the threshold. The GP contract, like the National Service Framework and most national guidelines, was unambiguous that anyone with Stage 3 CKD – an eGFR of 60 or less – should be investigated and followed up. But, for the GPs, the questionable validity and consequences of pursuing that line led to a tussle over what the actual threshold should be. As the meetings progressed, we saw the clinicians continually clarifying, comparing, balancing and reformulating who and what would count as a case of renal failure. In short they were negotiating[5] their own individual and collective norms of practice alongside those advocated by central guidance. As a result they arrived at a general understanding on how to alter the way they managed the condition, while leaving sufficient flexibility to allow for individual judgement within acceptable (if imprecise and implicit) bounds. The statements in Table 8.1 précis some of the arguments deployed for raising or lowering the threshold for Stage 3 CKD, and each statement can be seen as rooted mainly in one of the four groups of roles that we discussed in Chapter 2.

The outcome was nothing as simple as a single threshold, nor even an explicit decision pathway. There emerged a written CKD policy – but what really counted was a collective mindline that continued to evolve. Some of the partners when asked later didn't even know where to find the CKD policy document on the system (Appendix 2), perhaps because it barely scratched the surface of the actual decision making, for example around the difficult question of when to 'exempt' a patient from the CKD 3 category. They knew the outcomes of the discussions, though, the collective mindline. And it mattered to patients: depending on the balance of forces in its formulation, hundreds of local people would either be identified, labelled and managed as having Stage 3 CKD or not. In that sense, the organizational contingencies of practice were shaping the very existence of Stage 3 CKD,[6] a point to which we shall return later.

Three months after the third meeting, at which a CKD policy had been agreed, the CKD statistics came up as part of a general review of progress towards achieving Lawndale's contractual requirements (Box 8.1). They showed that 100 per cent of patients with Stage 3 CKD had met those requirements – an excellent result from the managerial perspective of maximizing income from the contract. However, Barry, who was still leading on CKD, reflected that they had been careful

Table 8.1 A précis of some of the arguments in the Lawndale GMS contract meetings for raising or lowering the threshold for defining Stage 3 CKD

Domain of practitioner as clinician	Domain of practitioner as manager	Domain of practitioner as health promoter/disease preventer	Domain of practitioner as guardian of professional standing
Arguments for excluding most patients whose eGFR technically indicates Stage 3 CKD			
We are already giving the right care to most CKD patients because of the good follow-up on their related illnesses.	It won't be practicable to carry out all the required new tests.	'We have only had one death from CKD in the last 10 years!' so this isn't a priority.	The guidance takes little note of the realities of primary care practice (e.g. there has been no GP consultation over local guidelines).
Results of routine screening will unnecessarily alarm patients.	We need to avoid unnecessary workload – both within practice and elsewhere (e.g. the laboratory service and hospital nephrologists).	It's generally agreed that the US basis of eGFR makes it unhelpful for an elderly UK population. Low scores in Stage 3 are especially dubious. So why comply?	
	Results of routine screening will overburden resources with little or no resulting health improvement.		
Arguments for including most patients whose eGFR technically indicates Stage 3 CKD			
We fail patients with high creatinines in ways that aren't even mentioned in the QOF and in other guidelines (e.g. medicines management). So let's focus on those, not just QOF items. (*Also an argument for refashioning the QOF criteria*)	With training we can find ways within the rules to recode patients with eGFRs of 30–59.	Our CKD prevalence seems comparatively low – we may be missing too many renal patients.	We will become better at generally managing patients with renal disease if we take this seriously. It is our duty to do so.
Maybe we currently fail to identify renal patients who therefore miss out on important follow-up care.	Ensuring that we identify and register all renal patients will secure QOF points and payments.		

to exclude a lot of patients and that the real prevalence 'may be higher' than the figures suggested. 'And we wanted to do this for the patients, not the money', he said. Jean expressed similar concerns, because from a clinical and public health perspective they might well be underestimating the real prevalence by excluding patients whose CKD should be better managed.[7] She was, though, partly reassured by Clive, who through contacts within his wide national networks knew that – despite all the exclusions – Lawndale's prevalence rates were in fact slightly *higher* (i.e. they were excluding fewer patients) than national QOF figures about to be published. So the discussion – now in September 2006, six months after the first contract meeting about CKD – reverted to a negotiation of details about whom to screen, when and how, and what codes to use in what circumstances. It was a continuation of the same role-related tensions that had all along shaped the way in which the clinicians were refashioning and refining their collective and individual views on how to define, identify and manage renal disease.

By April 2007, national comparative data issued by the NHS Quality Management and Analysis System showed that Lawndale's resultant prevalence of just under 3 per cent for eGFR levels 3–5 was indeed in line with other practices around the country. Although much lower than the 5–10 per cent prevalence predicted in the contract documentation, Lawndale's figure was actually one-third higher than the national prevalence figure of 2.24 per cent.[8] In other words, practices throughout the country were, as Clive had already hinted, excluding possible CKD patients even more frequently than Lawndale was, which suggests that the processes we had observed were being replicated and the thresholds for renal disease were being similarly negotiated and renegotiated throughout the country.[9]

The influence of such collective decisions on actual individual practice varied. We were not able to research this directly, since we did not have the chance to see how the doctors dealt with early chronic kidney disease in individual patients. But Barry, who was by now taking the lead on diabetes as well as renal disease and hence had the responsibility for monitoring practice in both, found that his colleagues were all conforming remarkably well to their agreed management plan for CKD. He told us that this contrasted with diabetes, for which it had been difficult to avoid a lot of variance. Perhaps, he volunteered during a taped interview, this was because 'targets have changed so much over recent years with diabetes that there's quite a difference between the different aged GPs and what they've been used to in the past. But since this [approach to CKD] is new we all started off at the same level.' In other words, as Clive also later volunteered, because practitioners had trained at different times during the evolution of diabetic practice there was, as a result, much more choice and accepted variation in the way they could approach diabetic patients than there was for CKD.

In our terms, this was a facet of the variable relationship between individual and collective mindlines. It had been comparatively easy to forge a collective mindline of what they saw as a relatively rare condition whose treatment had not changed very much over the years and where there was not much pre-existing variation in individual mindlines. For a common disease, however, that over time had evolved quite markedly in its definition and complex management regimes, each doctor was coming to the discussion with a different mindline built up over a different period. In such a case, one would expect any collective mindline to have relatively limited overlap with each GP's individual one; such a mindline would therefore have to be looser because of the ingrained strength of the differing mindlines that the GPs had grown over their asynchronous professional careers. In effect, in such a situation, the GPs had allowed looser boundaries around acceptable practice or, put another way, had agreed to disagree about some of the details in the collective mindline. Nevertheless, those boundaries were there and, if they were transgressed, then it was understood that the transgressor could be pulled into line, as we saw in the prologue.

Collective sensemaking

❖   *Mrs Astupile, who came into Oakville hospital as an emergency just before midnight, is a continuing mystery. Chrissie takes a long history; so do Craig and Surinder. Faints, chills, night sweats, pains . . . By 1.30 a.m. they have ordered 'a bunch of labs' while they ponder and look things up on a range of different websites. It just makes no sense. 'She's hypotensive so she needs all the help she can get. Normally a haemoglobin of 9.5 wouldn't bother me but I'm gonna order guaiac stools', says Chrissie as she writes up Mrs Astupile's eighteen(!) sets of drugs and her investigations. At 2.15 she has another thought: 'With yeast in her urine I'm gonna get blood cultures also. She's so weird. Jeez I don't even know what the question is!' They discuss her intermittently throughout the night as more results come in and as their online researches find more possible ideas that fit the picture. They swing from one possible diagnosis to another but as the night wears on Mrs Astupile seems to settle and so do their differential diagnoses. By the time they present Mrs Astupile to Josh around 8 a.m., she's become once again a very clear story of orthostatic hypotension with a mild urinary infection and a lot of those extra investigations that seemed so important during the night now begin to look a tad over the top. 'You gotta have the midrodrine', Josh says to her. 'Yup I'm listenin to ya!' replies Mrs Astupile, smiling, and she goes home that afternoon.*

❖   *At a Lawndale 'critical incident meeting' the GPs are discussing a case of community-acquired pneumonia that has given rise to a complaint about a late referral to hospital. Jean mentions some guidelines that substantiate her robust defence of the actions that one of the partners took. A few minutes later when Peter asks her what those guidelines are she replies that they are from the British Thoracic Society (BTS) and impressively reels off several of the things they stipulate, even down to the detail of the exact threshold of oxygen saturation (<92 per cent, she says) at which one should refer the patient to hospital. She mentions that this is part of a range of criteria that give the patient a score (which I later learn is the 'CURB-65 score') that helps to decide the seriousness of the case. 'Oh yes I think I vaguely remember them now you mention it', nods Peter. Others agree and add some further points. All are relieved that the partners involved in the case had apparently acted exactly as required by the guidelines – although I don't recall anyone else mentioning the CURB-65 score. I ask Jean later how come she knew the BTS guidelines so well when the others (who had acted in* *line with them but didn't specifically seem to recall them) did not. 'I made a point of looking them up when we got our pulse oximeter', she says.*

I later look up the BTS guidelines (all forty-four difficult-to-navigate pages of them) and, although in principle Jean may have been correct, as far as I can tell the oxygen saturation figure (of <90 per cent) refers to the threshold for discharge from hospital. The indication for admission to hospital is the CURB-65 scores that Jean had alluded to, but which does not include oxygen saturation. I can find no reference to an admission threshold for oxygen, which is what the GPs actually needed to know here. Yet they had, it seems, for all practical purposes correctly interpolated it and do certainly seem to have handled this case of pneumonia logically and correctly.

❖ *At a GP contract meeting about the management of coronary heart disease, they are discussing a proposed protocol dealing with CHD prevention, which states that the practice nurse should refer to the GP anyone with a cholesterol of >5 mmol/l or if they are not on a statin without good reason. 'So what do we do', asks one of the GPs, 'if it's 5.1?' 'Or 5.7?' Most of the doctors chip in here animatedly with a flurry of slightly varying cholesterol levels and dosages of various drugs that they routinely work to. Each seems to be reeling off their mindlines and justifying them. No one seems way out of line. The researcher's field note reads: 'Some checking and comparing. All done in a minute or two. No quoting of evidence. I can't begin to keep up. Blimey, this time I wish I'd had a tape recorder!'*

❖ *Following a review of prescribing carried out by a nurse specialist from the primary care trust, the GP contract meeting focuses on a medicines review of non-steroidal anti-inflammatory drugs (NSAIDs). Clive says he's stopped using Cox 2 inhibitors. 'We're still using meloxicam', says Peter. 'There seems to be a swing against them', comes the reply. During a two-minute rapid-fire discussion they speak about the pros and cons of various NSAIDs, especially Cox 2 inhibitors, in short sharp phrases that no one who doesn't already know the issues would have been able to follow, and which finishes with 'But it is gastro-protective!' and the riposte: 'Hmmphh – at forty times the cost!' The next question is whether they should regard these as 'drugs of limited clinical value' (which the PCT is contractually requiring them to review), given that the PCT's analysis suggests they use them too freely. Tony questions the analysis. Clive calls it 'cobblers'. Nick is more conciliatory; beginning with, 'It's not bad clinical practice and it's not a lot of money', he gives a reasoned, balanced and fairly detailed review of the analysis. 'We all have our favourites', he concludes. The others chip in with a number of reasons why the use of these NSAIDs is justified, despite the official line that they are of limited value: 'There are plenty of studies out here that show they work.' 'It's better to prescribe some of these not because they have a pharmacological effect but because of their placebo effect or because they reduce the use of more worrying NSAIDs.' As the conversation draws to a close Jean jokes, 'Oh dear, after this discussion I feel guilty about using them. But I'll still prescribe them.' 'Well I don't feel guilty!' answers Clive, 'maybe we should feed this back to the PCT, who don't seem to take any of this into account.' They agree to restrict themselves to a smaller group of NSAIDs and then to adjust that list in the light of patient experience. They move onto another, similar five-minute debate about drugs for Alzheimer's disease.*

When something occurs that suggests they need to amend their mindlines – be it an unusual experience or a new scientific development, a minor tweak or a radical challenge[10] – clinicians have to try and make sense of that new information before they decide what to do. Karl Weick (1995, 2001), whose work has pioneered over the past twenty years the understanding of collective 'sensemaking' in organizations, highlights the way in which such sensemaking is anything but a linear and rational process, but is inherently a complicated social, multidimensional and often retrospective process.[11] Sensemaking, he argues, always involves an anomalous new perception that does not fit the usual picture, but it is often also triggered by uncertainty and ambiguity due to information overload, complexity, and the urgent need for decisions and action.[12] People do not gather all the information, weigh it up and then arrive at a judgement. If anything, Weick suggests, they decide first and cogitate afterwards, often by fitting the phenomena into a new or modified narrative (p. 116) that helps it to make sense. As he is fond of saying, 'How can I know what I think until I hear what I say?' – or indeed see what I do. A classic example is the detailed study that Harold Garfinkel made of the way jurors arrived at their verdicts in a US courtroom; he found that they reached rapid conclusions, which they then retrospectively justified by weaving selected elements of the case into a story that made sense to them (Garfinkel 1967). Similarly, when a patient and a doctor are together trying to make sense of a set of symptoms, they may reach a conclusion and then fashion a story that fits the selected features that fit their conclusion. ('My rash must be an allergy', the patient concludes [p. 121] and then looks for the culprit, a new shower gel, and ignores the fact that her allergic skin reactions have never looked like this one before.)

Such processes of retrospective reattribution of meaning never end; no sooner have we justified an action or dealt with a challenge to our usual frameworks, than another hits us. ('But what about these strange new hot flushes and now the sharp pains in the legs? Maybe, just maybe, the rash is more than a simple allergy', thinks the patient, and decides to go to the doctor.) Making sense of new perceptions is based on a continuously

> rolling hindsight. It is a continual weaving of sense from beliefs, from implicit assumptions, from tales from the past, from unspoken premises for decision and action, and from ideas of what will happen as a result of what can be done.
>
> (Pugh and Hickson 1996: 118)

We allocate meaning to our actions and our environments by continually reconstructing the narrative, retelling the story to ourselves and to others, so as to substantiate, validate and reconstruct our worldview. ('It was only later that I read on the web that sharp leg pains are a recognized symptom of meningitis', the patient would subsequently say once the diagnosis of meningitis had made sense of all the symptoms – rash, hot flushes, leg pains – and she was retelling the now very coherent cautionary tale to friends.)

Sensemaking entails arriving at a particular decision, say, to consult the doctor with this strange set of symptoms, or to refuse to follow up patients with an eGFR of 59, or to begin using glitazones for patients with diabetes, and this in turn entails forgoing the attractions and advantages of whatever we have chosen not to do. The discomfort that we may then feel if we cannot justify our judgment is due partly to 'cognitive dissonance' with what we feel we perhaps should have done. Thus a GP faced with children's nasty sore throats that seem to demand greater generosity with antibiotics than the guidelines advise will tend to 'increase the number of cognitive elements that are consistent with the decision' (Weick 1995: 12). So she selectively perceives the things that fit with the decision to prescribe, and ignores those that do not. She tells herself that she can often detect early signs of exudate, or that the children only come back a few days later if they withhold the antibiotics, and ignores the research evidence that says patients who are given antibiotics, even though they have no discernible curative effect, are more likely to come back expecting them every time they have a (viral) sore throat (Little *et al*. 1997). Such views can also be reinforced when the collective mindline is being aired, as in the dialogue about NSAIDs, when their initial stated heterodox views ('Cobblers!', 'It's not bad clinical practice') led to their justifying an ostensibly reasoned refutation of the PCT auditor's conclusions. Weick presents evidence to suggest that, once a conclusion is reached, most of the cognitive effort goes into justifying rather than testing why it made sense that way.

It is part of all social interaction to be held accountable for what one does, and people therefore learn to know what others would expect of them. Their decisions must look good not just to themselves but also to their interlocutors, be they real or virtual. The silent conversations in their heads with imagined judges 'may become the mirror in front of which individuals primp, evaluate, and adjust the self that acts, interprets, and becomes committed' (Weick 1995: 21). This tendency, which he calls the 'social construction of justification', is an important aspect of sensemaking; people's sensemaking is to a large extent shaped by what they believe their networks of peers might think is appropriate. (What will the patient think of me? Would my trainer have approved? How will I explain this to my partners/the PCT?) In short, people often make decisions based on the perceived majority view – or the collective mindline – and then retrospectively select out and reconstruct the facts to fit the decision, thus reducing any cognitive dissonance. For the clinicians we observed, this was especially true if they thought that colleagues and teachers whom they respected might disapprove. Hence in the collective discussion on NSAIDs, where the same principle applied, they needed to justify themselves to their patients but also to the authorities ('Maybe we should feed [our explanation] back to the PCT . . .').

In the rapid-fire discussions on CKD, most of the GPs had already seen patients whose eGFRs were close to the threshold and had already acted either in accord-ance with the new requirements or – much more often – not. They each seemed therefore to come to the discussion about how to deal with this challenge to their practice with a mindset based on those earlier decisions, which they believed to have been justified. The collective sensemaking at the practice meetings was ret-rospective in the sense that they often appeared to be looking back on how they had instinctively responded, and explaining to themselves and to each other why they had done so. One could see the discussion around the table as partly a way of rationalizing (sometimes quite explicitly as patient records were pulled up on the screen and discussed) why those actions had indeed made perfectly good sense despite the new guidance. Weick would argue that this had been more likely to happen because the group was able to have a high opinion of the quality of its work. This gave them more confidence to reinforce their feelings of self-efficacy than might have been the case had they been called upon to change practice that they knew to be substandard. If they had suspected their performance was poor, the retrospective sensemaking might have veered more towards a change of practice rather than a justification of the status quo. For example, Lawndale's robust response to the new information about renal disease contrasted with the situation back in the late 1980s when, we were told, in response to rising pressure to audit one's care, coupled with a wave of new guidance about best practice in diabetes, Jean had audited Lawndale's diabetes care. The poor results had shocked them all and had led not to retrospective justification but to immediate action and improvement, and a much greater willingness to learn and continue learning about the best ways to manage diabetics.

On the one hand collective sensemaking can be a useful check that becomes part of a justifiable consensus, such as Lawndale's collective decision to change their mindlines on diabetes in the 1980s, or to hold hard on NSAIDs or early renal disease in the 2000s. On the other hand, Weick reminds us at the outset that such collective sensemaking can lead to serious errors, such as 'it can't be, therefore it isn't' (Weick 1995: 1). For example, in 1943 John Caffey, after struggling to make sense of children's radiographs in which there were multiple fractures but the parents gave no history of injury, suggested the possibility of the battered child syndrome. So strong was the profession's collective denial to such an unexpected and horrifying thought that it was some twenty years before the syndrome was accepted as real. It was rejected out of hand for so long because plausibility, Weick asserts, is a more important part of sensemaking than accuracy.[13] Yet by 1976, when the balance of power in this argument had shifted, there were an estimated half a million cases being recognized annually in the USA alone. 'Sense may be in the eye of the beholder, but beholders vote and the majority rules' (Weick 1995: 6). The way people make sense of new ideas (as with the group meetings in Haymarket [p. 137]) depends, in other words, on the power relations that accompany the presentation and perception of the new information[14] and how it is negotiated by the community concerned.

Irving Janis's (1972) concept of 'groupthink', based on his study of the US foreign-policy decision making that resulted in fiascos such as Pearl Harbor, the Bay of Pigs invasion and the Korean War, describes why group decisions can go dangerously awry. By being too cohesive, too firmly led, too cut off from outside influence or independent expertise, and too pressured to arrive quickly at a definitive conclusion, groups can persuade themselves collectively to believe fallacies or make decisions that they would never have countenanced as individuals.[15] This seemed not to occur at Lawndale, presumably because the practice meeting was neither too cohesive nor firmly led; on the contrary, it was heterogeneous and relatively democratic both in its multidisciplinary membership and in the non-controlling style of its leader.[16] Anything but isolated, Lawndale was continually bombarded with admonishments and advice from, for example, local consultants, the NHS hierarchy, patients or the pharmaceutical sales representatives; the practice meeting showed itself well able to critically (if informally) appraise new evidence when members deemed it necessary. Above all the members of the group always had a chance (either collectively at a later meeting or individually when subsequently seeing patients who, for example, might or might not fulfil the criteria for early CKD) to reconsider the consensus. The Lawndale meetings therefore fulfilled Janis's main criteria for *avoiding* groupthink. Yet this does not mean that there was no mutual influence or pressure to conform to what they collectively thought was best practice. Far from it. We were witnessing an unmistakably social process that was shaping their views and leading them to what Weick would call 'generic sensemaking' – a new collective mindline (about NSAIDs, CHD prevention, CKD) that anyone working in the practice would henceforth be able to pick up on and be expected more or less to follow.[17]

How precisely does such a collective view inter-relate with the individuals' views? That question has for decades been a focus for social psychologists, symbolic interactionists and ethnomethodologists and we will not explore it here.[18] Suffice to say that, as the participants expressed their ideas, they were also listening to each other because, despite their natural individuality, they each knew that they should be acting as a group. As a group edging towards a collective view they could all work with, each person had to build upon their own representation of what the others thought (and, recursively, what they themselves thought the others thought they thought).[19] In contributing their own ideas whilst simultaneously making sense of what the others were saying, they were subordinating their ideas to that emergent collective view, and negotiating a firmer place for their own view as a part of the collective whole.[20] As Weick and Roberts's (Weick and Roberts 1993; Weick 2001) work on the collective mind suggests, each participant is 'heedful' of the others, so that what they contribute and take from the discussion entails their being simultaneously aware of a range of each other's concepts, constraints and motivations that lead to that thought or action. This mutual heedfulness, they argue, forms the basis of any interactive discussion or action. (Nick's discussion with the patient in the 'cholesterol consultation' [p. 40] illustrates how he needed to be heedful of the patient's views and of all the other relevant organizational and social factors that shaped the way he proceeded.) To be heedful, Weick stresses, is also to be continually thinking, feeling and learning, willing both to apply and to adjust one's thinking (mindline) for current and maybe future use. As one becomes less heedful, the act becomes more repetitive, merely habitual and more likely to lead to failure.[21]

If Weick is right, the processes we observed may have required the individuals to recapitulate in their own mind what they were hearing while recursively constructing and reconstructing their own thoughts (and mindlines) on that basis. Hence, while the doctors were arguing their own case for the best way to deal with early CKD, they could also be taking into account what the others were saying, so that as a group they edged towards a collective decision, even though they retained some of their differences. The upshot was to allow Barry to take note of the others' views to produce a suitable policy that they could all work to. However, what mattered was not what emerged (such as the agreed protocol, which was rarely explicitly referred to and was soon forgotten about) but the nuanced ability to act so that each could feel that what they were doing was heedful of what the others think should be done, tempered by their own opinion of how their various views should inter-relate. In other words, when each called upon their own mind-line they were also aware of aspects of each other's views that might modulate how they practised, which in turn might impact on their subsequent collective interactions. We need not delve further into this difficult area of social psychology, but simply wish to suggest that the collective mindline is not so much an entity as a social process of continual mutual heedful interacting between those who share it (Rapley 2008).

That social process served a number of functions that went beyond the simple reappraisal or upgrading of their individual mindlines. As they wrestled with CKD the members of the group were also bolstering, or even redefining, their own identity (pp. 143, 151) – not only how they wanted to be seen by others but also their own self-perception of the kind of doctor they were. Jean's arguments were usually reinforcing her firm commitment to being an exceptionally conscien-tious, empathic GP. Clive's contributions often reaffirmed how well plugged in he was to the nuances of medical politics and how shrewd he was in dealing with NHS bureaucracy. Barry was bolstering his image as a quiet but thoroughly knowledgeable doctor, Nick as a wise and pragmatic leader, Tony a bit of a lateral thinking individualist, and so on. All of them were also at the same time want-ing to maintain Lawndale as an exemplary practice. The act of making sense of the CKD threshold was therefore closely bound up with their sense of their own and their organization's identity, which was particularly apparent at a time when, as a result of the financial and political fallout following the new contract and QOF agreements, general practice felt under fire from politicians and the press. They were reasserting, and justifying, their power and autonomy to deal with their patients as they, not the government, saw fit (p. 1).[22]

When the group were making sense of the new requirements for kidney disease they were also collectively, as Weick would put it, enacting (i.e. bringing about) a particular kind of environment – one in which they could score maximum QOF points while still being fair to the patients, themselves and the practice. We subse-quently learnt of other practices that had enacted quite different environments, for example by simply delaying any involvement with the new GP contract. Such practices and practitioners, by interpreting the situation and behaving differently, found they were operating in a world completely different from Lawndale's, but which they had actually helped to bring about for themselves.

There were also more specific, routine ways in which the Lawndale GPs enacted the environment that they then had to react to. Setting the CKD threshold at any given level would result in more or fewer patients making return visits to have their eGFR monitored, and in higher or lower levels of income for Lawndale to deal with the consequences. So making sense of the situation and reacting accordingly was not (and never is) a simple matter of reacting to a given environment, but itself iteratively, recursively, contributed to shaping that environment. (There is no escape; even leaving the threshold unchanged would have an impact on the numbers of patients attending cardiac or diabetic clinics.) Another simple example is the decision to prescribe – or not – antibiotics to children with simple sore throats. If the local convention is to be generous with such prescriptions, then more and more patients will expect them (Little *et al.* 1997); consequently the GPs will find themselves justified in saying that there is no point in following the evidence to withhold antibiotics because the patients demand them and will keep coming back until they get them, so we might as well prescribe them straight away! This vicious circle creates a greater workload, increases the medicines bill, and allows the GPs to justify and make sense of the decision to prescribe as though constrained by an external environment beyond their control, when in fact their actions are helping to create that environment. Indeed Weick (2001: 176–203; Daft and Weick 1984) even goes so far as to suggest that the way groups ('cognitive communities') interpret and hence enact the environment has more of an impact on the environment than vice versa.

In summary, by heeding each other's knowledge, views and experiences the members of the community of practice were building and reinforcing a collective mindline that not only shaped their practice, but shaped their world. Together, they were 'co-constructing' how they practised, what kinds of practitioners they were, on which patients with what diseases they were practising, and in what sort of organization and what environment they did so.[23]

From community of practice to collective capital

The capacity to be part of this co-constructing activity was hard won; eligibility to participate required not only years of training but also to have achieved respect and trust as a member of that community of practice. Having attained that position, however, the practitioners had access to many powerful resources that have been likened to a form of 'capital', which, once accumulated and fostered, yielded dividends not only for the practitioners, but also for their patients and the NHS organization. Le May has suggested (le May 2009b: 9–14) that communities of practice can generate many types of such capital – social, human, organizational, professional and patient[24] capital. The term 'social capital' includes the improved relations and networks that allowed the Lawndale practitioners to rapidly take advantage of their connections with trusted networks (Putnam 2000) and hence work more efficiently and effectively (Nahapiet and Ghoshal 1998; Lesser and Prusak 1999). It also includes the structural opportunities (such as formal and informal meetings or intranet links) that Lawndale practitioners had for networking within and beyond their group, and having the capacity to assess the degree of trust that they could place in each other's assessments of new knowledge or unusual events. Trust and respect (which included knowing each other's foibles and weaknesses) allowed them to make the most of their collective ability to make sense of departures from routine practice and to generate and share useable knowledge-in-practice-in-context.[25] Another evident resource was the 'human capital' such as the range of different education, training and experiential knowledge that the members of the community imparted to each other and to the collective mindline.

So, for example, experienced GPs guided recent recruits in the-way-we-do-things-here, the 'diabetes lead' kept people apprised of the place of new drugs, bright young registrars explained new techniques, the practice manager clarified the new contractual requirements, the nurses brought practical *nous*, or the long-serving phlebotomist brought local knowledge about the patients and the practicalities of the laboratory service. The collective knowledge and altered practice that resulted from these exchanges could be described also as 'organizational capital' that enabled Lawndale, staff and patients, to benefit from a better-run surgery, whether as a result, say, of abstract changes in attitudes and mindlines, or physical innovations such as new clinics, equipment, protocols, or more practice income that led to better resources.

By being part of their communities of practice at Lawndale, the practitioners also enhanced what le May has called their 'professional capital' (le May 2009b). This refers to such resources as the *knowledge and skills* embodied in their individual mindlines and the *sociocultural practices* embodied in their collective mindlines and in their shared values and ethos, their agreed ways of behaving, practising and communicating, their use of language, vocabulary and jargon (Fairclough 1992) and their shared history of learning. The *formal and informal networks* of colleagues, along with their subtle awareness of their strengths and weaknesses, were also part of their professional capital, which relied also on their accumulated sense of the *written and unwritten rules* that permitted them to partake profitably in interactions with colleagues that could improve their own and each other's professional prowess. Like their fiscal counterpart, these more abstract forms of capital were both self-selecting and self-perpetuating in that the practitioners needed to have a substantial minimum amount even to take part, but once able to do so they were well placed as professionals to capitalize on them to enhance their individual and collective standing. But membership of that community also, as we have seen, gave them the power to co-construct both the content and much of the context of their practice. It is to that process of co-construction that we now finally turn, for that is what links clinical mindlines to their social and organizational context.

Chapter 8: Summary

While discussing their work together, clinicians formulated and refined 'collective mindlines' that acted as templates against which to check their individual practice. Collective mindlines are complex, flexible, context-specific virtual guides to practice that cannot be made fully explicit but are incessantly being validated through the interactions between clinicians. We present a detailed example of how a particular community of practice redefined incipient chronic kidney disease such that they could make collective sense of the competing social, clinical, professional, organizational, financial and ethical considerations that faced them. Such collective sensemaking was actually reshaping the clinical environment in which the clinicians practised.

9 Co-constructing clinical reality

This chapter deals with broad-brush questions about the relationship between clinical knowledge and its social origins. Overt examples are by the very nature of social construction not easy to see in brief vignettes, but to give some background to that discussion we start with examples where social and organizational context seemed to be shaping knowledge-in-practice-in-context.

❖ *During a long discussion at the Lawndale GP contract meeting to optimize the way patients with coronary heart disease should be reviewed, there is the usual twin thrust of improving quality of care plus meeting the contractual requirements to gain points and hence income for the practice. Whilst the former is clearly providing the main driving force for the debate on how best to ensure that every patient is reliably recalled and properly checked with minimum inconvenience, some of the discussion is shaped by the latter – as when the meeting begins talking about how best to target a group specified by the contract: 'the 150/90s, who are an important group of patients'. The term continues to be used liberally. One wonders whether, if the contract didn't have that particular (fairly arbitrary) blood pressure as the cut-off,[1] but, say 155/85 instead, then suddenly 'the 155/85s' would have been labelled and focused upon as 'clinically important'.*

❖ *We are at an Oakville team meeting about a project designed to provide guidance based on activity data in order to help physicians modify their current practice. The team are discussing the findings of a recent audit and how it compares with current best practice. They are designing and refining a newsletter that will be sent to hospital physicians giving the data about current practice and suggesting new guidelines. As they go through it line by line, comments fly from the clinical scientists and their assistants: 'They'll get pissed at us if we say that.' 'That will be misunderstood.' 'That should hit the spot.' . . . The eventual product is agreed – a pristine and objective set of figures, graphs and 'key points'. None of the data in the eventual product are untrue, but it is clear that they are not simply data; they are very subtly negotiated data that have been subjected to judgements based on an intimate knowledge of the factors that affect practice.*

❖ *On the Oakville round, not long after they have discharged Mrs Astupile (p. 157), they are looking at the chart of a patient referred from another hospital. There are apparently five sets of comprehensive biochemistry ('comp.') results. 'Jeez those guys are so dumbass. How many comps does a fella need in three days for chrissake?' demands Craig rhetorically. 'Is it anything to do with the payments system?' I ask disingenuously. 'You betcha!'*

❖ *It is a rather tetchy lunchtime Urbcester practice meeting, attended just by the GPs. (There are no nurses, practice manager or others such as receptionists at their meetings although, as it turns out, they would have held the key to a lot of today's discussion.) The GPs are getting irritable about the rota and the allocation of patient slots. So that they can fit in all the patients that want to see them (and so hit government targets as well as improve patient satisfaction), the PCT has insisted that the practice have two types of bookings: ten-minute consultations for chronic conditions and their flare-ups, and seven minutes for new, acute cases. The GPs are very unhappy about this restriction. Such arguments as 'A lot of my sevens need much more and sometimes the tens are quicker because we know them' continue for quite a big proportion of the meeting, revealing increasing dissatisfaction about the whole principle, which is linked to several swirling undercurrents about the difficulty of establishing any continuity of care, about teaching medical students, about getting accredited to train GPs, and about the allocation of workloads. There is also evident irritation at the way the 'sevens' and 'tens' are being administered by receptionists who do not understand what is involved. The focus shifts to such administrative problems, away from the other underlying concern that continuity of care will be further undermined by this initiative. Nothing is resolved; Urbcester patients will continue to be 'tens' or 'sevens'.*

I notice that Frances in surgery that same evening, when seeing a 'seven' towards the end of the surgery, is far less inclined to deal with the patient thoroughly than she was with previous 'tens' who actually seemed to have less serious symptoms, but with whom she dealt with fully. But when she sees that 'the seven' has had previous treatment for his indigestion (and therefore can be called chronic and dealt with as a 'ten') she recommends that he come back and see his usual doctor. Having been a 'seven', and therefore dealt with one way, he can now, as a 'ten', be managed another way. 'Better for you and for us as doctors', she says, harking back to the problem of continuity of care that had vexed her at the lunchtime meeting. Shortly afterwards, at the end of a difficult and long surgery, she breaks down in tears about the stress of having to work like that and my observation session turns into a counselling session.

When common sense gets to be a *habitus*

Mindlines are so fundamental to a clinician that to fellow practitioners the majority of their content, which they have all built up in similar ways throughout their careers, seems to be simply 'common sense'. But it should be clear by now that there is nothing simple about the way in which health professionals get to the stage where they just cannot envisage any other way of seeing and acting except as the clinician they are. Clifford Geertz has observed that for all individuals in all cultures, common sense is very difficult to pin down, yet has a number of key properties that are worthy of further study (Geertz 1983: chapter 4). Like a suburb of a sprawling city where a pedestrian usually gets to the main highway by going down minor side roads, short cuts and sometimes dubious alleyways, common sense is often messy and internally inconsistent and yet it has what Geertz calls a 'natural-ness', 'practical-ness' and straightforward-ness that, while it may be unmethodical and complex, is immediately accessible and self-evidently recogniz-able to those who have acquired it but very hard to explain to those who have not. Mindlines appear to us to have very much that feel to them. Where formal clinical knowledge is akin to a set of maps depicting the main roads of the clinical 'city', it is that common-sense nature of the mindlines that helps clinicians navigate the actual disorderly terrain where the main roads are often blocked and the back routes are attractive and you need to know where the muggers hang out.

When clinicians arrive quickly at decisions that 'just make sense' but which they can't explain (Chapter 3), it is arguable that part of their inarticulacy is due to exactly these attributes of the 'clinical common sense' that are the hard-won basis of their professional capital (p. 165). The French anthropological philosopher Pierre Bourdieu (1992, 2006 [1972]) has also observed that when we see someone perform successfully within their culture (Bourdieu uses as an example the way members of Algerian Kabyle society use gift exchange such as camels for brides to enhance their social standing, but it could equally apply to the way doctors or nurses use clinical knowledge in practice) we see them doing so in ways that go well beyond the 'rules' that anthropologists or their informants can abstract from the process. To watch a clinician manage a patient competently is to watch much more than the application of a set of rules or guidelines. It is an act of extraordi-nary sophistication and complexity based on a lifetime of learning (but then, so is gifting a camel). As Bourdieu suggests from his study of the Kabyle:

> [O]nly a virtuoso with a perfect command of his 'art of living' can play on all the resources inherent in the ambiguities and uncertainties of behaviour and situation in order to produce the actions appropriate to do that of which people will say 'There was nothing else to be done' and to do it in the right way. We [as researchers] are a long way too from norms and rules . . . [in] . . . the 'art' of the *necessary improvisation* which defines excellence.
>
> (Bourdieu 2006 [1972]: 8, his emphasis)

Witness the way in which discussants anticipate each other's moves (like a boxer, he says) with dummies and ripostes, ducking and weaving in response to the merest flicker from the opponent who may themselves be feigning a move – in a series of actions that can never be exhaustively listed and codified, but which nevertheless are explicable by a strategy that both participants share and understand. It has taken them years of learning and training, of exchanging ideas and practices, of reinforcement and development within their communities of practice to arrive at their ability to do that. Discourse analysts (Cicourel 1987; Elwyn *et al.* 1999a) have shown that even the shortest discussions between doctors and patients or between clinical colleagues are also characterized by twists and blocks, elisions and pauses, allusions and counter-assertions, euphemisms and evasions, etiquette and banter, ritual and game playing. What hope has an outsider, asks Bourdieu, of understanding such a process simply by trying to crystallize out of it a set of rules, even were it possible for the members of the community themselves – if pressed and given enough time – to account for every move? Even the best analysis would produce a set of rules that cannot by definition deal with every new and varied instance, as the practitioners do. Or, if it did, it would do so only by having embraced *all* the presuppositions taken for granted by the practitioners and which cannot normally be expressed. Moreover such a comprehensive tome would be incomprehensible as a set of rules to anyone but the insiders who don't need to be told the rules because they already understand all those unspoken presuppositions. In which case one wonders what hope the outsider would have of modifying that practice by trying to impose such a set of rules from outside that community. Catch-22 for guidelines again (pp. 5, 30, 94).

This is why clinicians cannot be expected simply to ensure that their mindlines be nothing more nor less than evidence-based guidelines committed to memory – and also why it is not possible for practitioners to explicate fully the content of their mindlines. Producing a codified, crystallized version of the mindline would immediately make it into a different kind of entity altogether, and one that would fail to fulfil the functions of a mindline. However much it allows for flexibility of decisions, a guideline is an entity that is fixed and codified in writing. A mindline, in contrast, is not a *thing*, but a *process*; it provides not only a set of propensities to act in appropriate ways in given circumstances, but also a large range of well-tried contextual modulators for all likely occasions. (Think, for example, of Nick's 'cholesterol consultation' [p. 31], or the negotiated outcome of the CKD debates which resulted from the intricate negotiations between the various positions sketched in Table 8.2). The minute one tries to crystallize such interactive thought processes into a tangible entity one loses their very essence – their processual nature, their personal adaptability and their flexible logic – all the features that enable them to be applied in real situations that vary from the context-free codified, simplified, rigidified propositional knowledge of 'if this then that' guidelines and textbooks.[2]

Mindlines also have a much deeper and more pervasive function than merely guiding the diagnosis and management of patients: they both embed and express professional norms and values. They embody the clinicians' conformity to the collective precepts and principles of their relevant communities of practice, past and/or present. Mindlines are therefore, as we have seen (e.g. in Chapter 8 in the response to new edicts about CKD [p. 152] or NSAIDs [p. 158]), an important means by which a health profession develops and maintains its identity and its standing. As such mindlines do not simply provide immediately accessible patterns of information and possible actions; they link individual practitioners to the profession as a whole. They mediate the values of those whose opinions the clinicians respect and wish to emulate. By putting those collective views of appropriate clinical behaviour into practice each clinician then purveys and reinforces those views. Moreover, if and when they subsequently discuss their practice with colleagues, they will be feeding those views back into their communities, perhaps with new adjustments, continually reinforcing but also modulating the collective mindline.

As long ago as the 1970s, Bourdieu was among the first to argue that such collective norms comprised a form of social and symbolic capital – and we would add professional capital (p. 165) – built up by a community such that its members could practise their lives in ways that meet the demands they faced. He coined the term *habitus* to describe the manner in which people in a community learn, ineluctably and indiscernibly over a lifetime, to think and act in the ways of their wider group(s). The *habitus* acts as the collective and practical (i.e. practised) embodiment of the group's norms (Bourdieu 2006 [1972]). When the Lawndale GPs collectively transmuted the contractual definition of chronic kidney disease (p. 156), their discussions embodied not only the practical exigencies of their managerial and clinical roles, but also – at all sorts of levels – the values and norms underpinning the roles they identified with. At one level their discussions followed the well-honed conventions of practice meetings: who speaks when, how, with what influence, and so on. At another they embodied the constraints and requirements of the organization: how far can one defy the NHS hierarchy, challenge hospital experts or step out of line with other GPs? At yet another level they were reinforcing their ethos as a primary care team by asserting such principles as GPs being allowed to provide what they themselves, not outside agencies, consider to be the best care for their patients, or to maximize the benefit for their practice, and so forth. So, using Bourdieu's analysis one can discern that, by developing collective mindlines about CKD or NSAIDs that defied the externally imposed norms and reinstated clinical judgement, they were also reinforcing and perpetuating the status, authority and power that enabled them to practise. No surprise, then, that they were resistant to following new protocols that did not stem from their network of trusted colleagues whom they could recognize as being part of their own professional group, and as sharing their norms, their *habitus* (Mutch 2003).

So while the development of the *habitus* is a collective response to the challenges of practising as a part of one's community, it also helps to develop and maintain that community.[3] But there is a further important twist in this Bourdieu-derived analysis, which is that, while the *habitus* is a response to the environment, it is also itself the product of that environment.[4] The ethos and practices that shaped what the Lawndale clinicians said and did had been inculcated by the particular context in which they had acquired their *habitus*. It was precisely because they had 'grown up' in the modern NHS that they had learnt the tricks of treading the careful line between sacrificing autonomy by complying with the requirements of the NHS hierarchy and risking sanctions by defying it, or that they valued patient benefit more than personal financial reward. A discussion about managing early CKD, just like one on the advisability of guaiac stools, blood cultures and 'an adrenal work-up' in a patient such as Mrs Astupile (p. 157), would take a very different tone in Lawndale (or indeed Westchurch Hospital) from the one seen in Oakville. Whereas the *habitus* embodied in such discussions would reinforce the ethos from which they arose (the Lawndale GPs were perpetuating the ethos of UK primary care, just as the Oakville physicians might perpetuate the US healthcare values), that ethos had itself arisen from their social, political, professional, economic, organizational, cultural and historical context. So, in short, there is reciprocity between the way people behave and the context in which they do so – they are mutually constitutive.

From clinician to society or vice versa? Structuration

Clinicians may be strongly influenced by their social, organizational and cultural environment but they still have the freedom to act, within limits, and thereby alter that environment. This brings us to the old sociological chicken and egg question: does society determine individual behaviour or vice versa? In trying to understand EBP, should we follow those who study grand social structures to see how they impact on individual behaviour or those who insist that we aggregate micro-studies of individual people's behaviour to explain society?[5] Anthony Giddens characterized this dichotomy in the late 1970s as the structure/agency (society/individual) debate, and – berating both sides for their respective tunnel vision – attempted to overcome the dilemma with a compromise synthesis he called 'structuration'. This was an influential[6] attempt at a 'third way' to explain how people's actions are shaped by their society and culture while at the same time individuals can act to change things (Giddens 2004 [1984]). The structuration thesis has been criticized both for its overambitious intentions and for the lack of precision about how the relationship between individual people (agents) and society (structure) works in detail, but it nevertheless commands considerable currency among social scientists and provides a productive framework for thinking about the problems with which we are concerned here – namely how individual clinicians both conform to and contribute to the broader professional norms of knowledge-in-practice-in-context. Or, more specifically, it may help to understand how healthcare 'structures' shape the mindlines and practices of clinical 'agents', which in turn impact on those very structures.

Let us assume, argues Giddens, that instead of thinking that *either* people's actions result from social forces beyond their control *or* individuals can always choose their own behaviours, we can accept a 'duality' whereby every action has components of both. This seems a sensible assumption. The reason that Clive decides to prescribe antibiotics for someone's viral sore throat may partly be due to broad socioeconomic forces that drive him unwittingly to do so (the paradigm of western scientific medicine, the economics of the pharmaceutical industry, the influence of patient pressure groups, the power of government exerted through NHS contractual guidance, the shortness of consultation times, the cultural ethic of trying every possibility even where there is little evidence of benefit, and so on). But he does also actually have a choice; social structure cannot fully determine social action. After all, just down the corridor, Jean, faced with a very similar patient and subjected to those same 'invisible forces', chooses not to prescribe. Yet both their decisions might have been predicted (psychologically and statistically) and are within what is considered acceptable in modern NHS practice. Neither Clive nor Jean, for example, prescribed prayer or leeches, both of which would have been perfectly acceptable in other cultures and eras (and would probably work just about as well on viruses as antibiotics do). Structuration theory gives us ways to explain how individuals absorb unconscious, tacitly understood routines of behaviour that generally remain unquestioned as long as they remain within accepted bounds. Years of socialization have made people deeply aware of how far they can safely stretch the norms. They have no need to monitor their own behaviour consciously unless they think, based partly on what they assume those who matter to them would think, that they might be overstepping the mark (cf. Weick's 'primping' in the mirror of imagined judges [p. 160]). In that case they adjust their behaviour, find some way to rationalize it or, occasionally, deliberately challenge the norm. (Even then such a challenge is likely to fall within some other presumed set of alternative opinions held by a subgroup they can relate to.[7]) By reflexively reinforcing or rejecting each other's behaviours and beliefs people affect their own and others' ability to reinforce or reproduce, or perhaps resist or replace, the accepted norms. Hence their individual actions help to develop and maintain the social structures. They may indeed act freely, but the freedom is unavoidably shaped by the principles and conventions of their society, which in turn are maintained and developed by the accumulation of individual actions. It is this continual process of reciprocity between structure and action that Giddens calls 'structuration' (Giddens 2004 [1984]: 191) or 'the duality of structure' (ibid.: 25).[8]

How far people can step outside the norms is crucially linked to discrepancies in their *power* to exert influence (e.g. the ability to control resources), which in turn is linked to the status they have acquired (or lost) over time through the very kinds of interactions that we have been describing.[9] Depending partly on that power, the influence of their actions can and often does have consequences far beyond what they are aware of – consequences that among other things help to structure the wider forces that in turn influence their own future actions. So, for example, a GP such as Peter had the power to choose which hospital his patients went to and might favour referring those with diabetes to Northton General rather than Westchurch. By repeatedly doing that, he might reduce the hospital's income and hence inadvertently contribute to the closing down of other services he values at Westchurch Hospital, thus unintentionally limiting his own future referral choices. Clive also had another type of power through the many regional and national committees he was on, where, for example, by making evidence-based medicine zealots the butt of his humour, he might unwittingly lend support to those who share his scepticism for central guidelines but not his high standards of care. Without realizing it, both might be having unintended effects far from their immediate spheres of influence.

Distant influence on people's actions is a key feature of structuration. People who are remote in time and place (not just Peter inadvertently undermining Westchurch Hospital or Clive unintentionally endorsing incompetence in distant practices, but also the policy makers who drafted the GP contract, renal researchers in the USA, former teachers, Florence Nightingale, Abraham Flexner . . .) play their part through what Giddens calls their 'co-presence'. They may act through relatively concrete, overt institutions and mechanisms that are able to influence people's actions (he calls them 'codified structures' and they might include written regulations, guidelines, curricula, the RCGP's award schemes, the Nursing and Midwifery Council's registration system, NHS contracts, the research and publishing industries . . .). But those structures and codified rules, argues Giddens, have a relatively limited role in guiding people's actions compared with other major influences. First there are deeper intangible 'social principles' that the formal structures represent (professional ethics, the relative status of health professions, the hidden curricula of student culture, the power politics of health service organizations, the economics of healthcare . . .). Social principles such as these cannot be seen directly but only inferred or fleetingly glimpsed through the way people and institutions behave. Second people's actions are mediated by what he calls their 'practical consciousness' – something sociologically akin to the Freudian psychological idea of the unconscious – in which people are deeply knowledgeable about the social conditions of their actions but cannot express that knowledge in words. It is this (tacit, ineffable) practical consciousness, says Giddens, that becomes the final common pathway by which the social structures and principles become built into daily routine activity.

These three different social theories of Geertz, Bourdieu and Giddens all point in the same direction.[10] Geertz's 'common sense', Bourdieu's *habitus* and Giddens's 'practical consciousness' all describe internalized social processes that are much more powerful determinants of behaviour than inadequate maps, 'rules' or 'codified structures' that society produces expressly for the purpose. And all three social theories seem to us to describe something akin to our finding that mindlines inform clinical practice and its practitioners in ways that a codified guideline simply cannot. The three analyses also open up ways in which we can explore how clinical mindlines might be shaped by, and contribute to, wider social structures. But, if we are to trace the social origins and influences of knowledge-in-practice-in-context, we must first establish the possibility that clinical knowledge may indeed be socially constructed.

Social construction and deconstruction: what a performance

The social sciences literature is suffused with talk of the social construction of medical knowledge but most clinicians still find the idea alien. Surely, they insist, medicine has largely progressed precisely because we have stripped away the value judgements and subjective social mishmash to get to real scientific facts. That traditional view, though, has been strongly challenged since the 1970s following a growing body of analysis of the ways social structures influence our whole interpretation of reality (Berger and Luckmann 1966). That work showed unequivocally that humans inevitably create the reality that they experience through a process of socialization – a finding that is being increasingly confirmed by studies of infant and child development as well as adult behaviour. How else but through our families, upbringing and social institutions do we learn to interpret and respond to 'the sum total of "what everybody knows" about a social world, an assemblage of maxims, morals, proverbial nuggets of wisdom, values and beliefs, myths and so forth' (ibid.: 83)? The way we come to see the world is due to this 'primary socialization', which for specialized groups such as professions is later overlaid with 'secondary socialization', Berger and Luckmann's term for the socialization processes we described in Chapters 4 and 5. But the twist is that we then see 'the products of human activity *as if* they were something other than human products – such as facts of nature, results of cosmic laws, or manifestations of divine will' (ibid.: 106, their emphasis). We take these 'facts' to be our objective world, embedded in our language and our behaviours; there is no other way for us to experience reality. We assume that the view of reality that our processes of socialization have collectively and historically created *is* the only possible objective reality. We have 'socially constructed' our society and all that it contains, and our social order – such as the power invested in social institutions and experts – inexorably legitimizes and perpetuates that construction.

This view was widely taken up in the social sciences from the 1970s onwards and, in parallel with the rise of a body of post-positivist history and philosophy that questioned the nature of science (e.g. Kuhn 1964; Lakatos and Musgrave 1970), social scientists were inevitably led to scrutinize scientific knowledge and develop a social constructivist perspective (e.g. Barnes 1974; D. Bloor 1976; Young 1977; see also Barnes *et al.* 1996). Throughout the 1970s and 1980s, the more they looked at science, the more they found it to be dependent on its 'external' social context, and the more they looked at the 'external' context of the science, the more they found it to be inseparable from its 'internal' content. They demonstrated how scientific communities had overarching ways of investigating and seeing the world (paradigms) that shaped their entire view of their subject – paradigms that were clearly historically and culturally contingent. Theory after scientific theory was shown on closer examination to be ineluctably rooted in social values and in economic forces that linked science and technology inextricably to the world of commerce and politics.

Naturally, medical science came in for scrutiny too, and revealed time and again that, however objective and scientific doctors thought they were being, 'moral values, social attitudes, or political prejudices are deeply embedded in their knowledge – shaping, structuring and indeed constituting it' (Gabbay 1982: 23).[11] By the 1980s early 'social constructionists' were 'refus[ing] to regard medicine and technical medical knowledge as pre-given entities, separate from all other human activities. Instead [. . .] medicine can be seen as a highly specialized domain of social practice and discourse, the limits and contents of which are set up by wider – but not separate – social practices' (Wright and Treacher 1982: 10). This approach, which has been described as possibly *the* most important strand within the sociology of health and illness (White 1991), has led to a spectrum of interpretations (Elston 1997; Nettleton 2006). One can take a soft line and argue simply that our knowledge of the body and disease is coloured and modified by social or ideological interests. This was the view taken by Eliot Freidson (1988) who in his classic analysis of the medical profession argued that medicine creates, for example, the social role of illness by defining what is sufficiently deviant to be accorded the status of a disease. But, he crucially continued, doctors inevitably build their social and moral assumptions into that role, and hence into the very definition of illnesses and their management. For example, whereas we have good scientific evidence about the cost-effectiveness of drugs to delay the progress of early Alzheimer's disease, whether or not the disease is diagnosed and the drugs prescribed is determined by economic, political and humanitarian pressures. The moral values of the clinical professions can therefore influence how the 'illness' (what the patient experiences) is defined and dealt with even if the underlying science of the 'disease' (the pathological changes that lead to the experience of illness) remains value free. In other words, according to the 'soft' version of social constructivism, the science remains pure even if its application is often overlaid and distorted by social considerations.

A stronger line would be that the very substance of our knowledge about disease can also be shaped by outside interests. For example it has been argued that the interests of the pharmaceutical industry and others have led to the invention of a new and dubious disease category, 'mild cognitive impairment', which once 'identified' and 'diagnosed' requires treatment (Moreira *et al.* 2009). (Or, as Marshall Marinker [1973: 28] pithily characterized the same principle in a different age with different pharmaceuticals, 'It seems to me you are case of diazepam. You'd better have some anxiety.') Particular targets for such critiques about the external structuring of medical knowledge have been disease concepts about mental illness and obstetrics, both historical and contemporary, in which the most extreme view has been the suggestion that much of the illness and disease recognized by those specialties has been a questionable accumulation of the medicalization of professional dominance, moralizing and social control (Turner 1995).

An even stronger line would be that the way we classify *all* diseases is socially contingent on how and why we are doing the classifying (Bowker and Star 1999), but the strongest line of all would be that not just diseases but *everything* that we think we know about medicine, even when dealing with unquestionable and life-threatening physical diseases such as heart failure or cleft palate, is a culturally specific fabrication (Silverman 1983). By that view it is not just fringe categories such as 'mild cognitive impairment', but core concepts such as Alzheimer's disease (Fox 1989), even the central nervous system itself, that are socially constituted interpretations of reality. Under that radical version of social constructivism, our modern notions of dementia, like the old idea that hysteria resulted from the womb wandering around the body, will one day be completely superseded by a different paradigm brought about by a different set of social, technical and ideological constructs. And there will never be an objective way of knowing about reality outwith those different paradigmatic representations. The strong view – often linked to the work of Michel Foucault – is therefore that there is no medical reality save that which powerful discourses conjure into existence.[12]

In an ethnography of ENT surgeons in the mid 1970s, Michael Bloor drew similarly radical conclusions (although he pointed out that his ideas had a respectable philosophical pedigree dating from the eighteenth century). He noted how the surgeons continually reformulated their criteria for performing adeno-tonsillectomies in the light of a host of considerations, such that:

> the theoretical construction of a disease entity is essentially arbitrary and value-laden and since any disease entity is in effect a general name which can refer to a wide variety of different particular conditions.
>
> (M. Bloor 1976: 43)

The surgeons not only varied from each other but each also recast their own general concepts differently over time and from setting to setting. One could not, therefore, ever pin down any specific disease entity that they all subscribed to. Bloor concluded from his observations that, although there might be a general term for a symptom, sign or disease (e.g. 'tonsillitis'), the surgeons could function in practice only by reconstructing it each time they applied it to a new patient or used it in communication with different colleagues. 'Thus, variation in medical assessments is a natural consequence of the structure of medical knowledge' (ibid.: 59).

Paul Atkinson's ethnographies have also shown how doctors bring medical facts into existence. His study of haematologists, for example, revealed in detail how their moment to moment discussions about microscopy slides, charts and other matters involved negotiations, nuances and disagreements that fashioned what they took to be the diseases that they were treating. He calls the process the 'narrative reconstruction of clinical cases', which is shaped by the often ritualistic ways in which the doctors work and talk. The social processes he described shaped, developed and reinforced the way the doctors worked and talked together, but at the same time constructed the diseases the doctors believed themselves to be dealing with (Atkinson 1995: 89). Among the students he studied in Edinburgh too (p. 81), Atkinson dissects the way in which 'clinical . . . "reality" is artfully stage managed and constructed in such a way as to reproduce particular *versions* of medical work and a particular form of medical culture' (Atkinson 1981: 22, his emphasis) that presents the students with a construct (e.g. of what constitutes a 'case') that they both engage in and perpetuate during their time on the wards.

Using historical accounts of asthma Gabbay came to similar conclusions when he found himself in a state of 'historical paralysis' because no two past accounts of the 'disease' could be compared:

> Far from medical knowledge about asthma having consisted of proven, timeless objective facts, it has appeared under scrutiny to be composed of limited interpretations of the complex phenomena of illness. The nature of those interpretations is formed by the world, a social world, in which the physician and patient happen to live; it also contributes to the formation of that world.
>
> (Gabbay 1982: 43)

Such a strong view of the social nature of clinical knowledge would be consistent with the 'mutualist' view held by many sociologists, anthropologists and psychologists that *everything* we think we know – science too – is the result of our 'intersubjective' interactions with each other, and moreover that it often entails the mutual development of a narrative understanding (see also Chapters 6–8) of the phenomena we all need to deal with (Carrithers 1992). The problem, however, is that the views of 'strong' social constructivists are also the product of *their* social circumstances, and we can find ourselves in an abyss of infinite regression.[13]

One need not go that far to accept that clinical knowledge is socially contingent and that the day-to-day interpretation and practice of medicine and the other health professions is at *some* level a social construct. Even for 'soft' constructivists there still remains the challenge of understanding precisely how the undoubted links between medical knowledge and its social context are actually forged. From that perspective, our challenge is now to consider how mindlines link to the social and organizational context of practice. This was not a question uppermost in our minds, however, when we began our ethnography. We had set out to explore how clinicians use research-based knowledge in practice, not to delve into the social construction of that knowledge, so our ethnographic methods of investigation were therefore not designed to deal with the latter. There were occasional clues, such as the 'important patient group of 150/90s' or the way Frances in Urbcester seemed to take a completely different *clinical* approach to the 'seven' minute patients and the 'tens', even when they had similar symptoms of severe indigestion. Was this an indirect result of the tensions between her deeply held values in favour of appropriately long consultations and continuity of care and the contrary values of organizational pressures to split patients arbitrarily into 'sevens' and 'tens' and allocate them to whichever doctor is available on the rota? Did those tensions plus the administrative problems of inadequately trained receptionists (who moreover were excluded from the thinking behind it all), plus the doctor's psychological stress, plus the time of day, all contribute to the classification and management of the patients? Perhaps. But drawing conclusions from such serendipitous findings as these would be unduly tentative as we had not set out to record our findings so that we could investigate the social constructivist aspects more deeply. To help illuminate the way that clinical knowledge might be socially constructed we must therefore, for this last part of our analysis, turn to an example taken from a previous study in which JG and others investigated how doctors in a particular social and organizational context improved the way they dealt with heart failure or, as we would now describe it, developed a new collective mindline. Our account is based on the simplified retelling of the story that appears in Box 9.1 (Dopson and Gabbay 1995; Dopson and Fitzgerald 2005: 159–162). Our approach to this study will borrow heavily from so-called 'actor-network theory', to suggest the ways in which people, organizations and even inanimate objects (all of which in Box 9.1 we *italicize*) interacted to construct the new mindline.[14]

A network of action to change collective mindlines in heart failure

What – apart from an object lesson in how to implement evidence-based practice – do we learn from the story in Box 9.1? There are three very important conclusions relevant to our development of the idea of mindlines. First, it is very difficult to separate the context from the action and the knowledge. There is no obvious place where the social structures can be separated from the agents or actors. Was the project team part of the context or part of the action? How about the Queens

Box 9.1 **An account, using actor-network theory, of the development of services for congestive heart failure in 'Heartshire'**

It is 1997. The *hearts* of 10 per cent of elderly people in the UK are failing to pump blood effectively. *Doctors* manage them with established methods such as *diuretics* (costing the NHS *over £360m per year*). *Drug companies* are producing new *ACE inhibitors*. *Inventors and manufacturers* produce a new kind of instrument (*echocardiographs*) for measuring heart failure that can help guide the use of ACE inhibitors. *Researchers* (with the help of *research funders, industry, health service providers, patients, universities, journals*) show that the use of these new techniques unquestionably improves care. *Department of Health civil servants*, anxious to meet *political targets* and demonstrate NHS improvements, call on *national opinion leaders* to endorse the *research findings* to guide improvements in practice. *Royal colleges, R&D centres* and *medical journals* are strongly promoting evidence-based practice. The resulting *guidelines* and *exhortations* to a large extent fall on deaf ears; many *GPs* cavil at such external interference. But they are coming round to the idea that *clinical audit* – still in 1997 seen warily by many doctors as a suspect innovation – is a Good Thing. Audits are showing that some *patients* do well on old-fashioned diuretics but some continue to die unnecessarily. *The NHS management hierarchy* exerts pressure through *performance targets* for improving the proper use of the new drugs.

Meanwhile *public health doctors* in Heartshire, anxious to assert their role in improving health, produce a document showing that thousands of life years might be gained locally by conforming to the new guidance. *Cardiologists* at the *Heartshire Hospital* are mightily frustrated by the lack of action to set up a much needed echocardiography service. Local *GP opinion leaders* argue for two main changes to combat serious defects in services for people with heart failure: (1) use more ACE inhibitors and (2) establish an open echocardiography service directly accessible to GPs. Others argue that echocardiography should be obtained only through cardiology out-patients. Those keen to improve the service begin to examine *the research evidence* closely and find little clarity about clinically important details such as the dosages of ACE inhibitors or the type of echocardiography provision required. There are many meetings. *Local managers* remain unconvinced about resourcing an echo service. GPs are increasingly complaining about the current poor provision of echocardiography and public health doctors and some *key hospital doctors* are arguing for open access. They see that the *Queens Trust* is offering *funds* to help implement evidence-based practice; they apply and are selected to run *The Heartshire Project* on ACE inhibitors and echocardiography. Although there is no research evidence to suggest that echocardiography should be by open access, they wave the (metaphorical) *banner of evidence-based practice* – possibly because all the local leading clinicians agree that an *open access echocardiography service* is for the best. They all respect *the chief cardiologist* and, if he says such a service is needed, who is to argue? To prove the need they ask the GPs to do an *audit of heart failure care*; the GPs oblige and show it to be inadequate. This locks the GPs into the campaign – they want improvements, but they also see the chance to take charge of the service. The *hospital management team*, initially concerned about ceding control (and funds), nevertheless agrees to a primary care-led service. It would gain them kudos in the relentless top-down drive to meet targets. The *local pharmaceutical representatives*, who have good relations with *the cardiology department*, spot an opportunity to boost ACE inhibitors and offer to fund the new echocardiography service. With that and the Queens Trust funds to pay for a dedicated *project manager* in the public health department, The Heartshire Project is finally under way. But the *rank and file GPs* still need to be brought on board.

The public health team, experienced and shrewd, decide against *educational events, local guidelines*, or *contractual arm-twisting* – all of which they think will merely provoke an abreaction. They choose instead to exploit *good professional networks* and 'work with the grain'. They work through *practice managers, nurses* and *popular opinion leaders* so that when the GPs come to (small, routine, local, informal) educational events they are already 'warmed up'. Once the GPs are engaged in the Project they receive not the usual high profile *mass mailings* associated with such projects, but personalized *'bite-sized' communications* (an important innovation introduced by the Project manager) about progress. *The Project team*, who have now succeeded in getting GPs to take seriously an information pack that outlines the evidence, achieve widespread commitment to an audit of the developing service. They have also engaged *patients* directly through information leaflets and the local *Community Health Council*. The patients are reminding doctors about the evidence.

By 1999 The Heartshire Project is one of the few real successes among nearly fifty such Queens Trust projects around the UK. Elsewhere, many have made little impact; they have run into disputes about the evidence, inter-professional rivalries, bad blood between key players, funding difficulties, poor management, ineffectual education events, misguided publicity programmes and so on and so on. In Heartshire, though, all but a handful of over seventy GP practices are signed up to the new echocardiography service. They are keenly auditing the service and show that more than three-quarters of them are now using the new referral protocols for echocardiography, prescriptions for ACE inhibitors have risen by around a fifth and diuretic use has fallen by a third. The collective mindline has been changed.

Trust, the hospital consultants, the GPs, the patients, the managers or even the Department of Health? In terms of their impact on changing the mindline, were they context or key actor? The answer is surely that they were all both, and that they were all continually and inextricably related.

The second conclusion is that the Heartshire GPs radically shifted their practice as a result of a wide and densely woven web of interconnected actors and actions, circumstances and attitudes, events and objects.[15] Would the GPs have altered their mindlines if the cardiologist had been determined to keep control? If the drug company had not paid for the echocardiograph? If the health authority had made heavy-handed contractual demands rather than hiring a project manager? If the project manager had been incompetent? If alienating mailshots had thumped onto their desks? If the ACE inhibitors had produced unpleasant side effects in the early patients? Judging from the other Queens Trust projects, the answer is no (Dunning *et al.* 1999; Dopson *et al.* 2001). Following the work of Bruno Latour, Michael Callon and others (Latour 1987, 1999a, 2005; Callon 1986; Prout 1996; Timmermans and Berg 1997; McGrath 2002) we would argue that the dense web of *actors* (as *italicized* in the story) all contributed in some way to the Heartshire GPs' mindlines on heart failure.[16] We have given this example because it was a case study in which all the actors in the story could be studied, something our Lawndale ethnography was not able to do. But the Lawndale discussions that shaped their collective mindline about heart failure (p. 33 and p. 141) were clearly a melange of considerations about many of the 'actors' that were seen in Heartshire: the PCT, the GP contract, electrocardiographs, echocardiograms, local specialists, practice computers, guidelines, questionnaires, referral and appointment systems, reporting systems, drugs, advisory committees, research reports, audits and so on.[17] Neither is it difficult to imagine how the eventual CKD mindline, and therefore the medical management of hundreds of possible CKD patients in Woodsea, was influenced by Whitehall mandarins, US renal researchers, UK nephrology conferences, local guidelines, royal college working parties, primary care trust managers, budgets, guidelines, audits and so on (Box 9.1). Although we are not in a position to delineate exactly how these interacted to influence the eventual outcome, it would be difficult to argue that any was without impact, especially if one applies some of the elements of Giddens's structuration theory. When one follows the path taken by the idea[18] through actors such as these, one encounters Giddens's 'codified structures' (e.g. a guideline committee, the Quality and Outcomes Framework, a practice protocol), his 'social principles' (e.g. evidence-based medicine, clinical freedom, cost containment) and the 'co-presence' of 'agents' (such as leading international nephrologists and local patients' relatives), all of which could be seen as influencing the negotiation of the local CKD threshold at the Lawndale practice meetings. The idea of heart failure, or kidney disease – or, more properly, what was said, written and done about these conditions – seems to have been batted about like the ball in a pinball machine.

The third conclusion is that the story does not deal with one entity, heart failure. The pinball's path is much more complicated than first appears because on closer inspection it morphs with every interaction. Scientific facts about the disease have been fated to be transformed into many different things by the statements and actions of those who referred to them (Latour 1987). Moreover we find that this pleomorphic pinball seems to exist in many states at once, even though any one actor at any one time can usually envisage only one of those states. Every actor gives a different meaning to the disease, as Annemarie Mol (Mol 2002a,b), Marc Berg (Berg and Mol 1998) and others have demonstrated elsewhere.[19] For the patient, heart failure can be an awful, gasping, life-threatening existence; for the clinical researcher it is a carefully defined set of entry criteria to a randomized trial; to the pharmaceutical drug developer it is a set of intracellular interactions to be interrupted; to the echocardiographer it is a collection of images portraying blood flow; to the manager it is a problem that doctors need to tackle if health service targets are to be met. To the GP, we would suggest, it is a set of patients who resemble a particular set of illness scripts that need to be dealt with according to a particular set of mindlines. For some doctors this meaning may include a deep appreciation of cardiac physiology and pathology; for others it may be more pragmatic – a set of signs and symptoms that have some dimly recalled logical connection and respond to diuretics and other treatments (that by 1999 – in Heartshire at least – at last included ACE inhibitors[20]). As Mol would put it, each type of actor 'performs' a different version of the disease; or putting it another way, each has a socially constructed interpretation that helps them to make sense of the illness and guides what they do, which in turn helps to define the disease. So when the actors come together, when clinician meets researcher, opinion leader meets policy maker, or doctor meets manager, or patient meets doctor, they need to negotiate what they mean by that disease and how it can be dealt with. Given the potential complexities of those interactions and the likelihood not just of misunderstandings but of completely differing ways of construing the subject under discussion, it is a wonder that any generally acceptable decisions are ever reached. Nor is it usually possible to appeal to any one final arbiter, since even the scientific view of the best option for treatment often has many different and differing interpretations when applied to individual cases. Annemarie Mol has provided a detailed analysis of these fearfully complicated matters in an arterial clinic, where the different actors construe the problems of intermittent claudication (roughly speaking, the restricted ability to walk because of blocked arteries in the leg) in incompatibly differing ways. It seems to be an irretrievable conundrum. As Mol wryly observes, the hospital brochure helpfully suggests several telephone numbers for patients to call when deciding which treatment to opt for but there is no number that the professionals or researchers can call, for there is no final arbitration as to which is the definitive way to construe the disease (Mol 2002b: 249).

The EBP movement would contend, of course, that the final arbiter for practitioners is the codified, propositional, formal research-based knowledge about '"the disease and its treatment"'. (Let us designate that level of understanding with triple quotation marks.) They may not suggest a telephone number but they do suggest that clinicians look up, say, the Cochrane database, the research literature or the guidelines for the definitive answer. Underlying that contention is the philosophical assumption that the (context-free) scientifically received view about "'the disease'" (or "'the treatment'") is the gold standard. Yet our findings have highlighted that in practice that may be a false assumption. We have found that knowledge-in-practice-in-context, represented by the collective mindline as negotiated among the relevant communities of practice, is the actual arbiter about how to deal with the "disease and its "treatment". (Let us designate this level of understanding with double quotation marks to make the distinction.) The "disease" (collective mindline) is of course strongly informed by the "'disease'" (formal knowledge), but, because it is also highly contextualized and takes account of the conflicting roles and goals of practice, it is a different construction.[21] Who is to say which construct the clinician should use when faced with a patient who brings another set of illness constructs and contexts (Table 9.1) that the two of them must negotiate as they jointly make sense of what is wrong and what to do about it?

Patients

We finally bring our argument to the dyadic interaction between a clinician's mindlines and the patient's understanding of their illness.

❖   *Lara's patient is a senior teacher from Urbcester College who has been enduring a serious professional trauma in his job. He – presumably a 'ten' (p. 167) – is already on tablets for his blood pressure, and may well need tablets to quell his constant anxiety, but he won't consider them because 'they may numb my thinking and I need all my wits about me'. 'How would you feel if I started pushing you on that?' she says. He admits that the counsellor that he has been seeing has told him 'it is possible to be too strong' in these situations when it could be better to accept support. He thinks for a while and says he will consider the pills. Lara backs off. Then he requests a flu jab even though he is under sixty (the age when influenza vaccinations become automatic on the NHS) because he is prone to chest infections, he says. Lara ducks the decision for now and says, 'Ask the nurses – they're the bosses.' Finally Lara turns to his blood pressure problem. As she checks it he jokingly criticizes her technique. They laugh. 'Your BP's always been hit and miss', she says, getting serious again. 'There are no hard and fast rules but it's higher than I'd want it to be.' She suggests a beta blocker. He asks about side effects and jokes about cold feet in bed, and then more seriously queries if a slow heart will make him tired when (thinking of his crisis at the college) he needs to be alert, and whether once started the new pills will need to carry on for ever, which clearly concerns him. She is honest and says where he may be right and where not. 'Want some thinking time?' 'Yes, I'd prefer that.' They agree a date to discuss it further. I ask Lara afterwards why she chose not to push him harder to take either lot of tablets. 'Just coz I sort of know him. There comes a time when "today's the day!" but today wasn't quite it. I know the boxes aren't ticked [i.e. she hasn't done all that is technically and contractually required], but you can see why. I can't just push him – and I know he wouldn't listen if I did. He* started on antihypertensives yonks ago and he just ditched them. And I have to admit I still don't know why.'

❖ Ben is in the office next door seeing a recent Slav immigrant. 'I take pastemol. I kolt. Haul body pen. Dip pen. Not slaffen.' Ben asks her in slow, clear English, 'What do you think is wrong? What could I do to help?' – which is typical of his style; let the patient lead. 'You doctor. You look!' comes the riposte. He eventually concludes that she has flu with widespread joint pain that keeps her awake and has tried paracetamol to no avail. He examines her carefully. 'I think it is an infection. It will get better soon. No need for antibiotics. I will give you stronger pain killer', he repeats deliberately and emphatically, hoping she may eventually have understood.

❖ Lara sees an articulate young Jamaican woman with asthma, a chest infection and thyroid disease. There is a long discussion about what effect she thinks 'the brown inhaler' (corticosteroids) and 'the blue inhaler' (salbutamol) are having. The woman has almost run out of inhalers and has been using her son's to make sure she didn't. As they check the peak flow and discuss past and present results, the figures fly back and forth between them: 370 . . . 450 . . . 350. 'If it goes below 300 at night we need to know', Lara tells her. They talk about antibiotics and decide to start her on a course. The patient asks in passing about 'the thyroid test'. As they talk around it, seemingly in circles, Lara suddenly realizes that the woman is taking 50 mg of thyroxin, not the prescribed 150 mg. The patient admits 'I just don't like taking tablets.' In fact she had stopped taking it at all for a while but then felt worse and started back on 50 mg. She has been fearful of the thyroid pills making her hyperactive again. The tone of the discussion relaxes but the content intensifies. They pore over the screen together, looking at her thyroid test results, and another set of numbers is batted around. Lara is calm and persuasive, the patient is softening. They chat about how her kids are doing at school. They compromise – 50 mg and 100 mg on alternate days and retest in a month, when she is here anyway seeing the asthma nurse.

❖ Back at Lawndale Audrey sees one of Nick's patients and explains to him in simple terms that he may find 'it's a bit difficult for fluids to wash their way down'. 'Oh yes', says the patient knowledgeably. 'My achalasia often does that and actually the peristalsis even stopped completely this morning.' Audrey rapidly adjusts her consultation style!

❖ Jean is seeing a seventy-year-old ex-shopkeeper with long-standing asthma. The conversation sounds like two doctors talking: rapid, full of technical jargon, elliptical and straight to the point.

❖ A mildly diabetic patient, who has an impressive knowledge of how to monitor and control his blood sugars by dieting, seems firmly in control and to be simply checking back with Peter as they carry on a highly technical conversation. But then it becomes clear that the patient has misunderstood food labelling and also believes that if he moves from pills to insulin he will have to give up driving for a living. The nature of the consultation changes as Peter explains more about the relevant physiology and pharmacology before they agree a new management plan.

Table 9.1   Distinguishing different (interdependent) levels of constructs about illness and disease

Conceptual level	"'Disease'"	"Disease"	'Disease'
What it is	Context-free, research-based theoretical, formal (a.k.a. codified, canonical, propositional) knowledge	Collectively developed knowledge-in-practice-in-context (collective mindlines)	A clinician's personal knowledge and beliefs about a clinical condition (their individual mindlines)
Who holds it (e.g.)	Theorists, researchers, textbook authors, examination candidates, EBP systematic reviewers	Communities of practice	Individual practising clinicians
Where it is found (e.g.)	In textbooks, formal lectures, exam papers, research papers and reviews, protocols, guidelines	In discussions between clinicians, 'story-swapping', local practice 'protocols' and routines	In the clinician's mind, where it develops implicitly and continually throughout their career
How it is manifested (e.g.)	As definitive statements about current knowledge and the state of the art (e.g. textbooks, reviews, and leader articles in journals)	Revealed by discussions and disagreements and by routines; partly captured and reified in local 'protocols'	Although often tacit it is revealed through clinical decisions and their expressed rationalizations
When it is used (e.g.)	In lectures, courses, exams, research, systematic reviews, guidelines committees	When seeking local pragmatic ways to deal in context with practical problems	Whenever a clinician is faced with a clinical problem

Notes: (1) These constructs are just some of the main possible constructs that might be distinguished. (2) They are interdependent and mutually constitutive, in that, e.g., "'disease'" and "disease" shape each other. (3) They refer to real phenomena, but only as experienced/

❖   *An eighty-two-year-old lady with swollen legs tells Peter 'I'm wondering if it's the lymph system. Somebody was telling me they knew someone who went to Westchurch and was given some instructions about exercises and pressure points. I'm hoping to do something like that about it – or maybe special shoes. I was told it's varicose veins but I don't think so because I haven't got any, have I?' Peter looks carefully and agrees she hasn't. They have a laugh about the special stockings that she tried but which were not fashionable enough for her. He suggests a store that sells nicer ones. While he examines her chest and checks her blood pressure, they discuss her diuretics, and she says she doesn't want to increase her water tablets. She shows*

Illness–disease	'Illness'	"Illness"	"'Illness'"
The negotiated construct of a particular instantiation that the clinician and individual patient can work with	*A person's knowledge, beliefs and experiences of their (or their charge's) clinical condition; 'the patient narrative'*	*The common beliefs about a clinical condition held by a person's network(s)*	*The general public's belief (Zeitgeist) about a clinical condition*
The clinician–patient dyad, who continually 'negotiate' what they understand the illness–disease to be and how to act	*A person who feels unwell or who is receiving attention from a clinician*	*Those who influence the person, such as family, workmates, friends, patient organizations*	*No one and everyone (i.e. it is diffuse and heterogeneously distributed but nonetheless very pervasive)*
In the consultation process of (joint) sensemaking and decision making	*In the person's perception of their experience, or that of their responsible carer*	*In what is said in discussions among, e.g., family, friends, workmates or patient groups*	*The media, health books, fiction, public dialogue; political and policymaking circles*
As the content of discussion, e.g. the explanations and stories shared, the choices and decisions made, the actions taken	*The person's behaviour, utterances and actions concerning their clinical condition*	*As stories, images, myths and ideas expressed, e.g., in the form of metaphors; by the group's behaviours*	*Media articles, TV programmes, films, novels, urban myths, political statements, public policies, health campaigns*
Throughout the consultation and its aftermath	*When consulting (or not) a clinician or taking (or not) their advice and prescriptions*	*Whenever the clinical condition is being discussed*	*It informs most discussions about the condition, whether public or private*

perceived/envisioned. (4) The term disease or illness includes what it is and how to manage it. (5) Our study did not directly give us empirical data about the illness constructs, and the italicized columns are therefore merely speculative suggestions.

him how she massages her calves (in the wrong direction, which he doesn't notice). He explains about gravity and venous return and 'sluggish circulation', and talks about keeping moving and raising her legs whenever she can. She comes back to the 'pressure points' idea and asks him about acupuncture. He promises to 'ask around' and see if it might help and meanwhile recommends that she goes to the nurse the moment she sees the slightest damage to the skin. I reflect how this whole consultation has been a (still unfinished) joint search for common ground, a shared narrative, to make sense of the problem so that they can agree what best to do about it.

❖   At coffee Audrey, having just sketched out her usual routine for a patient with hypertension, tells us a story from her husband's practice where word got round town that pineapples were good at lowering blood pressure. No idea where it came from but it made it harder to keep patients' blood pressures under control until they were 're-educated' into sticking to their blood pressure tablets as prescribed rather than scoffing lots of pineapples. Part of her routine for hypertension is to always be on the lookout for similar myths that might stop 'compliance'.

❖   Clive happens to see two depressed patients in a row. The first is a middle-aged man worried about a recent anxiety attack. Clive explores it in some depth, getting him to open out, and then he explains about the 'chemicals in the brain'. They discuss various options. No prescription. The second is an elderly lady patient who is losing her eyesight and has had a recent family/financial trauma. Clive knows her well and does not engage. She doesn't seem to think she is depressed as such – just that she can't cope and wants to talk about it; but he seems to have decided almost straight away that there is little he can do to help in these circumstances other than prescribe an antidepressant. Several times as she starts to relate her woes, he deftly cuts her off and steers the conversation firmly back to the antidepressants track. I later point out the remarkable contrast between the two consultations, but Clive claims he has a pretty regular way of dealing with mild to moderate depression. (He reels it off so fast for me that I don't manage to note it down. I recall that it includes three stages of acceptance and discussion leading to antidepressants only if necessary after at least a ten-day period, when over a third of people no longer feel they need them.) He also compares and contrasts rapidly for me the pros and cons of the three main antidepressants he uses and I ask how he arrived at that shortlist. Having heard a respected local psychiatrist say in a lecture that almost all antidepressants are pretty similar in their effects, Clive now just sticks to the three he knows and has got to know more about their effects and side effects through accumulated experience. I ask what would change his mind. 'Certainly not some trial done by psychiatrists on very different groups of patients', he snorts, 'which is what most of the "expert" opinion is inevitably based on.'

❖   Jean very sympathetically discusses possible treatments with a mildly depressed lady around fifty-five years old who feels that antidepressants are a sign of 'giving in'. They agree to try, in ascending order depending how it goes, oil of evening primrose, St John's wort, hormone replacement therapy, antidepressants. 'Whose pecking order was that? Yours or hers?' I ask afterwards. 'Both – probably more hers.' Jean says she has learnt a lot about herbal remedies for mild depression from general reading and from patients themselves. She tells me that some 80 per cent of patients have got some kind of psychological component to their complaint; a lot of patients are depressed perhaps without realizing or admitting it because there is a stigma about it and they are worried about addiction to antidepressants. Asked how she copes with such a high load of psychological problems, she replies 'It's common sense really.' She denies any particular training in psychiatry or even in primary care mental health. Jean has read some textbooks but frankly they aren't much help, she says. And then she goes on to explain how she tends to handle mild depression, what the options are – including medication, local counselling and her own attempts at counselling – and it becomes clear that, although she may not claim to have very much formal knowledge, she is a pretty expert 'amateur' whose 'common sense' is actually very sophisticated and honed by years of learning.

Although the clinician's mindline and its social origins may be abstract and virtual notions, when the clinician and the patient interact the mindline must produce a practical, concrete outcome. For it is at this point that we see the final co-construction: the clinical action. That action results from the negotiation[22] between the differing meanings that the clinician and patient attribute to the patient's illness.[23] The clinician has in mind the 'disease' and its 'treatment' (their individual mindline, for which let us now use single quotation marks); and the patient has their view. Obviously there are always differences between them (Kleinman 1988; Herxheimer and Ziebland 2000; Gabriel 2000), but what those differences were in the consultations we observed we are unable to say because we did not interview patients and can therefore only indirectly infer the constructs that they had about their illnesses.[24] We will therefore draw here upon the findings of a different study that JG was involved in (Johnston *et al.* 2007) in which seventy-nine patients and their supporters and thirty-two GPs were interviewed to explore in depth their views about just one illness, mild to moderate depression.

Unsurprisingly the study found a wide spectrum of views about the place of antidepressants. Participants varied as to where their views lay on almost every set of dimensions one might care to think of when trying to understand the nature of mild depression and its treatment: where the boundary lies between feeling sad and being depressed; whether depression is a mainly biological or a social phenomenon; whether it is genetically or environmentally caused; if it tends to recur throughout life or tends to be a one-off occurrence; if it stems from early life experiences or current ones; whether external pressures or internal psychological problems are the more likely cause; whether it is an extension of the human condition or a distinct disease; whether it betrays a moral weakness or a biochemical imbalance; whether counselling is likely to help; whether the doctor should help the patient live with the depression or help them get rid of it; whether doctors have any useful part to play or not; and so forth. There was no obvious pattern: among both patients and GPs there were some who tended towards, say, a biological explanation and the use of pills and others who focused on the psychosocial and tried to avoid antidepressant prescriptions. The point here is that it was inevitable that, when a doctor and a patient met, there were always likely to be considerable differences in at least some aspects of their perceptions of the very thing the consultation was about (as with the depressed elderly lady who wanted to talk when Clive had decided there was no point).[25] Even when there is little overlap between their differing views, the management of the problem rests upon how they succeed in negotiating those differences, as with the woman with acne (p. 114), when Audrey explained about the benefits of going to the gym as a first step towards treating the depression that the woman had not thought she had. On each occasion, therefore, there has to be a negotiation (often unawares, p. 138) between the two constructs, the outcome of which depends on the differences across the many dimensions of each party's understandings of the phenomena of the illness, and their mutual ability to alter their prior views (Figure 9.1). The examples of Peter's knowledgeable diabetic patient, who had nevertheless misunderstood about food content and the risk of insulin, and Lara's Jamaican asthmatic with hypothyroidism show that this is by no means confined to relatively imprecise conditions such as depression.

We have seen how the doctors' mindlines are a social construct. But the patient's views are of course also a social construct – he or she will have acquired them through their life experience, their family history, their friends, their reading, their exposure to media discussions of depression and so on, and these in turn may be influenced by wider forces such as the views of politicians, psychiatrists, celebrities, the pharmaceutical industry, self-help and other books, and so forth. He or she has acquired their view of the disease through what Berger and Luckmann (1966) call the 'primary socialization' of general upbringing and social experience (p. 173). That construct is derived through its own elaborate web of actors and interactions, equivalent to that of the Heartshire actor-network example (Box 9.1), and is shared among their own communities of practice – for example of family, friends and neighbours who have experienced similar problems.

Thus, when doctor and patient meet, they are not just bringing divergent concepts of the illness; they are mediating two explanatory models (Kleinman *et al.* 1978) comprising quite different social constructs[26] each of which is tightly bound into the collective view of their respective communities of practice and the wider web of sources that feed and shape that view (represented by the two large, layered triangles in Figure 9.2). At the very least (p. 162), the doctor must be 'heedful' (Weick and Roberts 1993) of the patient's views, as well as all the factors that will shape how they apply their mindline on this particular occasion. The outcome of that interaction, their co-constructed view of what is wrong and what to do is what we shall call the illness–disease (represented in Figure 9.2 by the star shape formed by the overlapping tips of the triangles), which will depend on how they negotiate their two socially embedded constructs. (For particularly enlightening detail on the social rituals, ploys and organizational institutions that shape that negotiation see, for example, Strong 1979; Silverman 1983, 1987.) In a firmly doctor-led encounter, the patient's constructs are merely swept aside. After all, the doctor's construct is robustly supported by a dense web involving respected experts, royal colleges, textbooks, guidelines, Nobel laureate neuroscientists, the Department of Health, global pharmaceutical giants and the long-accumulated power and authority of the profession and more. With such a powerful web of support, when Clive was minded to impose his view on the depressed lady then the patient's web was no match for it. At least not until perhaps she got home and recovered her confidence in her own worldview, maybe boosted by experiences that did not accord with his newly imposed view of her depression or by swapping stories with her own community of practice that help reinforce her original views so that she didn't take the pills. In contrast, one patient in our depression study (Johnston *et al.* 2007) told the interviewer: 'When I went to see one of the doctors for the first time, um, he basically tried to say [. . .] that I wasn't depressed. Um, and sort of his view was that a person who is depressed is what I see as sort of very far down the scale, you know.' She then related a triumphant story of how she talked it through with her partner, who 'sort of said that's not good enough

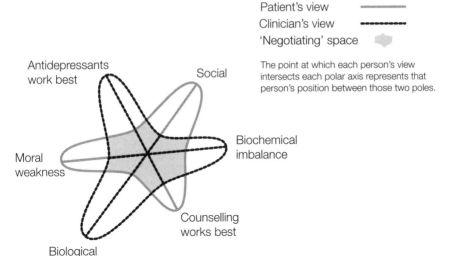

Patient's view ————
Clinician's view ••••••••••
'Negotiating' space

The point at which each person's view intersects each polar axis represents that person's position between those two poles.

Antidepressants work best

Social

Biochemical imbalance

Moral weakness

Counselling works best

Biological

Figure 9.1 Three of the many dimensions that shape the negotiating space in a depression consultation.

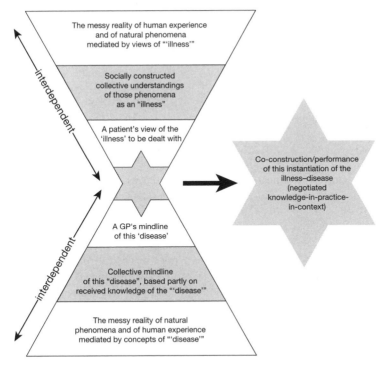

The messy reality of human experience and of natural phenomena mediated by views of '"illness"'

Socially constructed collective understandings of those phenomena as an "illness"

A patient's view of the 'illness' to be dealt with

interdependent

Co-construction/performance of this instantiation of the illness–disease (negotiated knowledge-in-practice-in-context)

A GP's mindline of this 'disease'

interdependent

Collective mindline of this "disease", based partly on received knowledge of the '"disease"'

The messy reality of natural phenomena and of human experience mediated by concepts of '"disease"'

Figure 9.2 The emergence from two sets of social constructs of a co-constructed single instantiation of an illness–disease in a consultation.

really. [Laughs] He was ready to march back to the doctor's with me.' The couple did so the next day and fortuitously saw a locum GP. She got her antidepressants.

GPs are now strongly encouraged by the profession to always attempt a patient-centred consultation, taking the trouble to elicit the patient's own views, concerns and expectations. This helps to build a shared view of the problem and a firm, well-understood commitment to managing it (Elwyn *et al.* 1999a,b; Elwyn 2004; Griffin *et al.* 2004). In an ideal consultation it is vital that the clinician explore the patient's construct in order to find some common ground upon which to build the negotiation, which may or may not be a shared narrative (Launer 2002, 2006). Achieving that overlap is much easier if the clinician is working from their mind-line rather than a formal protocol or guideline. One reason for this is obviously the flexibility of mindlines compared with protocols – helped of course by a mindline's being not a thing but a process that can duck and weave through the inevitable tensions and negotiations. Another is that, as we clearly found in the depression study, clinicians are by no means restricted in their thinking to their clinical knowledge. The GP, like everyone else, has undergone primary socialization. She too has suffered family and personal experiences of sadness and depression, read the newspaper articles about Prozac, seen the TV shows featuring famous depressives, talked with friends about their experiences of healthcare and formed her own non-professional views that also inform her mindline (Gattuso *et al.* 2005). The secondary socialization (Chapter 4) that has taught her how to think about brain chemistry and to behave as a doctor does not and cannot completely replace the constructs, the *habitus*, that she has developed simply as a member of society through primary socialization like everyone else (p. 173). Her mindline is therefore inevitably informed by those underlying views, and as such is a much more likely source of common ground with the patient than are the received views expressed in textbooks and guidelines.

In all but the most doctor-led of encounters, therefore, the final instantiation of the patient's illness–disease, whilst of course containing elements of the received view ('"disease"') and collective mindline ("disease") as carried in the clinician's mindlines, emerges as a negotiation between their own clinical mindline ('disease') and the patient's construct ('illness'). Sometimes, as with Jean and the asthmatic ex-shopkeeper, the patient's and doctors' models are almost indistinguishable. Other times they may use stories as boundary objects to help their negotiation (p. 120). Sometimes the co-construction succeeds, sometimes not (Sharf 1990; Clark and Mishler 1992; Eggly 2002). Where it does succeed it may not always be a good thing: it may fall foul, for example, of what Armstrong (1983) has described as a doctor–patient space that intrudes with ever more pernicious surveillance into the very being of the patient.

Be that as it may, the patient and clinician emerge with a particular formulation, more or less shared, of what is wrong and what to do. The unique version of the illness–disease that they have co-constructed and performed then feeds back into the continuing development of their own (and hence their community's) constructs. It contributes, in other words, both to how the patient manifests their illness in future and to the mindline that the clinician uses when next managing this or any other patient with a similar problem. Moreover, the episode may become a story to be told to others, making it easier to find its way into the discussions among the clinician's community of practice and thence into the collective mindline. If similar experiential evidence accumulates, the collective mindline will inevitably diverge from – and may even eventually subvert – the received view that is codified in textbooks and guidelines.[27] When that happens, who knows whether the clinician is right or wrong to follow the collective mindline? And if they do, who is to say they are ignoring 'the evidence'?

Chapter 9: Summary

We explain how several influential social theories help illuminate the deeper aspects of clinical mindlines, exploring how, for example, collective mindlines exemplify many of the features of the *habitus* (Bourdieu) and of structuration (Giddens). Such theories describe social processes that are much more powerful than any formal measures aimed at controlling (or even describing) individual and collective clinical behaviour. They also permit us to understand how mindlines might be shaped by, and contribute to, wider social structures. We present several worked examples that illustrate the way clinical knowledge and practice are socially constructed and interact with patients' constructs to inform mindlines.

10   Conclusions and implications

Summary: what have we concluded about practice-based evidence?

❖ *(Chapter 1)* We used ethnographic methods to see what we could learn from observing the way that high-quality clinicians actually use knowledge because we wanted to understand how research evidence, as advocated by the evidence-based practice movement, might be better incorporated into their practice. After several years of ethnography, mainly in primary care, supplemented by observations in teaching hospitals and a great deal of reflection and reading around the many academic disciplines that touch on the topic, a much clearer picture seems to have emerged that may help to explain why the EBP movement has had such a difficult time in persuading front-line clinicians to espouse its methods.

❖ *(Chapter 2)* Our early observations confirmed that clinicians tended not to make direct use of guidelines, systematic reviews and other formal sources of knowledge or research evidence while practising, but neither did they ignore them. In fact they seemed to acquire new ideas from a very wide range of sources. They needed to because they needed a very wide range of types of knowledge to deal with everyday practice. We quickly realized that clinicians, especially in primary care, constantly needed to resolve many competing roles and goals, balancing, for example, the therapeutic, preventive, managerial and wider professional aspects of their work. The resultant tensions continually shaped much of what they did, but were rarely addressed by the formal knowledge promulgated by advocates of EBP. The instantly accessible tacit guidelines in the clinicians' heads – their mindlines – were much better suited for that purpose, not least because they encompassed many more factors relevant to the competing tensions, but also because they did so with a practicable plasticity based on collective experience.

❖ *(Chapter 3)* The next question, therefore, was how do mindlines work? This led us to review what is known about the way clinicians think, which has been widely researched in the last forty years or so. Experienced clinicians do not usually need to apply deductive logic but instead tend to recognize patterns, often apparently instantaneously. These have been variously referred to as illness scripts, heuristics and rules of thumb, but those terms refer only to the clinical aspect of the practitioners' work, and not the other roles and goals that they simultaneously need to deal with. Nor do they include the skills, norms, attitudes and infrastructural demands and constraints that shape every clinician's thinking. Mindlines, which are a much less reductionist concept than has previously been used to describe clinical pattern recognition, are able to incorporate all of these much wider but equally important aspects of practical knowledge. Moreover it is these additional components that constitute the difference that has long been recognized between the (variously labelled) formal, canonical, propositional, codified knowledge advocated by the EBP movement and the tacit, personal, practical, 'phronetic' knowledge that professionals use to deal with the messy reality of practice. We refer to the latter as knowledge-in-practice-in-context. We concluded, then, that mindlines may well be highly adapted to clinical practice in ways that codified knowledge and simple illness scripts can never be.

❖ *(Chapter 4)* This next led us to explore how mindlines are acquired and updated during training and beyond – which we did partly through the literature and partly by observing the training of students and junior doctors. We concluded that, from their earliest training, clinicians are continually absorbing an inseparable mix of basic sciences, technical skills, practical knowledge, soft skills, cultural values, socialized attitudes, institutional norms, routinized behaviours and so on, and doing so usually in an inextricably practical context as they undergo what is to all intents an apprenticeship. These and other forms of knowledge are being continually built into their mindlines in such a way as to lose their original identity in the resultant knowledge-in-practice-in-context. There is an analogy between mindlines and a fine sauce being blended from its many original ingredients, or (to echo the famous 'garbage-can' theory of decision making) the manner in which disparate garden and kitchen waste thrown into a bin can result in excellent compost. All three result in something unrecognizable from the original material deposited, something safe and fit for purpose only if the right material, however incongruent, is processed in the right way.

❖ *(Chapter 5)* Drawing upon influential educational models we examined how, throughout their careers, clinicians acquire the expertise that allows them to act with what we call the 'contextual adroitness' that is missing not only in beginners and trainees, but also in established experts who are new to a particular role or organization. Even when they have achieved contextual adroitness, however, clinicians must constantly absorb changes in the environment, including new information about best practice, and we therefore went on to investigate how that happens. Using models drawn from the field of knowledge management, we concluded that new information goes through a series of social processes before being internalized in the clinicians' mindlines. They gather new ideas from many varied sources (of which research evidence is but one) and then (usually collectively) share and discuss these, combining them with their own and each other's tacit and experiential knowledge before either incorporating them into their local policy or internalizing them (or not) into their mindlines.

❖ *(Chapter 6)* Much of that discussion takes a narrative form. Stories and anecdotes, social psychologists tell us, are the most effective, efficient and deep-seated ways by which we all communicate; they are often much more powerful than the kind of rational discourse to which clinical scientists aspire. We therefore delved into the nature of narrative discourse (storytelling) and showed how fundamental it was to the 'social life' of clinical knowledge, not only in communications between clinicians but also with their patients.

❖ *(Chapter 7)* This moved us onto the role of communities of practice, groups of people who share practical interests, problems and passions and talk informally to each other about them as a way of sharing and learning knowledge-in-practice-in-context. We found many examples of such communities and/or loose professional networks both within and outwith the group of clinicians we were observing. Much of the development of their clinical mindlines appeared to take place through the medium of those communities of practice. Clinicians were processing new information, assessing its value, and incorporating it into their mindlines (usually in transmuted form) or rejecting it. It was through their informal chat that the clinicians gave clinical knowledge the 'social life' that was an essential part of its eventually being used or discarded.

❖ *(Chapter 8)* One crucial outcome of the communities of practice was the formulation of *collective* mindlines that were providing a flexible, bounded, implicit local touchstone for practice norms. Through their informal discussions, the participants were engaged in ceaseless mutual refinement of both their individual and their collective mindlines as they tried to make collective sense of the incessant challenges to their current practice from, for example, anomalous experiences, unexpected events or new ideas, techniques and evidence. This socially based process of constantly crafting and reformulating of mindlines seemed well suited to resolving the shifting requirements that shape the way clinicians practise as professionals. As a result, both their knowledge (e.g. concepts of a disease and its management) and their practice, and hence clinical outcomes, could and did change as the clinicians collectively 'constructed' and reconstructed their knowledge-in-practice-in-context.

Moreover that social process was also instrumental in helping the clinicians assert control over their own identity and activity as professionals.

❖ *(Chapter 9)* Finally we ventured into some swirling sociological and philosophical waters to try and understand the significance of the way this 'social construction' of disease and clinical practice was occurring. Using social theory to examine the ways in which mindlines are essential to the way in which individual clinicians link with the 'social forces' that shape health services, we found that this linked closely also with the way mindlines are important in maintaining the roles and status of clinical professions. Most importantly, they provide the mechanism – in ways that formal knowledge does not – that allows them to deal with each individual instance of what we call the illness–disease that clinicians and patients co-construct during each clinical consultation. We distinguished the illness–disease from its representation in the knowledge-in-practice-in-context of individual mindlines ('disease'), from that in collective mindlines ("disease"), from "'disease'", the referent of the codified knowledge of clinical science and canonical evidence. The fundamental differences between these formulations, and between the ways that different actors (clinicians, patients, researchers, policy makers) construe the disease and its appropriate management at different times, make it inevitable that formal guidance (which is chiefly about "'disease'") largely fails to connect directly with actual practice (which deals with "disease", 'disease' and illness–disease).

Our analysis of mindlines therefore made it difficult to escape the conclusion that the current assumptions of the EBP movement are misguided about both the nature of evidence and the context of its use. Adding new pieces of research information to mindlines and expecting 'knowledge transfer' to occur is like adding leaves to the compost bin and expecting to see them on your flower beds next year.

There is, however, a twist in the tale: mindlines don't exist. As astute readers will have gathered, mindlines are not *entities* at all. The word is just a shorthand reminder of the complexity of the social and psychological *processes* that one is trying to alter when implementing research findings, promoting guidelines or promulgating EBP. But that does not mean that, because we have found mindlines to denote something that 'we cannot speak about, we must pass over [them] in silence' (Wittgenstein 1974 [1922]: 74). Nor should we, now having climbed it, 'throw away the ladder' (ibid.). On the contrary, there are patients to treat, clinicians to educate, health systems to improve. There are no actual mindlines, but by the same token neither are there any definitive "'diseases'", only a bewildering confusion of 'disease' and "disease" constructions, a cacophony of conflicting narratives and illness–diseases; and yet there continue to be ill patients, knowledgeable clinicians and unceasingly variable clinical practice. We would therefore rather that everyone used whatever ladders are available to help them be mindful of all the evidence both *about* practice and *for* practice. But we must begin by examining the robustness or not of our ladder.

What do we still need to find out?

Ours has been an initial foray into complex areas many of which have not been applied to this field before. Our fieldwork has been limited to a few sites, and our analysis, as we freely admit, has inevitably been partial in every sense of that word. There has probably never been a research report that does not conclude that more research is needed[1] and there is certainly much to be done to both test our findings and take them much further. As we hope this book has demonstrated, there are many kinds of research in many disciplines that should help us to understand better the part that mindlines play in the practical uptake of new knowledge, and we shall give just a few examples here, some of which have yet to be applied to healthcare in the ways that we envisage.

- First and foremost, of course, because we recognize that our analysis is only preliminary, there is the need to replicate our study with other types of practices and organizational milieus, including secondary care (hospital), and with clinicians of different professions, ages, career stages, competence levels and consultation styles. There is also a great deal more detail needed, using other observational and interpretative research methods, before we can really understand the precise ways in which clinicians seek out new knowledge and what they and their patients then do with it. (For examples of the research methods used in organizational research see Orr 1997; Boden 1994; Choo 1998: chapter 2; Czarniawska 1998.) There will also be a need to review and synthesise (as we have only barely begun to do) the findings from the many disciplines relevant to this analysis, so that there may be better use of theory in the design of methods to promote research use (Davies *et al.* 2010).
- More research needs to focus on the social and organizational aspects of innovation and knowledge transfer, rather than the individual uptake of research evidence (Lam 2000; Greenhalgh *et al.* 2004, 2005b; Kitson and Bisby 2008; KT08 Forum 2008).
- The question of the nature of healthcare 'evidence', which has already been partly explored (see, for example, Upshur 2000, 2001; CHSRF 2005a,b), and also of 'context' (e.g. McCormack *et al.* 2002) and the relationship between them (e.g. Dobrow *et al.* 2004) needs further rigorous philosophical and pragmatic exploration. Philosophers might also help to unravel the epistemological and ontological muddle of the morphing pinballs of '"disease"', "disease", illness–disease and so on, since that problem – what is it that the evidence is actually *about?* – lies at the very heart of EBP.

- There is much that we could learn from an anthropological perspective about the 'culture' of EBP (Kleinman *et al.* 1978). For example, what meanings and symbolic values do clinicians and others attribute to different kinds of knowledge and belief (Helman 2000: 33)? What rituals are associated with the way knowledge and beliefs should be discussed (ibid.: 33–38) or with the social 'grammar' of what kinds of knowledge are deemed to be suitable for what occasions (ibid.: 39), and how do these impact on the way people deal with new evidence? (For an international perspective on such matters see also Payer 1996.)

- There will be merit in examining from a sociological and social policy perspective what one might call the 'political economy of clinical knowledge', by which we mean the ways in which the evidence base is structured by its political and economic aspects, for example who has the power to tell whom what to do and why, how the various interests in promotinwg different kinds of evidence collude and collide, how their resources affect their influence, the costs and benefits of EBP; and how the complexities of different types of evidence are – or should be – weighed against each other (Pawson 2006).

- Sociologists, actor-network theorists and historians could also contribute much to our understanding of the social, organizational, professional, political, economic, ethical, cultural and historical origins of EBP (e.g. Latour 2005) as currently practised and how that may militate against the changes that may be needed (see, for example, Harrison 1998; Trinder and Reynolds 2000; Pope 2003; Timmermans and Berg 2003; and, for a parallel approach from the education sector, Tomlinson 2001).

- From a psychological and educational perspective we need to know much more about the potential methods by, and extent to, which mindlines might be elicited and made explicit by individual as well as group reflection – for example using methods pioneered by Garfinkel (1967) and also used by Argyris and Schön (1974), who used the techniques of close, interpretive observation coupled with active reflective commentary to elicit the differing models of organizational behaviour that characterized theory-in-practice. And as Fish and Coles (2005) remind us, there is much research still to be done to understand the educational consequences of developing practice-focused knowledge as opposed to imparting canonical knowledge and competencies.

- Once such work and its synthesis, borrowing methods from these and other disciplines, has helped clarify the processes by which clinicians use knowledge-in-practice-in-context, health service researchers and trialists might be better placed to design intervention studies such as trials that are designed both quantitatively and qualitatively to test new methods of introducing sound, high-quality, practice-based evidence. Nevertheless, we hope that it is not premature to begin to tackle the final question to which we now turn (Box 10.1).

Box 10.1 Reflective summary points for improving practice-based evidence

- Move beyond the rhetorical debates about what EBP is or is not and pursue the practical question of how the best evidence of all kinds might best be combined, internalized and used in the best ways.
- Acknowledge that health care *and* knowledge transfer are complex, diffuse, organizational processes rather than simplistic linear rational ones.
- Work with the grain of practice and encourage the discussion, debate and modification which ensure that evidence is refined appropriately into knowledge-in-practice-in-context, rather than criticize practitioners for non-implementation of decontextualized evidence.
- Encourage opportunities for learning and sharing knowledge that build on the social processes instrumental to the development of collective and/or individual mindlines and practice.
- Promote organizational structures and routines that value and support the exposure of tacit knowledge and the use of various forms of knowledge-in-practice-in-context through the social processes necessary for knowledge uptake and mindline development.
- Introduce research evidence succinctly through sources actually used and trusted by practitioners, and actively engage local communities of practice, expert practitioners and opinion leaders in processing new evidence through active grassroots dissemination and discussion.
- Encourage critical appraisal of *all* sources of evidence, not just research or research syntheses.
- Ensure that standard setting involves those expected to meet targets rather than being imposed unilaterally by those unfamiliar with the relevant knowledge-in-practice-in-context.
- Work *with* clinicians at every stage of their development to grow their mindlines wisely, rather than focus on inculcating 'competencies' *into* them.
- Actively promote closer, more realistic relationships between the worlds of research and practice and research, education and practice. Get active practitioners and other relevant parties involved in all stages of research to ensure that research findings of value are generated which then slip effortlessly into knowledge-in-practice-in-context.

What can we do to improve practice-based evidence?

We, as researcher–authors, cannot now do much more. Our work was driven by a desire to improve the way research findings are put into practice. What we found was that research evidence may not – and indeed cannot and should not – be taken up unquestioningly without being subjected to collective scrutiny by communities of practitioners who understand its practical realities because they live them daily as, for example, practising clinicians, policy makers, managers, educators or health service users. So, however much we as researchers would like our work to be used, how ironically inconsistent we would be if we now tried to dictate how it should be put into practice! If our conclusions are to change anything, it will be because not we the writers but you the reader who is engaged in the practical realities will have worked through the implications of our analysis.

To resolve this paradox, therefore, all we can do is to encourage readers to reflect (collectively, of course, among your own communities of practice . . .) on the feasibility of applying our findings in general, and the notion of mindlines in particular, to help practitioners use new evidence more effectively. It is in that spirit that we offer some pointers (summarized in Box 10.1), many of which feed into existing debates from which we provide a few very selective references to encourage the reader to explore them further. Our, we hope, provocative questions (which sometimes appear mutually contradictory; no one said this was straightforward!) merely betray *our* opinions. What matters, though, are *your* reactions and those of your own communities of practice.

- If knowledge-in-practice-in-context is something people do, not something they have (i.e. it is performative, not substantive), then a fundamental change is needed in the prevalent assumptions about the nature of evidence and knowledge for policy and practice. *Evidence* is not just research-based knowledge that one either has or does not have. Knowledge *transfer* is not just a matter of handing someone a parcel of new evidence, however easy it is to open and however carefully chosen the contents. Knowledge *translation* is not just a question of someone from one world with some new evidence getting someone from a different one to understand it. Knowledge *utilization* is not just about applying or failing to apply evidence when one has found it. They are all complex social processes of *knowledge transformation*. Maybe therefore it is time to move beyond rhetorical debates about what EBP is or is not and whether it is a Good Thing or not[2] and pursue the practical question of how the best evidence of all kinds might best be transformed, internalized and practised in the best ways.

- Is it not time to finally renounce the unhelpful view of healthcare provision as a mechanistic system in which innovation and knowledge transfer is a linear, rational process? There is a great deal of academic work to draw upon, which several authors have recently reviewed, pointing in more complex but ultimately much more promising directions (Van de Ven *et al.* 1999; Dopson and Fitzgerald 2005; Nutley *et al.* 2007; Kitson 2008; Lemieux-Charles and Champagne 2008; Crilly *et al.* 2010). Using the insights from the many relevant disciplines will, however, require all parties to be prepared to learn about the approaches of academic disciplines that are unfamiliar to them.

- Good clinicians do not simply accept, ignore or reject new evidence. How they receive it almost inevitably involves three major components (Choo 1998):
  - a collective social process to try and make sense of the new information and contextualize it;
  - the (again usually collective) reformulation or transformation of research knowledge as it is combined with other knowledge to become knowledge-in-practice-in-context; and
  - some degree of further negotiation of individual practical decisions on each occasion that the knowledge is used.
- New knowledge, it seems, is almost always discussed, contested, debated, combined, before it becomes (or not) part of a clinician's mindlines, and we have seen why that is necessary. Can strategies for knowledge transfer not be designed that explicitly recognize and work *with* that grain rather than (as now) ignore it and expect clinicians simply to accept new ideas because other authorities say they should (and pressurize or berate them if they do not)? An open and interactive approach may be more likely to achieve a satisfactory outcome than a didactic or coercive one.[3]
- Our work suggests not only that practitioners glean new information about best practice from multiple sources, but also that they often require many confirmatory sources (including trusted colleagues) to triangulate it. Does this not at the very least require strategies for introducing research evidence through a wider range of media than at present? Should not those who hope to impart useful information ensure that it is distributed along more of the channels that practitioners actually use and not just the learned journals, official guidelines and websites that the EBP movement, academics, managers and policy makers would prefer them to use? (See, for example, Box 5.1.) A leaf taken from the marketing departments of the pharmaceutical industry (e.g. the use of opinion leaders, well-placed articles and advertorials in non-peer-reviewed professional magazines) might be worth considering, for example.
- On the other hand, the clinical world is awash with guidance and policy initiatives. Assuming there is no democratically acceptable way of stemming this bewildering flood, is there some way in which it might be funnelled, filtered and focused? One possible way to achieve this might be to use specially convened local multidisciplinary/multisectoral groups (which may become communities of practice) to preprocess the new guidance. This would not only solve the problem of channelling the ideas more appropriately, but also mean that before important new information reaches individual clinicians and their communities of practitioners it would have been processed through what some have called 'respectful dialogue' (Nutley *et al.* 2007; le May 2009b) between different communities (clinicians, policy makers, patients, researchers, for example).[4] The aim would be to ensure that the specialists, researchers or policy makers who are hoping to introduce new evidence, but do not have the relevant contextual understanding, engage in intelligent dialogue throughout the innovation process with those who live and understand the

context – rather than, as so often happens now, simply disseminate the evidence or attempt to use techniques of persuasion or coercion.

- Should more effort not be devoted to multifaceted approaches that (i) include both centralized (context-free) and localized (context-specific) evidence, (ii) have a practical and realistic view of what constitutes relevant and legitimate evidence and (iii) recognize the role played by the relevant actors with differing power within the networks involved in implementing evidence? (See, for example, CHSRF 2005a,b). It might also be a way of moving towards what Greenhalgh and Worrall (1997) have called 'EBM Mark III . . . Context Sensitive Medicine'. More effort not only to understand the kind of sources and discourses that practitioners use when processing new knowledge but also to take account of their conflicting organizational roles and goals would help in 'translating' relevant evidence to meet the needs of the various parties involved. Similarly, values, past associations, familiar rituals and many other elements of emotional, moral and practical reasoning also play a part, and need to be understood and taken into account (Van de Ven and Schomaker 2002). Rather than deluging (supposedly) passive individuals with information they find unhelpful, this would entail engaging locally influential actors, who are best placed to provide the detailed and sensitive prior analysis of the local context and the intelligent and facilitative leadership that would ensure apposite, active and appropriate integration of evidence into local systems. (See also Dopson *et al.* 2001; Nutley *et al.* 2007: chapter 10).

- If well-founded advice from colleagues is as crucial to learning and the spread of innovation and best practice as our findings suggest, should we not explicitly structure and fund that activity (e.g. as part of a job profile)? Should we not focus (as the pharmaceutical industry has successfully done for decades) on training opinion leaders both in the detail of the evidence and in the ways of communicating it? The aim must be to ensure that those sources (expert practitioners, local opinion leaders and the collective mindlines they so strongly influence) are not misinformed either about the context-free codified evidence, or about the local detail of context-specific knowledge, or about the strength and validity of colloquial evidence (CHSRF 2005a,b). Might it not also be useful to educate opinion leaders (at all levels – see Locock *et al.* 2001) about the nature and functioning of knowledge networks and communities of practice? Armed with such knowledge, opinion leaders might be more effective in interacting with their clinical colleagues both to promulgate best practice in their own field of expertise and also to learn about the limitations of such practice in cognate fields and different contexts, and hence be more able to relate to those they are hoping to influence.

- Should more not be done to develop and inculcate methods of critically appraising *all* the types of evidence that are melded into mindlines? Even syntheses of different kinds of research evidence are rare (Oliver *et al.* 2005). At present there is an extraordinary imbalance between the efforts that the EBP movement expends on improving the critical appraisal of research and research syntheses, and the almost none on appraising experiential evidence, the views of opinion leaders, narrative evidence from colleagues and so on (le May and Gabbay 2010: 394–396). Yet we have found that clinicians use the latter types of evidence at least as much as the former because the bounded rationality of turbulent practice makes it more efficient to base decisions on accumulated mindlines and/or the views of trusted experts who share one's understanding of the context (Rich 1991), than to consult formal 'evidence' that does not. Clinicians' 'information-seeking heuristics' – the short cuts they have learnt to use – could be developed and strengthened (Box 5.1). A culture of constructively critical enquiry and knowledge exchange might be helped, for example, by developing and rewarding the use of techniques by which clinicians can back up and check up their advice to and from each other as a specific activity.[5] Given that clinicians are always having to appraise knowledge in areas and from sources where they may not personally be fully expert, should there be more of a focus on developing the generic skills of 'interactional expertise' that will enable them to make sound judgements about information coming from outwith their immediate expertise (Collins and Evans 2007)? This may also yield more immediate dividends than the current focus on detailed, scientific critical appraisal skills.

- We have argued that, once clinicians become aware of new guidance or other information, it is collective, social processes that are instrumental in processing and combining it into internalized knowledge-in-practice-in-context. At the very least might it be worth establishing and facilitating communities of practice among practitioners who do not currently work in that way.[6] Given that learning and the development of mindlines is such a fundamentally social process, should the focus of formal learning not be more on collective group processes and less on individual acquisition of knowledge (Timmermans and Berg 2003; Nutley *et al.* 2007)? This would entail the implementers of EBP 'recognizing the primacy of practice' and of 'professional artistry' (Fish and Coles 1998: 297) and engaging more explicitly and in a more facilitative way in the processes of collective critical reflection than they do now (which is very little). Much could be done to help practitioners learn from each other and process new ideas together, perhaps starting by going back to the principles set out by Reg Revans (1998 [1982]) and Michael Balint (1964 [1957]). (See also Gabbay 1991; and especially Launer 2002.) However, if those groups work within different, mutually exclusive communities of practice, it is highly likely that knowledge will 'stick' at the boundaries of their groups (Brown and Duguid 2001). Therefore it would make sense both to foster inclusive, multidisciplinary communities of practice and to develop better means of cross-boundary flow (e.g. making use of 'boundary objects', 'boundary spanning' and other techniques) to help foster communication between them.[7] There may be many ways to achieve this, depending on local circumstance, but knowledge brokers may have a key role to play here (Lomas 2007; Dobbins *et al.* 2009).

- The SECI spiral (Figure 5.2) suggests that a large component of people's knowledge about innovations and best practice comes from surfacing and sharing each other's tacit knowledge. Yet most health systems concentrate instead on trying to feed clinicians with explicit, canonical knowledge and to suppress tacit knowledge. It would surely repay the effort of developing ways of eliciting the richness of tacit knowledge and of making the combination of both types of knowledge more open to scrutiny. Such a process would recognize and encourage the vital part played by general chat and story swapping, but would also insist on, and provide both the techniques and the culture that allow, rigorous questioning and appraisal of the views put forward. There may even be ways of using communities of practitioners to develop expert systems to guide clinical practice in primary care, emulating the success that Scarborough and Swan (2002) report from their work in the hospital sector.[8]

- On the other hand, there is a worrying link between our findings and the existence of variations in clinical practice, in that local collective and individual mindlines can enshrine and perpetuate what are sometimes deplorable variations. That indeed was one of the triggers for EBP in the first place and has led to the increasing regulation and proletarianization of healthcare. Mindlines can spread collective folly. Unfortunately, though, the mantras of EBP do not equate to communal wisdom. It might therefore be worth the effort of developing techniques to capitalize on and to moderate the mindline processes that we have uncovered so as to strengthen the incorporation of both canonical and practical knowledge. It should be possible, for example, to cultivate skills both for eliciting tacit knowledge and for incorporating relevant research knowledge so as to critically evaluate and integrate them more robustly in existing mindlines than is currently often the case. Formally acknowledging and encapsulating both kinds of knowledge may prove more productive than the unhelpful war between clinical freedom and bureaucratic – even if it is 'scientific-bureaucratic' (Harrison and McDonald 2008) – regulation. If mindlines are to be safe and fit for purpose, we need to develop robust processes for linking the illness–disease via the mindlines to the research knowledge about the '"disease"' (and vice versa), so that mindlines reflect not collective folly, nor coercive scientism, but communal wisdom.

- If we accept that the judiciousness of clinical actions can be assessed only by those who understand the full contextual relevance and applicability of the research evidence, is it logical to judge clinical practitioners externally by auditing them against the 'gold standard' of context-free research-based evidence? Perhaps standard setting should be done in conjunction with those expected to meet the targets (or at least their representatives) rather than unilaterally by those unfamiliar with the relevant knowledge-in-practice-in-context. Might target setting and monitoring not be more appropriate if it were done by collective and critical reflection involving people who are not only mindful of the research evidence but also of other forms of evidence, and of the specific context (Ericsson 2009)?

- On the other hand, if the only assessors of practice are like-minded clinicians, there would be a high risk of a 'closed shop' if not outright groupthink. Our findings also point, however, to many routes by which one could safeguard against that. Clinicians in communities of practice have wide networks among clinical and non-clinical colleagues and among their patients. The conclusions drawn by any 'closed' clinical community of practice must be 'testable' by others who are not part of that group, such as local opinion leaders, managers, patient groups and the researchers who produce the evidence. Not only would this avoid any danger of groupthink, but the dialogue would do much to enrich and inform all parties. How can they best be included in such 'deliberative processes' (CHSRF 2005a)? The answer would depend on the local culture and even on the personalities involved – one cannot impose a single model any more than was possible to do so with the difficult early introduction of clinical (especially multidisciplinary) audit (e.g. Gabbay *et al.* 1990). One can, however, insist on the principle.

- If, as we and others have found, collective and individual learning (and teaching) is going on whenever clinicians interact with others (be they colleagues or patients), does our work add weight to the many repeated but all too often still unheeded calls for the education of health professionals to be focused less around the formal curriculum (Fish and Coles 2005) and more around acquiring the practical skills of knowledge-in-practice-in-context and of learning to be sensibly critical of all sources of information? Would mindlines not be more reliable if the continual learning processes that develop them involved well-honed skills in automatically assessing and systematically appraising whatever is being learnt and why? In short, should the habits of 'action learning' (Revans 1998 [1982]; Gabbay 1991) coupled with broad critical appraisal skills not be stressed from the very start of clinical training and continually developed thereafter? If so, then education methods, including continuing education, might be better able to develop practical knowledge in ways that work *with* clinicians to grow their mindlines wisely, rather than the current educational trend of trying to inculcate 'competencies' *into* them. Or, to put it another way, perhaps clinical education should be designed around, and aimed at improving, the way that clinicians actually learn-in-practice-in-context.[9]

- We have seen that knowledge-in-practice-in-context is intimately linked to organizational structure and function. Knowledge management, too, is not simply a technical matter, but an organizational and cultural one. How, then, can one expect knowledge transfer to be optimal if so little regard is paid to the organizational development that needs to accompany it? (See, for example, Crilly *et al.* 2010.) For example, there is little point in exhorting GPs to completely change their management of Stage 3 CKD unless the structures are in place to allow them to do so in ways that work for primary care. EBP may benefit from more explicit attention to context at every stage of knowledge implementation, rather than treating context as the final hurdle for context-free evidence to negotiate (Greenhalgh and Worrall 1997; McCormack *et al.* 2002). Not only is this fundamentally necessary but it has been shown to be pragmatically useful not least because it is well recognized that one way of altering personal routines is to alter the organizational routines in which they are embedded (Evans and Haines 2000).

- There remains the question of designing better ways to produce new knowledge that is relevant to practice, for that in itself will make it more likely that it is used. It has been widely argued that needs-led research (in line with current trends in the research for healthcare commissioning by organizations such as the UK's National Institute for Health Research and the Canadian CHSRF) needs also to become more 'socially distributed'. This means shifting the balance from what has been called 'Mode 1' science (the established model of a-contextual, aloof, narrowly focused and purist research) towards 'Mode 2' science, (actively contextualized, transdisciplinary, organizationally diverse, heterogeneous, socially accountable and reflexive), which would certainly be a way of producing knowledge that is more easily incorporated into mindlines (Gibbons *et al.* 1994). It might also involve moves towards what Fox (2003) has called the 'collaborative and transgressive' research needed for practice-based evidence, for which he envisages breaking down the current divisions between research and practice and encouraging practice-based and practice-led research. Such research should usefully complement positivist (e.g. trials-based) single intervention studies and so help overcome the serious limitations on their external validity and generalizability that currently render their results unhelpful for many practitioners. We do not regard these types of science as being in opposition; far from it. Both are needed, but we hope that the bodies of work we have reported here confirm the value of interpretative research, which has tended to receive a far smaller (but now increasing) share of healthcare research funding than positivist research (Cooksey 2006; Baker *et al.* 2009; O'Neil 2009; NIHR 2010).

- Finally, although the possibility of generalized, codified knowledge that is also context-specific is an oxymoron, research closely linked to the needs of practice and policy – what Van de Ven and Jonson (2006; Van de Ven 2007) call 'engaged scholarship' – is more likely to be absorbed within the collective mindline. The contextual nature of practical knowledge is also an incontrovertible argument for much closer engagement between researchers and, for example, practitioners, policy makers, patients and provider organizations at every stage of the production of research evidence. Producing context-rich, practically helpful research evidence will need much more than the token, often unrepresentative, 'users' currently found on the advisory panels of many research projects. It requires genuine engagement at all stages of a project – identifying and prioritizing research questions and agreeing the methods (e.g. outcome measures that are useful to the users), through to planning the dissemination and implementation (CHSRF 1999; Lomas 1997, 2000, 2007; Ginsburg *et al.* 2007; Oliver *et al.* 2007; Kitson and Bisby 2008; Dobbins *et al.* 2009). Moreover, it is well recognized that practitioners involved in research are more likely to understand its implications and promote its use, which makes it more likely to be incorporated into the mindlines of the communities of clinical practice with whom they work.

We hope that these suggested practical implications of our findings will have stimulated the reader to further discussion and argument, for – as our work has suggested – it is only through you and your communities of practice that innovations and improvements will become absorbed into practice.

Appendix 1   An example of a Lawndale practice guideline

Insulin: tips for Lawndale clinicians

Types of insulin

- There are many types and brand of insulin available but it would make sense to become familiar with a few in the Practice.
- Insulins can be broadly divided into 2 types – human and analogue. Analogue insulins are generally more expensive but have a more user-friendly profile of action and the long acting versions are less likely to cause hypos than human insulins.
- Insulins can also be categorised by duration of action into rapid acting, long acting and mixtures of the two (premixes, also known as biphasic).
- Common, locally used examples are:
  - Analogue rapid – NovoRapid, Apidra
  - Human rapid – Actrapid
  - Analogue long – Lantus, Levemir
  - Human long – Insulatard
  - Analogue premix – NovoMix 30

Insulin regimens

- Once daily basal insulin is the simplest regimen and involves one injection a day of a long acting insulin such as Lantus. It is ideal for type 2 patients new to insulin, patients who need their injections to be given by a carer and those who have a regular eating and exercise pattern.
- Basal-bolus involves Lantus once a day with 3 injections or more of a short acting insulin to coincide with meals. This regimen is closest to what the body normally does and allows flexibility of dosage and timing to match planned eating and exercise. It suits active patients who may work or do sport. Blood sugar control can be excellent but it does entail frequent blood sugar monitoring and at least 4 injections a day.
- Premixed insulins are usually given twice a day and offer some of the benefits of a basal bolus regime without the need for frequent monitoring. Titration and dose adjustment is more complicated.

Insulin devices

- There is a huge variety of glucose meters available. I advise patients to try a selection at the pharmacy (Heather also has some) and buy one that suits them. We prescribe the test strips for the meters – there is an excellent table in Mims that lists which strips are compatible with which devices. There is also a pictorial guide at the back of Mims.
- Insulin is normally injected with a pen device. These are either pre-filled and disposable, or refilled with a cartridge. The pens hold the insulin and a twist dial draws up the required number of units of insulin. Most pens give up to 60 units per injection.
- There are dozens of pen devices available and choice is mostly a matter of patient preference and which are compatible with their insulin(s). Particularly good pens are:
    - Innolet – designed for the visually impaired and those with poor manual dexterity. Provides Levemir or Mixtard 30. Disposable. Novofine needles.
    - Solostar – prefilled with Lantus or Apidra. Takes BD microfine needles.
    - NovoPen 4 – re-usable pen that takes cartridges of NovoRapid, NovoMix 30, Mixtard 30, and Levemir. NovoFine needles.
- Needles – 8mm length most often used. BD microfine or NovoFine.

Practicalities of insulin storage, injecting, and sharps disposal

- Insulin in pens and cartridges will be fine at room temperature for up to 6 weeks.
- Spare insulin should be kept in a fridge but not frozen. Should be removed from fridge at least 30 min before injecting.
- Premixed insulins need resuspending in cartridge by rolling the pen between hands for 1–2 mins.
- Best injection sites are abdomen (fastest absorption), thighs and buttocks. Injection sites should be used in rotation.
- Insulin should not be injected through clothes.
- Needles should only be used once. Sharps boxes and needle clips are prescribable and, locally, collected by the council (contact tel 01*********).

The patient commencing insulin (type 2)

- Continue metformin unless contra-indicated. Sulphonylureas can be continued. Pioglitazone is licensed for use with insulin.
- Normal daily insulin requirement is 0.5 units/kg body weight (ie 35 units for 70 kg patient) and a safe starting dose for long acting insulins is one third of this.
- Lantus is often commenced at 12 units a day and titrated upwards in 2 unit increments every 2–3 days until fasting morning blood sugar is 4–6.

- For basal bolus regimens half the daily insulin requirement is given in long acting form and half as short acting. The short acting insulin is best commenced at two thirds of the predicted amount, divided up over 3 meals according to carbohydrate intake, then titrated upwards according to blood sugar profile.
- Premixed insulins are commenced at two thirds of the predicted daily requirement with the dose being divided equally between the injections. Doses then titrated upwards in 2 unit increments to give a fasting glucose of 4–6.

Insulin dose titration (for those established on insulin)

- Human insulin can be switched to analogue on a dose for dose basis.
- Generally safe to increase or decrease insulin doses in 2–4 unit increments (or about 10% of the dose).
- A profile of blood sugar readings at 4 or more different times over a typical day is a useful starting point (eg pre breakfast and after each meal).
- If pre breakfast glucose high then consider increasing basal insulin.
- If postprandial readings high consider altering timing of oral medication or add/increase short acting insulins.

Insulin and travel

- Don't leave in suitcase when flying – will freeze and be denatured. Take spare insulin, needles etc. in separate bag.
- Coolbag/pouches available for transporting insulin in hot countries.
- Carry extra snacks.
- If crossing time zones, adjust injection times to coincide with meals. Long acting insulin injection time can be altered by an hour a day for a few days prior to travel. If travelling west, insulin dose may need decreasing by up to 20% as days are relatively shorter. If travelling east may need more insulin and more snacks.

Insulin and intercurrent illness (advice for patients)

- Keep taking insulin – dose might need increasing or decreasing depending on blood sugars.
- Try to continue normal meals but, if unable, replace meals with carbohydrate-containing drinks.
- Drink extra fluid.
- Measure blood glucose more often than usual (at least 4 times a day).
- Check for ketones if Type 1 or lean Type 2 if glucose above 15.

Injection site problems

- Rotate injection sites regularly (alternate weekly between left and right body sites, rotate sites within same area inject at least 1 inch away from previous site).
- If site lumpy then stop using until softens and attention to rotating sites.
- If local reaction (redness, irritation, stinging) problem often settles with perseverance. If not consider switching insulin or device.

Appendix 2 Practice chronic kidney disease (CKD) protocol (extract)

1. Background and definitions

CKD classification

Stage 1 (Normal renal function)   eGFR >90 and other evidence of kidney damage
Stage 2 (Mild impairment)   eGFR 60–89 ” ” ”
Stage 3 (Moderate impairment)   eGFR 30–59 (3A 45–59, 3B 30–44)
Stage 4 (Severe impairment)   eGFR 15–29
Stage 5 (Established renal failure)   eGFR <15

$$\text{eGFR (ml/min/1.73m}^2) = 186 \times (\text{plasma creatinine}/88.4)^{-1.154} \times (\text{age})^{-0.203} \times (0.742 \text{ if female}) \times (1.210 \text{ if Afro-Caribbean})$$

- **N.B. We can essentially ignore stage 1 and 2** (as eGFR unreliable above 60) **and stage 5** (already known to nephrologists or needing urgent referral).
- eGFR not validated in patients aged over 70 and unreliable in patients with severe oedema, who are pregnant or who have amputations.
- Interpret eGFR with caution if patient ill, dehydrated or extremely muscular or lean and repeat if in doubt (on non-fasting sample but ask patient to avoid eating large amount of meat), do not diagnose CKD on basis of a single eGFR result.

2. High risk groups

CKD is mainly a cardiovascular disease. High risk groups include:

- DM, IHD, CCF, CVA, TIA
- Hypertension
- Peripheral vascular disease and AAA
- FH of hereditary kidney disease or stage 5 CKD

- Structural renal tract disease or renal calculi
- Systemic disease with potential for renal involvement (eg SLE)
- Patients on long term nephrotoxic drugs eg NSAIDs, aminoglycosides, lithium
- Unexplained proteinuria or haematuria
- Outflow obstruction, neurogenic bladder, urinary diversion

Patients in these groups need regular (at least annual) renal function monitoring (eGFR and urine for PCR). Most of this is happening already via annual reviews, medication reviews and opportunistically. The CKD lead will regularly run searches to identify others.

3. Coding

Doctor to add or amend CKD classification code as needed when eGFR results received, in context of patient age and appropriateness.

Where eGFR below 60, 'Renal function monitoring' problem folder to be created.

4. Stage 1 and 2 CKD

If new finding:

- Arrange repeat eGFR with urine dip within 2 weeks.

If on-going or unchanged on repeat:

- Has eGFR fallen by > 15%? If so consider referral.
- Do CKD review (see below) – will need CKD review code.
- Annual review of eGFR, ACR, BP, lipids, Hb and medication.

5. Stage 3 CKD (eGFR 30–59)

If new:

- Exclude acute illness.
- Repeat in 1–2 weeks on early morning sample with urine dip.

If on-going or confirmed on repeat:

- Has eGFR fallen > 5 in past year or 10 in past 5 yrs? If so, CKD is progressive – consider renal referral.
- Do CKD review (see box below).
- Arrange 6 monthly eGFR, BP and ACR.

6. Stage 4 and 5 CKD (eGFR ≤30)

Refer (see Northton renal guidelines).

eGFR should be monitored 3 monthly for stage 4 patients and 6 weekly for stage 5.

Consider other hormonal and metabolic effects of renal failure eg anaemia, bone disorders.

Many of these patients already under nephrology review.

CKD Review

- Medication – minimise use of nephrotoxic drugs eg NSAIDs (see BNF)
- Lifestyle advice – smoking cessation, weight loss, exercise
- BP – target 130/80 (140/85 for QoF), ACE or A2RB if over target
- Lipids – target < 4 mMol/L
- Urine (early morning) for ACR and dip

7. Exemption codes (for QoF)

#9hE1   CKD pt unsuitable
#9hE0   CKD informed dissent

8. Indications for nephrology referral

- Stage 4 and 5 CKD
- Heavy proteinuria (PCR > 100mg/mmol) or lesser proteinuria with haematuria
- Progressive decline in eGFR (> 5ml/min/1.73 sq m in a year)
- Inability to control BP despite 4 drugs at therapeutic levels
- Rare or hereditary renal conditions or suspected renal artery stenosis

References

1. NICE guideline Sept 2008 'Chronic kidney disease'

Notes

1 Introduction

1 We will use the term 'clinician', likewise 'practitioner', to describe both doctors and nurses, reserving the latter terms for instances where one or the other is specifically indicated. (NB a different, more specific usage of the term 'clinician' is also introduced in Chapter 2.)

2 This is not the place to enter into the debates about EBP. For a recent example of the continuing arguments, see for example Wyer and Silva (2009), Silva and Wyer (2009) and the succeeding commentaries in the *Journal of Evaluation in Clinical Practice* 15: 899 *et seq*. See also Smith (2008).

3 There are also other initiatives designed with similar aims, such as the Joanna Briggs Institute, an international organization that aims to 'facilitate evidence based health care practice globally through being a leading international organization for the translation, transfer and utilization of evidence of the feasibility, appropriateness, meaningfulness and effectiveness of health care practices' (http://www.joannabriggs. edu.au/about/home.php).

4 Since the gap between research and practice became a widely noted cause for concern (Haines and Donald 1998), there has been a very large number of studies attempting to reduce it. Evensen *et al.* (2010), reviewing 169 intervention studies designed to reduce the evidence–practice gap across nine sets of evidence-based guidelines, judged that only one-third were well designed, and even there the median participation rate was 60 percent. The UK's flagship programme of implementation research, which ran for about twelve years from 1994, was judged on review to have yielded limited benefits (Soper and Hanney 2007). Recommendations have recently been made to set up a more sophisticated programme of implementation research in the UK that takes greater account of behavioural and cultural factors, and that is underpinned by a greater attention to the underlying theories of research utilization and knowledge uptake (Eccles *et al.* 2009), which have been somewhat lacking in existing research (Stewart 1999; Dawson 1999; Davies *et al.* 2010).

5 Some may argue that, although we employed ethnographic *methods*, we should not claim that this was an ethnography as we were not totally immersed in the culture of primary care during our research in the way that an anthropologist might spend months at a time living in, say, an African village, cut off from the rest of the world. We are quite happy to concede this distinction but because (a) we have been attached on and off to our research site, Lawndale, for several years now, and (b) we have spent our entire professional lives immersed in the worlds of medicine and nursing, we do not consider it to be an important concern here. The point of total immersion is to achieve a 'thick description' of the sort that can distinguish the subtleties of, say, irony,

parody and allusion when 'the tribe' uses them (Geertz 2000), and we are more than able to do that.

6 JG in particular had long been steeped in the social sciences, having spent several years away from medicine as a full-time medical historian working in a department of history and philosophy of science, poring over eighteenth-century medical books to try to understand how medical knowledge was socially constructed. ACLM had worked with an anthropologist, Ann Mulhall, on several healthcare research projects.

7 For example, one of our stated research aims was to explore whether clinicians as they acquire and adapt new knowledge rely on 'communities of practice', a theoretical term that describes networks of people who informally share practical learning. (See Chapter 7.) Communities of practice and other forms of social and organizational knowledge networks seemed to us to be a likely mechanism by which knowledge is disseminated and absorbed in clinical practice. To fail to be constantly aware that the very act of posing this question with such assumptions might affect the way we saw things would have been at best to weaken the rigour of our study and at worst to conjure up social phenomena that we were expecting to see but were not there. (In the event, we leant over backwards so far that it took us nearly a year to realize that a key community of practice was staring us in the face; Chapter 7.)

8 ACLM qualified as a nurse in 1982 and began her nursing career working in primary and community care before studying for her PhD. Alongside these studies in 1986 she started to work as a specialist nurse for research and development responsible for the implementation of research across the non-medical disciplines of a district general hospital. The complexity of this enterprise led her to question the ease with which the mantra emanating from the previous decade's Briggs Report (1979: 370, 108) that 'a sense of the need for research should become part of the mental equipment of every practising nurse or midwife' could be achieved. By 1990 this eventually encouraged her towards a career change that allowed her to pursue these problems through teaching and research in a university setting.

JG qualified in medicine in 1974 and spent a short time in hospital and primary care in his early career. His public health research since the early 1980s has consisted largely of organizational case studies that examined how research was being implemented. That research, his subsequent role in health technology assessment, and his participation on many national and international bodies concerned in one way or another with evidence-based practice kept him close to the thinking both of clinicians and of health service policy makers and managers.

9 We had both had a number of salutary experiences of NHS-based projects in which the original topic of research had all but disappeared under the shifting sands of NHS policy (Pope *et al.* 2007).

10 See note 14. Lawndale scored the full 1050 points in both the first two years of the Quality and Outcomes Framework (QOF). The national average was 959/1050 points (91 per cent) in 2004–5 and 1011 (96 per cent) in 2005–6.

11 We will return in Chapter 10 to the difficult question of how one might ascertain the extent to which they manage patients in accordance with the research evidence.

12 The partners at Urbcester were a relatively young group of forward-thinking, committed GPs with large teaching responsibilities at the local medical school. The practice was in a rather ugly and run-down 1970s building on a bustling, grimy, noisy, cosmopolitan main road. The waiting room was large, impersonal and dingy, with receptionists behind glass windows, peeling walls and a warren of dark, slightly grubby corridors leading to the doctors' surgeries. But the intellectual atmosphere was lively and rigorous, the relationships with patients were warm, and the style of practice highly patient-centred and generally regarded as being of exemplary quality. Several of the practitioners taught evidence-based practice. Oakville Hospital is a large, imposing teaching hospital in the USA that is part of a medical school complex of high repute, which boasts more than 1000 faculty physicians. Doppton is a relatively

small UK medical school with an excellent reputation for teaching. It produces well over 200 new doctors each year.

13 In the first phase we were grateful for the help of two research assistants, Dale Webb PhD and Harriet Jefferson MSc, who conducted some early formal interviews, piloted the taping of meetings and helped us to plan the rest of the study.

14 The rationale of the General Medical Services contract, which we shall refer to throughout as the 'GP contract', is to allow GPs 'greater flexibility to determine the range of services they wish to provide' (Department of Health 2003) and to reward them for delivering services of high quality, which generally means practising according to current best evidence of clinical and – to some extent – cost-effectiveness. Since its introduction in April 2004, the GP contract has rapidly become a highly structured mechanism in which financial incentives are coupled with detailed standard setting that is rigorously monitored through the QOF in order to encourage practitioners to meet given standards. (Marshall & Roland 2002). The contract also includes organizational features of the practice such as record keeping, communication and management. As part of the contract, the Department of Health, in consultation with expert groups, focused initially on ten clinical domains (e.g. stroke, cancer, asthma, mental health) within which they had developed a set of standards that were assessable using a set of routine indicators, each of which carried a given number of points on a 'quality scorecard'. The more fully the standards are met, the higher the points and the greater the financial rewards (Department of Health 2006).

Building on the experience of the first year of the new GP contract, the subsequent version of the QOF contained a number of revisions. These resulted from recommendations made by an independent expert panel, which reviewed over 500 suggestions that had been submitted in response to an open call for evidence about the way the QOF had run in its first year. Among the six new domains that came into the QOF as a result of this process, such as dementia, depression and palliative care, was one that we will focus on in Chapters 5 and 8: chronic kidney disease.

15 Chapter 6 will make clear why we have chosen this narrative strategy as a didactic device.

16 The Vancouver style, usually found in medical texts, enables one to locate the place where any given reference is cited. ('I see they've referred to XYZ. I wonder where, why and how?') This is much more difficult with the Harvard style, which is used almost universally, as here, in social sciences texts. We hope that our novel device has achieved the best of both worlds, which also serves as an author index.

2 From formal knowledge to guided complexity

1 We were not in any position to compare their decisions with some 'gold standard' of evidence in order to judge the quality of their practice, but, as will become clear, this would in any case have begged the question of what a gold standard is in any particular circumstance. We will return to this question (p. 203).

2 For more on the variable degree to which research evidence underpins guidelines, see Cook *et al.* (1997); McDonald and Harrison (2004); Raine *et al.* (2004); McAlister *et al.* (2007); Djulbegovic *et al.* (2009a).

3 Readers who are unfamiliar with the nature of clinical guidelines are invited to type 'clinical guideline' followed by any clinical condition of their choice into a search engine. The results will vary from dozens of pages to short flowcharts. See also the NICE (http://guidance.nice.org.uk/) and SIGN (http://www.sign.ac.uk/guidelines/index.html) websites for examples of the centrally sanctioned guidelines in the UK.

4 '[G]uidelines . . . do not become an active part of a practice's infrastructure, yet linger in the minds of the professionals involved. Such guidelines are constantly and routinely re-appropriated in light of the organizational demands of the medical practice and the situational requirements of each new case. They are hard for the researcher

to spot, since they become part of a physician's or practice's ongoing work routines. Overall, however, instead of a radical change in behaviour, the aggregated effect of clinical practice guidelines seems to be a more nuanced, ongoing learning process of ignoring, partially adapting and partially implementing guidelines in a variety of ways' (Timmermans and Berg 2003: 99).

5   In Chapter 8 we will discuss further how guidelines contributed to such discussions.

6   The impact of the 'look and feel' of a document is of course well recognized. '[R]eaders look beyond the information in documents. [. . .] The investment evident in a document's material content is often a good indicator of the investment in its informational content. Physical heft lends weight to what it says' (Brown and Duguid 2000: 187).

7   We make a distinction here between an expert system that one consults to help solve a problem, and the computer-generated prompts (Figure 2.2) that reminded the practitioners to carry out certain actions relevant to the patient before them, such as ordering a blood test or recording smoking status. (We discuss these further in Chapter 8 as 'reifications' of collective mindlines.)

8   One methodological problem, which we will not address here because we did not focus on it in our observations, is that the use of IT was continually developing during this period. However, the change was gradual and imperceptible and, although we did not observe clinical consultations after 2002, we heard nothing over the succeeding time that altered the general principles that we report.

9   We discuss further in Chapter 5 the differences in the ways that beginners and experts use formal sources of knowledge.

10 Harrison and McDonald (2008) make the useful distinction between the 'internal' (i.e. individual, personal) adoption of external research findings, characterized by the 'critical appraisal model' of evidence-based practice (Figure 1.1), and the externally driven implementation of such research, for example by guidelines, protocols and contractual frameworks, which they call the 'scientific bureaucratic' model. They point out that the latter has been increasingly the model adopted by the NHS.

11 The picture is slightly different among primary care nurses, which we have not delved into here. It would seem that nurses also have mixed views, and although in general they are well disposed to more protocol-driven care, which paradoxically may enhance their profession standing (Rycroft-Malone *et al.* 2008; Harrison *et al.* 2002), nurses in general (at least in Scandinavia) may be nevertheless reluctant to pursue evidence proactively (Forsman *et al.* 2008; Boström *et al.* 2009).

12 For a useful recent discussion of this point see Montgomery (2006). A classic account of the development of the autonomy of the medical profession (Jamous and Pelloile 1970) suggests that the profession thrived because the proportion of 'indeterminate knowledge' to 'rule-based knowledge' was particularly high. In other words the inapplicability of scientific knowledge worked to the profession's advantage, for it required erudite judgement that they alone could give. For a further twist – the tension between evidence-based guidelines as a way of retaining *collective* professional autonomy versus their potential to undermine *individual* autonomy – see Armstrong (2002).

It is not just clinicians who need to interpret generalized top-down knowledge to suit each individual circumstance. Knowledge in most walks of life is couched in general terms that need to be applied to individual cases that often vary from the norm. An ethnography of Greek call centre operatives concluded that '[o]rganizational knowledge is the capability members of an organization have developed to draw distinctions in the process of carrying out their work, in particular concrete contexts, by enacting sets of generalizations whose application depends on historically evolved collective understandings' (Tsoukas and Vladimirou 2001: 973).

13 NB Kathryn Montgomery (2006) and Kathryn Montgomery Hunter (1991) are the same person.

14 This is related to the distinction between 'knowledge', which is a general possession, and 'knowing', which is a tool used to support specific actions in an organizational context (Cook and Brown 1999).

15 This is reminiscent of the Catch-22 (p. 5) in which GPs and consultants each assumed that the local asthma and glue ear guidelines were applicable to the kinds of patients seen by the others but not to their own.

16 Other possible reasons for ignoring guidelines may centre on the need for clinicians to assert their professional autonomy. (See note 12 above, and also, for example, Timmermans and Berg 2003). This will become clearer in Chapters 7–9.

17 This unfortunate term is echoed also in Nowotny *et al.*'s (2001) influential book *Re-thinking Science*, which similarly discusses the part played by 'flexibilization' in creating the need for more 'contextualized' knowledge and hence a new mode of science to which we will return in Chapter 10.

18 The aim at Lawndale was ten minutes per consultation and in a typical surgery Lawndale GPs might deal with up to twenty patients and maybe take some phone calls from patients too.

19 Our use of the term 'negotiated' does not imply overt discussions or haggling. (See p. 138.)

20 We briefly discuss the related notion of synthesizing 'context-free', 'context-specific' and 'colloquial' evidence in Chapter 10.

21 Others have approached the question of the clinical role from quite different and more philosophical directions, for example stressing the role of the GP as 'interpreter and guardian at the interface between illness and disease and secondly . . . as a witness to the patient's experience of illness and disease' (Heath 1995: 26). We are taking a more practical view at this stage but see also Chapter 9.

22 In this context (see p. 214 note 1) we use the term 'clinician' to specify the strictly clinical role of a healthcare practitioner. We will continue to use the term both in this sense and in the generic sense of practitioner, and hope the context will make it clear which sense is intended.

23 For the classic account of this phase of the consultation see Byrne and Long (1976).

24 For a different and more formal 'think aloud' approach to understanding the multifarious considerations that doctors take into account when making decisions about case vignettes see Lutfey *et al.* (2008), who found a wide range of factors were involved. Vogt *et al.* (2010) used repertory grid techniques to elicit the reasons why GPs might choose not to intervene in various situations and found that two key constructs were their views of the likely impact of the intervention (which is open to research evidence) and their view of the patient effort that might be entailed (which is not). They conclude that, if EBP is to succeed, then more attention needs to be paid to the ways in which GPs assess patient behaviour and attributes.

25 Health promotion, health education and health protection at a population level – such as healthy eating campaigns, screening or vaccination programmes – also involve primary care, but in the UK are the main responsibility of other agencies (Baggot 2004). We mention them here because many of the consultations that we witnessed showed elements of both primary prevention (before the disease occurs) and secondary prevention (to avert the development of a disease that has been diagnosed early) as well as tertiary prevention (ameliorating the effects of a well-established disease, which will not be discussed as such further here as it shares many of the features of clinical care).

26 The position for the practice nurses was somewhat different, since many of their clinics had been set up with health promotion/disease prevention in mind – for example for asthma, heart disease or diabetes. These were run in quite close accordance with protocols that had usually been arrived at by processes such as those we describe in Chapter 8.

27 When the new GP contract was introduced (see p. 216 note 14), practices could achieve 'QOF' points and hence income for the practice by recording patients' smoking status.

28 In the event they obtained all 1050 points, one of only two practices to do so out of some twenty in the area.

29 There is a sociological argument that such behaviour self-serves to further the material power of one's profession, (e.g. Johnson 1972, 1984) but here we are simply taking at face value the desire to enhance the quality of the profession and its members.

Other aspects of upholding or developing the standing of the profession might have been involvement in research, for example entering patients into clinical trials or initiating their own research, and involvement in teaching undergraduates, but we did not see the GPs doing either during our observations. Had we done so, those too would have represented yet another set of forces, to add to those discussed here, that would impact upon many of their decisions about patient care.

30 We are grateful to Jonathan Lomas for pointing out this parallel to us.

3 Clinical thinking and knowledge in practice

1 '[T]he aim of a skilful performance is achieved by the observance of a set of rules which are not known as such to the person following them' (Polanyi 1958: 49).

2 This term, introduced by the Nobel laureate Herbert Simon, denotes the synthesis of satisfying and sufficing that characterizes many decisions (Simon 1957).

3 This view is theoretically grounded in the sociological traditions of symbolic inter-actionism and ethnomethodology, which posits that people understand the world only through the meanings they ascribe to things as they interact with each other to interpret and reconstruct them. Deirdre Boden, for example, through careful analysis of the discourse of organizational meetings shows how 'people build layers of dis-cussion, debate and eventual decision on a given topic or activity, diffusing possible disagreement while moulding decisions through multiple occasions of interaction. Their conversational collusion is a matter of weaving, turn by turn, one agenda into another' (Boden 1994: 164).

4 We later found that Eraut had come to similar conclusions when 'mapping' head teachers' and social workers' knowledge and know-how. (Eraut 2004: Appendices 1 and 2).

5 'Here it is difficult as it were to keep our heads up, – to see that we stick to the subjects of our everyday thinking, and not go astray and imagine that we describe extreme subtleties, which in turn we are after all quite unable to describe with the means at our fingertips. We feel as if we had to repair a torn spider's web with our fingers' (Wittgenstein 1953: 46). The general difficulty of describing thought processes has rarely been better described.

6 In fact the hypothetico-deductive model – that one formulates an hypothesis and then makes testable deductions based upon it – is misleadingly naïve as a description of the scientific method, but that is a whole other story. For a good introduction see for example Chalmers (2003); Lakatos and Musgrave (1970).

7 The psychologist Robert Hamm suggests that scripts are stored neuronally as 'seman-tic networks' that link 'nodes', which must be active in order for them to be changed. The complex knowledge of scripts incorporates many nodes, he suggests, so that clinicians find it hard to change their practice because '[n]odes have to be active or in awareness in order to be amenable to change through the establishment of new links. One can learn a fact that logically implies one should do a new behavior in a situation, but this does not mean that the fact will be active enough to influence behavior when next in that situation' (Hamm 2003: 318). The distinction between 'knowledge' and 'knowledge used in a context' may therefore have a neuronal basis.

8 It is also much more circumscribed than the kind of frame suggested by Minsky's model; one might speculate that a clinical 'frame' would be expected to include additional material about complicating social or organizational factors, remembrance of how similar cases responded to treatments, or words of advice inculcated during training. (See note 13.)

9   See note 6 above – the naïve hypothetico-deductive model is also discredited among philosophers of science.

10 This is reminiscent of Imre Lakatos's classic account of the way scientists also behave, not by ruthless rejection of falsified hypotheses as Popper would suggest (Popper 1975), but by the development of auxiliary hypotheses that allow them to hold onto their core beliefs. See Lakatos (1970).

11 The notion is linked to the influential concept of 'bounded rationality', first used by Herbert Simon in the late 1950s, arguing for a 'behavioural model' as opposed to an over-rationalistic model of decision making (Simon 1957, 1983, 1991). The idea of bounded rationality, developed over recent decades in many areas of social sciences such as economics and organizational theory, recognizes that real decisions are never made with all the facts to hand. Indeed we are rarely dealing with more than a tiny fraction of the variables that might affect a decision. Put simply, bounded rationality denotes the way we cope with the everyday limitations to rational decision making due both to restricted information or time and to our finite cognitive capacity. It is, argues Simon, the only way organisms can survive in a complex world. We necessarily focus on what matters and we get by with the limited alternative solutions and facts that we can use, which are often in the form of heuristic short cuts. The problem, as Tversky and others have stressed, is that such thinking has been shown to be open to many kinds of pitfalls, including confirmation bias, which is that 'People who hold strong opinions on complex social issues are likely to examine relevant empirical evidence in a biased manner' (Lord *et al.* 1979). (Not us, nor you the reader, of course!)

12 Interestingly, Elstein and Schwarz have suggested that evidence-based medicine, which they describe as 'the most recent, and by most standards the most successful, effort to date to apply statistical decision theory in clinical medicine' (Elstein and Schwarz 2002: 732), is the best way to overcome such problems. One strong counter-argument is that even the very act of consulting the evidence is already prestructured by the clinician's experience and prior assumptions, which itself introduces biases and even heuristics (Timmermans and Angell 2001: 354).

13 Arguably our findings accord most closely with Minsky's frame model, but since that was a rather speculative theory and was not applied to medicine we can only guess that Minsky might have postulated that a clinical 'frame' would include the wide range of social, organizational and other features that we observed being brought into decisions.

14 Many writers on this subject suggest that this distinction goes back to Aristotle, who classified 'practical knowledge' – or *phronesis* – separately from 'scientific' and other sorts of knowledge and wisdom, but that is actually somewhat misleading. Although his distinction does indeed lay down the principle that we need to think about different kinds of knowledge in different ways, the fact is that Aristotle's *phronesis* deals with the practicalities of political and ethical decisions rather than the professional craft or tacit knowledge under discussion here (Aristotle 2000 [~350 BC]: 5–7).

15 Indeed Schön's thinking can be traced directly back to John Dewey, the highly influential philosopher, psychologist and educationist who had been expressing similar ideas at the turn of the twentieth century.

16 Argyris and Schön's concept of theory-in-use has certain elements in common with mindlines. Contrasting with what they called 'espoused theory' it stresses that people know much more than they can state, which can be elicited only by observing their behaviours. This basic idea, developed in its original form to explore contrasting models of organizational behaviour, led the authors in several other directions besides knowing-in-action and the place of reflective practice, which we focus on here. The authors also moved on to the highly influential notion of 'organizational learning' (e.g. Argyris 1991) based on the much earlier idea (first suggested in 1952) of single loop learning (i.e. learning that accepts the given parameters) vs double loop learning

(learning that challenges and changes them – the kind of learning that we advocate for EBP in Chapter 10.)

17 Although it is widely suggested that only 10–20 per cent of medical actions have a research basis to them, this figure has never been substantiated, nor has its source (probably in the mid 1970s) ever been pinned down. Ellis, Sackett and colleagues found, in contrast, that, of the medical interventions actually carried out by hospital physicians on 100 consecutive patients in Oxford, over 80 per cent were indeed based on 'high quality scientific evidence' (Ellis *et al.* 1995). (For a comprehensive review of this question see http://www.shef.ac.uk/scharr/ir/percent.html.)

18 More recent work (e.g. Chaiklin and Lave 1996) has developed this theme particularly in relation to the way in which people's *learning* is context dependent, and we will return to this theme in Chapters 4 and 5.

19 This argument applies also to hospital medicine. Patients over sixty-five years old account for 70 per cent of NHS bed days (see, for example, Massoud *et al.* 2003).

20 Montgomery discusses this at length, distinguishing the tensions in medicine between the 'lumping' of widely applicable generalizations or laws and the 'splitting' of particular individual variations within those laws. 'Knowing in clinical medicine requires negotiating both the uncertainties of particularization and the tempting comforts of generalization' (Montgomery 2006: 90). It is hardly a newly recognized problem: Montgomery reminds us that Aristotle made it clear in his *Metaphysics* that there cannot be a science of individuals. 'It is evident that there is no science of accidental being; for every science is of that which is always or for the most part . . . for example, that for the most part honey-water is beneficial for a patient in a fever. But science cannot state the exception to what occurs for the most part' (Aristotle 1975 [~350 BC]: Book E, Part 2, p. 105).

4 Growing mindlines: laying the foundations

1 UK readers will recognize the tutor is contrasting Paxman's notoriously tough TV interrogations versus Ross's relaxed chat show style.

2 We discuss this inability to express 'clinical common sense' further on p. 167.

3 The 'personal knowledge' postulated by Polanyi is, we shall argue, also 'social knowledge' – not only because it involves the products of a student's socialization, but also because its formation is mediated through social interactions.

4 The educational literature on professional practice is very wide indeed and we do not attempt here to enter the wider domains of, say, the critical reconstruction of practice through dialogue and discussion (although we do recommend as much in Chapter 10). Even within the much narrower focus of this chapter, this was not a systematic review, which would have taken several person years in itself. Our strategy was to use our networks of educationist colleagues to locate key texts and follow the leads therefrom, and to hand search the key journals in medical and nursing education for articles relevant to our findings. The referencing is merely illustrative, but is designed to help the reader to enter the relevant literature should they wish to do so. (We hope that the referencing is not, as one of JG's predecessors in Cambridge, Bob Young, used to argue, 'a public wank – ostentatiously displaying the means of production in order to scatter fruitless seed'. Yes he was Marxist.) Perhaps, if we are honest, our referencing plays the roles so brilliantly described by Bruno Latour in *Science in Action* (Latour 1987) as a game played to bolster one's argument against attack. We have also, more seriously, tried to follow the acerbic advice of Barbara Czarniawska (1998: 51–63).

5 For a useful account of nurses' use of biosciences in practice see McVicar *et al.* (2010).

6 There is (unsurprising) evidence that family practitioners' concepts of the scientific rationales for their practice are not only simplified but sometimes at odds with the scientific models held by researchers in that particular field. See, for example, Lacasse

and Leo (2005), who suggest that the scientific explanations given by doctors when treating depression are fostered and shaped by the kinds of (misleading and simplistic) explanations that the pharmaceutical industry aims both at physicians and at their patients to encourage the uptake of their products.

7 Tanenbaum (1994) has highlighted the distinction between the deterministic bio-medical/laboratory research model of thinking, reliant on cause-and-effect patho-logical mechanisms (as traditionally taught in medical schools), and the probabilistic outcomes-based model, reliant on the results of clinical trials (as advocated by the EBP movement). This would be likely to mean that the early laying down of mindlines needs to be overlaid with, and accommodate, a very different kind of thinking as the probabilistic clinical model develops over time in the clinician's mind. This in turn suggests that encapsulation may involve a degree of suppression to avoid the consequent tensions!

8 For up-to-date information regarding other health professionals see the following web-sites: Nursing and Midwifery Council (http://www.nmc-uk.org/); Chartered Society of Physiotherapy (http://www.csp.org.uk/); British Association of Occupational Therapists and College of Occupational Therapists (http://www.cot.co.uk/Homepage/); Health Professions Council (http://www.hpc-uk.org/).

9 Benner, Tanner and Chesla (1996: 193–231) describe this in relation to nurses as the 'social embeddedness of knowledge'.

10 This process has been referred to by some sociologists (e.g. Berger and Luckmann 1966) as 'secondary socialisation' and we will return to it on p. 173.

11 These days too, whether following the new integrated or the old sequential model, students need to deal with an overload of clinical information and to amalgamate it with an overload of underlying science (van Hell *et al.* 2008). Our observations and interviews suggest contemporary medical students faced with that dilemma also focus most on what is needed for their exams, not for their later practice.

12 We owe this simple classification to Colin Coles, who draws a distinction between 'the curriculum on paper' (timetabled events, lectures, tutorials, ward rounds etc. and the perceptions and intentions of staff), 'the curriculum in action' (what is actually deliv-ered) and 'the curriculum experienced' (Coles 1985; Fish and Coles 2005: 218; Coles 2010). These three curricula may or may not overlap with each other; for example superficial rote learning of the Krebs Cycle in detail for its own (or examination's) sake might be part of the experienced but not the intended curriculum. But Coles argues strongly that even the paper (i.e. intended) curriculum may not be appropriate, hence our recasting of his classification into that which is taught, learnt and needed, which also may or may not overlap.

13 It is no accident that the tradition of the 'Medics' Revue' is such a big part of UK medical school culture, and transmits a great deal of stereotyping and satirical com-ment about medical specialties and attitudes. But there is also a subdivision: for example all year-groups have their subgroups and cliques, even to the point of being caricatured by terms that we have heard such as the 'girlie swots', the 'rugger buggers', the 'lefty intellectuals', 'the clubbers', 'the jet set' and so on.

14 Moreover, methods are being developed to evaluate such skills formally (Hojat *et al.* 2007).

15 There is of course an even more pervasive underlying set of cultural values: the variation of values, norms and beliefs between countries, which inevitably means that mindlines will differ – sometimes greatly – between clinicians trained in, say, the UK and those trained in the USA. See Payer (1996) for an illuminating comparative account of often radically differing views about health and medicine between the USA, England, Germany and France.

16 The clinical training gives students an opportunity to try to balance experiential and theoretical, codified knowledge (apprenticeship vs scholarship). (See, for example, Bosk 1979: 84–94.) Ideally it allows them to exploit all four stages of the widely accepted

'learning cycle' as a way to link theory and practice and to make the most of their different learning styles that may favour different stages of that cycle. The stages are: concrete experience (doing things) leading to reflective observation (including watching things) leading to abstract conceptualization (thinking it through) leading to active experimentation (trying new things) and so round the cycle again. See Kolb (1984).

17 Atkinson describes how students are exposed to a very 'artfully stage managed' reality that teaches them to see 'objective' things that are often quite problematic constructs (such as debatable heart sounds) that form the basis of their subsequent knowledge. A similar process can be seen in the way in which the Oakville residents (p. 85) were encouraged to think in terms of the standard 'thumbnails', or were provided with carefully managed data to help change their practice We discuss in Chapters 8 and 9 the collectively constructed sensemaking that is at the centre of mindlines from the very start.

18 Jamous and Pelloile (1970) in their discussion of the establishment of the dominance of the medical profession in the early modern period stress the important role played by the indeterminate aspects of practice (as characterized arguably by the soft skills we have been discussing here).

19 This question could of course be answered at many different levels, which ideally would refer to a whole literature of educational theory going back at least to the work of Lev Vygotsky, which became highly influential when first translated from the Russian in the 1960s. He pioneered in the 1920s the notion that the way humans learn (by internalizing small advances while guided by more knowledgeable people around them) is inextricably linked to social development and the inherent sociocultural context (Vygotsky 1978). Also relevant is the highly influential work of Bandura (1986), which stresses the way people tend to learn in an apprenticeship style by modelling their behaviour in context from watching, imitating and being led to the next stage by the 'master'.

20 'Communities of practice', a term introduced in Lave and Wenger (1991) to describe groups or networks of people who informally share practical learning, will be discussed in much greater detail in Chapter 7.

21 We have always observed and been amused by the way that students and junior doctors, for example on ward rounds, gradually over a period of months acquire the mannerisms and speech patterns of their consultants.

5 Growing mindlines: cultivating contextual adroitness

1 The attending (physician) is the equivalent of a UK consultant (physician) and – for billing purposes – is obliged to do a ward round every day. The round at Oakville also has a teaching and training role.

2 For a discussion of the social control that goes on among surgical residents, see Bosk (1979: 101 *et passim*).

3 For a particularly graphic and illuminating account of how doctors learn skills, see Gawande (2006).

4 Some would go even further with this notion. The 'constructuralism' theory put forward by the cognitive psychologist Kathleen Carley, for example, suggests that *everything* that people learn is the result of social interactions undertaken in the pursuit of the tasks they need to perform, and that social knowledge continually underpins what we know (Carley 1986) (cf. Chapter 4, note 19).

5 For those interested in pursuing these ideas, see Benner *et al.* (1996), where she and colleagues (including the Dreyfus brothers) take both the analysis and the practical implications further.

6 Interestingly, Benner in turn uses the Dreyfus brothers' theories to structure her own analysis of the way nurses absorb their expertise, but this apparently circular mutual

support system nevertheless has great prima facie credibility and has been highly influential.

7   A 'consultant' surgeon is the UK equivalent of a US attending surgeon.

8   What the student may not yet have realised is that the answers to all these questions come from having the courage to admit ignorance and ask others who work on the ward (usually the nurses!), since such knowledge is usually shared anecdotally among a community of practice (Chapters 6 and 7).

9   One may therefore question why we have added Contextually Adroit as an *extra* stage at the end. Our answer, paradoxically, is that the very fact that Benner and the Dreyfus brothers have (wrongly in our view) considered the novice stage to be context free suggests that there are more, and more complex, dimensions to context at *all* the stages than they recognized. However it would overcomplicate things to add this dimension to their model, and this is not the place to delve into that debate (see also Collins and Evans 2007). So we have added the extra stage simply as a way of flagging it up as something worthy of more thought. We return to the place of context in Chapter 9.

10 Of course, depending on culture and personalities, that inter-reliance might be minimized. A particularly tough and competitive second-year resident in Oakville University Hospital, expert as a resident but still an advanced beginner as a physician, confided that he had learned to '*never* trust the other idiots' and always checked everything for himself.

11 Moreover there are other ways of thinking about the nature of expertise (e.g. Collins and Evans 2007) but they too usually build on the general consensus about the Dreyfus/Benner model of the development of professional expertise. Collins and Evans propose a 'periodic table' of many different kinds of expertise ranging from the ubiquitous skill such as language, through superficial factual ('beer-mat') specialist expertise, through to, for example, the 'technical connoisseurship' that – like most of the higher forms of expertise – involves tacit knowledge. Their most interesting innovation, to our minds, is the notion of 'interactional expertise', which allows a person who is not actually a true expert in the field to nevertheless be able to make sound judgements about it. Anyone who has ever, for example, sat on a guidelines committee, refereed research proposals, taught a subject they are not fully trained in, chosen a doctor, dealt with a medical complaint or done an ethnography will recognize it instantly.

12 This was the same speaker that gave the diabetes lecture referred to in this chapter's third prologue.

13 Although some partners had assumed she had used the national service framework (NSF), they were not surprised or concerned to discover later that she had not done so directly. After all – as more than one of her partners said – there was nothing new or surprising in them. ('I wasn't sure that the NSF was necessarily going to provide me with any more information than direct studies and guidelines and all the rest of it and it obviously is quite thick as well,' she admitted subsequently when interviewed. 'I probably should have done, but I didn't.')

14 It is important to note that the idea that knowledge is 'tacit' does not imply that it *cannot* be communicated. Far from it. Indeed Polanyi claimed in his pioneering explorations that 'tacit sharing of knowledge underlies every articulate communication' (Polanyi 1958: 209), even silent ones. We are, in other words, always communicating some tacit knowledge in some way or other. The problem is understanding how that happens, beyond his lengthy but ultimately vague analysis of 'conviviality' (Polanyi 1958: 209–226), so that clinicians can share their tacit knowledge more reliably (p. 203).

15 Although they do not mention it, there is also a clear link between Nonaka and Takeuchi's distinction of formal knowledge and tacit knowledge and the 'two modes of thought' – logico-scientific and narrative – (Bruner 1986) that we mention in Chapter 6, p. 115).

16 Nevertheless, GP practices and other healthcare organizations that need to succeed in a difficult financial environment might also benefit from a more professional approach to knowledge management.

17 For a useful review of knowledge management readings, see Prusak and Matson (2006). Nonaka and Takeuchi, while having been remarkably influential in the field of knowledge management, are not without their, sometimes trenchant, critics. For two critiques see Blackler (1995) and Zhu (2006). Nevertheless the basic model we put forward here seems to escape relatively unscathed.

18 This is a two-way process, in that the dialogue requires the listener to adapt the tacit knowledge so that it makes sense in his or her own context, which can alter the meaning of the tacit knowledge for both parties. In other words, the very act of communicating tacit knowledge can transform it and bring about new and different understandings of that knowledge both for the original 'owner' of the knowledge and for the recipient. (The old hand, while discussing a procedure with the neophyte, realizes something new about the way she herself does things.) One could argue that this transformation therefore entails a process of social co-construction of new knowledge, in that the social interactions between the individuals give rise to newly constituted knowledge for at least one and sometimes both parties. See Chapters 8 and 9.

19 We refer of course to educational courses, not golf courses, but on the other hand . . . (see Chapter 8).

20 We ourselves have experienced, both as clinicians and as ethnographers, the sometimes overt but usually subtle, subliminal but still powerful ways in which patients signal their approval or disapproval of the way the doctor or nurse is acting. This, as well as interactions with colleagues, is an important part of clinical socialization.

21 For this to happen effectively many key factors need to be in place, such as the existence of appropriate networks and groups who can access and process the knowledge (Rogers 2003; Cross and Borgatti 2004), their shared use of language and local jargon (Fairclough 1992) and their trust in each other's views (Nahapiet and Ghoshal 1998).

22 Language plays a vital part in this process, since it is used not simply to convey information but also to mediate social matters such as the relative power, values and group membership of the speakers and listeners. Therefore language not only structures what is understood by the participants but at the same shapes the relationships between them (Fairclough 1992).

23 For a detailed account of the complex processes that were entailed in the transfer and internalization of new 'best practice' in a hospital trust, but which makes no explicit mention of the SECI spiral, see Newell *et al.* (2003).

24 For an example of such transformations when GPs adopted new evidence about the use of statins, see Fairhurst and Huby (1998).

25 For further explanation of this topic, see p. 152.

26 This is the same speaker who had previously convinced Tony to cease asking for cholesterol levels to be done on fasting patients, as he had always done before (p. 95).

27 Another speaker very much in demand to teach about skin conditions was good, said the GPs, because he always kept it simple and practical. His slide-show talk involved no overt scientific evidence at all, just lots of information and advice based on authority and experience. It was riveting and had the trainees scribbling reams of notes and the senior GPs writing almost nothing down but presumably – as they told us they learnt a lot from it and talked about some of the points later – making mental notes.

28 As may become clear in Chapters 7 and 8, the social way in which knowledge was processed made it more likely that the same information would come forward in very different ways. The fact that all of them could introduce the group to new ideas from many different sources maximized the likelihood that the relevant sources associated with different learning styles (i.e. those with a tendency towards learning from experience, reflection, experimentation or theoretical abstraction; Kolb 1984) would enter the collective mix.

29 Clive subsequently audited their heart failure treatment after the agreed changes in practice had been put into place. The standards against which he audited their practice he derived from the NICE and SIGN guidelines for heart failure and from the Quality and Outcomes Framework of the new GP contract. He also checked a couple of research papers in the journals that they referred to. The audit showed that all the standards were met or exceeded.

6 The place of storytelling in knowledge sharing

1 We use the term 'anecdote' to denote a short, striking personal story told for effect. We use 'story' as the generic term, since all anecdotes are stories but not all stories are anecdotes. The term 'narrative' will be used to denote the way in which events and objects are ordered within a story.

2 This is also the case with hospital doctors. In a project designed to introduce day surgery into a hospital in the 1980s JG repeatedly ran into the same story about a patient who had had his haemorrhoids removed as a day patient and had nearly bled to death on the way home. This one story overcame all the statistics, research, national opinion leader views and cunning techniques that we had mobilized to try and sway the opinion of surgeons and anaesthetists to include haemorrhoidectomies in their day surgery unit (Gabbay and Francis 1988). Similarly, in 2010 ACLM found that a drug proven to be of benefit in neonatal intensive care was never used in one particular neonatal intensive care unit because of stories circulating about a single death of a child on that drug.

3 A related concept that Nonaka and Takeuchi have introduced is the Japanese concept of *Ba*, which they found crucial to sharing knowledge: it is a word that cannot be easily translated but refers to the place or context in which people share, develop or use knowledge – anything from the Lawndale coffee room to an audit meeting to a conference to a research team awayday to a website. An informal atmosphere where stories flow easily is an important part of *Ba* that needs to be cultivated, they insist, if knowledge is to be shared effectively.

4 See also note 1, where we distinguish stories, anecdotes and narrative.

5 Of course had JG's fellow casualty officer replied with a story in which another senior surgeon had behaved differently, it would not have been so straightforward and we might have needed to have a more complex mindline that depended also on which seniors were on call.

Benner, Tanner and Chesla (1996: 209–210) describe an even more memorable thirteen-line story told between nurses about a baby and monitor alarms. The result – the baby's death because the alarm was ignored – is retold repeatedly to others to prevent this happening again.

> The experienced nurse spends the rest of her career honouring the tragic experiential lesson she learned. She tells other nurses so that they will not have the same tragedy she has experienced. She no longer can ignore alarms; they have a powerful sense of salience and urgency that does not require thought. Stories of missing clinical cues, or missing the mark in taking care of patients, are told as a means of instruction and correction.

6 In one of the study sites for an evaluation of the implementation of research evidence in practice (Dopson and Gabbay 1995), we heard from clinicians that several of their GP colleagues began to take note of the place of triple therapy for *Helicobacter* only after seeing this story on a televised science documentary.

7 'Boundary object' is a term first introduced by Star and Griesemer (1989), which Star later used to describe the way different groups of 'actors' (in the original analysis it was professional scientists, amateur collectors and administrators at a zoological museum) manage to engage each other in productive activity despite the differences in their

worldviews. (See our discussion of actor-network theory on p. 177.) It has since been used by Wenger (1998) to describe how communities of practice interact (Chapter 7 note 3). We use it here to mean an entity that is accessible to two potentially conflicting ways of seeing events; in this case the views of the clinician and of the patient.

8 Mattingly describes how doctor and patient develop a shared narrative that may twist and turn as things develop, each tailoring their improvised version of the developing 'plot' to what they think the other will want to know (Mattingly 1994). This can be taken a step further and used therapeutically, for example by counsellors helping to co-construct a narrative that allows a patient to come to terms with their problem (Hermans and Hermans-Jansen 1995).

9 See also Witteman *et al.* (2007) for a discussion of the possible link between stories and clinical reasoning.

7 A community of clinical practice?

1 For a systematic review of the effectiveness of communities of practice see Li *et al.* (2009).

2 Lawndale held plenty of meetings. Once every month there was a clinical meeting, a staff training meeting, a finance meeting, a treatment room meeting, a reception-ists' meeting, an educational meeting (in the form of a lecture open to neighbouring practices too), a primary healthcare team meeting, an evening partners' meeting (off site, over dinner) and the QPA (later GP contract) meeting open to the whole practice. Every week there was an executive meeting of a subset of the partners. Every two months there was a meeting about IT and one about education; every quarter there was a staff meeting of which one each year was an awayday for all staff.

3 Wenger (1998) refers to this as 'cross boundary flow', but Brown and Duguid (2001) and others have pointed out that communities of practice also *inhibit* the spread of knowledge by restricting its flow beyond their members. Where communities of prac-tice become cliques or develop an exclusivity of thinking and practice, then they can indeed prevent the flow of knowledge beyond their boundaries. The old craft guilds (of which medicine was arguably one) are a good example, as is any situation where the members of different communities are in competition with each other, such as in commerce or sport.

4 We do not have evidence of whether these staff members were thereby restricted in their learning, but neither is there any evidence that they would have engaged in other, more formal learning processes. One had the impression that these were simply people who did not have the need or desire to learn about the matters being discussed at these meetings.

5 Of course it is quite possible that the national decision makers were themselves making non-evidence-based policy recommendations because they too were experiencing a similar process of negotiation and transformation of knowledge that sceptically over-whelmed any evidence base. (We couldn't *possibly* comment . . . !)

6 Note also how many different elements were being recruited to help them arrive at the appropriate conclusions – colleagues, textbooks, printed and online guidelines, phar-maceutical reps, patient leaflets and thence all the sources that in turn had informed them. Timmermans and Berg (2003: 77) suggest that protocols and guidelines act as 'glue' that ties together the ideas of all the various actors involved in shaping practice (see Chapter 8). For a further discussion of this point see the section on actor-network theory on p. 177.

7 Klein *et al.*'s model (2005) is based on a 2×2 matrix of deliberate, explicit *knowledge sharing* vs implicit, tangential *knowledge nurturing* on the one axis and *egalitarian* vs *stratified* (i.e. hierarchical) on the other. Knowledge exchange and development at Lawndale was usually a by-product of talking about work that took place between colleagues of whatever profession and seniority, hence it was largely 'egalitarian knowledge

nurturing'. At Oakville, in contrast, most of the meetings were of a 'stratified knowledge sharing' community, so called because the primary aim was to explicitly transmit knowledge, and to do so mainly from the senior to junior members of the community. We saw no obvious examples of stratified knowledge-nurturing groups, but the discussions among Doppton students preparing for a joint presentation (p. 70) entailed egalitarian knowledge sharing, the fourth possible category.

8 Co-constructing collective mindlines

1 Elsewhere in the same interview, however, when discussing the grey area of prescribing statins to elderly patients, where there was no clear evidence, she was aware that patients may have been started on them in hospital by *junior* doctors, and was therefore less willing to accept the hospital's lead.

2 Cf. Wenger's 'reifications of practice routines' (Wenger 1998: 57–62) – see p. 142.

3 J. Greenhalgh *et al.* (2008) gives an account of the way groups of clinicians weigh up tacit and encoded knowledge and McDonald (2002) discusses how multiple, differing clinical, economic and policy considerations impinged on a local emerging policy for managing heart disease. At a deeper and more general level see Douglas (1987) for an illuminating analysis of the interplay between institutional, collective thinking and individual thinking.

4 Our methods did not allow the kind of in-depth conversational analysis that Boden (1994) undertook, which enabled her to show how individual and organizational structures are 'co-determinative' of each other, such that 'individuals interact to institutionalize information'. However the general pattern of what we observed has much in common with her findings. As she argues, based on an in-depth analysis of an apparently rational (but actually highly contingent) administrative decision in a US hospital setting, 'the way organizational actors categorize and account for the world is not some woolly process of social construction, but a finely ordered and consequential alignment of differing perspectives, goals, and agendas' (Boden 1994: 57).

5 For an explanation of our use of the term 'negotiating' see p. 138.

6 We will distinguish on pp. 184–5 between, for example, 'disease' as perceived and discussed by a clinician, and illness–disease as a negotiated understanding of a particular set of real-world phenomena.

7 Lest this example give an impression that the Lawndale doctors tended to favour the managerial rather than the clinical (QOF points rather than quality of patient care), we should point out that in at least two other areas with controversial QOF criteria, chronic obstructive airways disease and depression, their collective mindline opened up many patients to care that the contract would have excluded.

8 For an interesting ethnographically based commentary on the process of data collection for the GP contract, and the impact that may have on what the figures mean, see Checkland *et al.* (2007).

9 Harrison and McDonald (2008: 32) distinguish three types of autonomy linked to the 'collegiality' of the medical profession, referring to the clinical freedom that comes with membership of the profession. The first is the 'micro level', the individual clinicians' control over the diagnosis and management of their patients, which has been increasingly challenged by the EBP movement, protocols and guidelines. The second 'meso level' is the collective right of the profession as a whole to determine how it practises (such as self-regulation, which has also increasingly come under challenge that includes the new GP contract). We would argue that collective mindlines, such as the one we have described here for CKD, play an important part in that meso-level struggle for control. In their collective determination of appropriate practice the GPs were asserting this meso level of autonomy, which in turn allowed them the micro-level autonomy of their individual mindlines. (Harrison and MacDonald's third 'macro level' is the taken-for-granted biomedical model of the disease, the scientific

framework within which clinicians work, which, whilst it clearly underpins the meso-level collective mindline, is also – we contend – challenged and shaped by it. See also pp. 184–5, where we draw a similar distinction between "disease" and "'disease'".)

10 Note that, without the external challenge, this reformulation of CKD would not have occurred. It was the Department of Health's attempt to standardize procedure that, for better or worse, precipitated the negotiation of new meaning and practice for CKD.

11 One might argue that Weick's work on collective sensemaking is focused on *organizations* and is therefore not relevant to individual primary care clinicians. But we contend that individual clinical practice is inter-dependent with the collective thinking of the clinical community and indeed neither could exist without the other. Moreover we agree with Magala (1997: 318) that 'meetings are like miniature models of organizations, they are, in sense, laboratories of sensemaking'. We maintain that the collective sensemaking that went on in meetings between colleagues is a major component of clinical thinking, and indeed much of our evidence comes from interactions that went on in discussions within communities of practice about how to organize clinical matters.

12 Weick argues that this partly explains why action is often followed, not preceded, by rationalization (Weick 2001: 176). ('Ready. Fire. Aim!' as he puts it.) This may be one possible explanation for the way that clinicians often reached decisions almost imme-diately in their individual decisions about patients, where complexity and the need for a quick decision were often met with decisions far quicker than the explanations for them. But in Chapter 3 we suggest that it is equally if not more likely that they did so because of their ability to call instantly on their individual mindlines. We were not in a position to judge whether they were retrospectively justifying conclusions they had jumped to but, when and if that happened in the collective setting, others were often quick to point it out.

13 This might be one way to interpret the reason for the CURB-65 example (p. 158) bringing such great relief to the troubled discussion. Even though it was not strictly accurate it was plausible enough to help them find their way through the problem. The CURB-65 may have acted in the way that Weick claims a map of the Pyrenees saved a group of soldiers who were lost in the Alps ('almost any old point of reference will do as a start'; Weick 1995: 54) – except that it turns out that, sadly, that wonderful example is probably an urban myth enshrined in poetry (Basbøll and Graham 2006).

14 When a skilled committee chair wants a decision to go in a particular direction but knows that maybe half the group disagree, he or she often ensures that the first few speakers on the topic are those who support the chair's opinion. More often than not, the others either fall silent or fall into line, resulting in a healthy majority vote in the favour of the chair's preferred outcome (S. J. Watkins, personal communication). See for example Asch (1951); Davis *et al.* (1988); and of course the notorious experiments conducted by Stanley Milgram on obedience and Philip Zimbardo's Stanford Prison experiment, both of which shockingly reveal the power of social conformity.

15 The irony is that the concept of groupthink has been widely and uncritically accepted by many disciplinary groups from managers to politicians, psychologists, organiza-tional theorists and health professionals despite a marked lack of empirical research to substantiate it (Turner and Pratkanis 1998).

16 It would be difficult to imagine any group of GPs fulfilling the criteria for groupthink! They tend to be a very independent-minded, sceptical profession.

17 An example might be the way that the discussions about spurious low potassium levels (p. 129) were reflected two years later in comments made by Tamsin, the trainee.

18 For a useful introduction see, for example, Outhwaite (2005). Our own view is essentially that when people are dealing with phenomena, their moment to moment interactions-in-context bring about their view of reality, which – as it is all that is available to them – to all intents and purposes *is* their reality, and moreover is a new

reality in which their recursive interactions have reconstructed the phenomena they were dealing with.

19 Our favourite definition of 'recursive' is: 'Recursive: See *Recursive*. And if you still don't understand, see *Recursive*.'

20 Boden (1994) has some excellent examples of the way in which the moment-to-moment detail of talk produces collective organizational views. See note 4 above, and Chapter 3 note 3. Her approach, like that of Weick, owes a great deal to Harold Garfinkel. The kind of collective mindline that emerges from the interactions at Lawndale would be, as he might have put it (Garfinkel 1967:106), *the-CKD-management-that-will-actually-benefit-the-patients-and-more-or-less-fit-the-QOF-requirements-and-be-easily-done-by-the-nurses-and-get-us-the-points-while-not-causing-undue-problems-for-us*, which they then set about retrospectively justifying within their personally held values as well as the official rules.

21 This need not imply that repetition and routine per se are detrimental to good practice – indeed they may well help to improve quality so long as they are judiciously applied. However, such routines are usually developed locally, often through the 'mindful' melding of organizational, group and individual activities that bear many of the hall-marks we have been describing here (Greenhalgh 2008).

22 There is a parallel here with Lipsky (1980), who suggests that 'street level bureaucrats' such as social workers and police reconstruct official policy in the course of their day-to-day interactions with their clients. When they make individual and collective decisions that bend the rules, they transform policy as seen from the top of the organization. Although most doctors and nurses are spared the rigorous rules and working conditions of the providers of those particular public services, the increasing bureaucratization and 'proletarianization' of clinical professions (p. 2) may intensify the potential for such parallels to be drawn. See Checkland (2004).

23 Although we will not explore it further here, this approach to understanding the collective nature of clinical decision making may have much in common with 'social cognitive theory', as proposed by Albert Bandura (1986). His very influential theory argues that human decisions rely on the continually interacting triad of the environment (which includes other people's thoughts, attitudes and behaviour), our own behaviour (which includes active reflection and evaluation) and our cognitive and other personal factors. All three reciprocally affect and determine each other.

24 We do not here discuss patient capital (the resource gained, for example, by involving patients in collective health service decisions, or by groups of patients in their own patient organizations) as it was not very evident in our observations at Lawndale. However, we will return in Chapter 9 to the part played by patients in the generation and utilization of clinical knowledge.

25 Compare the interactions at the informal dinner described on p. 132. The privilege of being able to participate in such discussions and learn from them is itself a form of professional capital.

9 Co-constructing clinical reality

1 If a practice managed to ensure that 70 per cent of patients with coronary heart disease had had their last blood pressure reading measured in the previous 15 months and that it was 150/90 or less, they could gain as many as 19 points (out of a total of 1050 for the whole QOF.)

2 '[A]ttempts to codify tacit knowledge may only produce knowledge that is: useless (if it is too difficult to explain); difficult to verify (if it is too uncertain); trivial (if it is too unimportant); redundant (if it is subject to continuous change); irrelevant to a wider audience (if it is too context dependent); politically naïve (if it is too politically insensitive); inaccurate (if it is too valuable and therefore secreted by the 'knower'). Tacit knowledge, therefore, cannot easily be articulated or transferred in explicit forms because it is personal and context specific' (Scarborough and Swan 2002: 9).

3 There are parallels here with Weick's suggestion that making sense of the environment also changes, or 'enacts', that environment (p. 163), or with Bandura's reciprocally interactive triad of behaviour, environment and thought (Bandura 1986). By their response to the GP contract or by choosing not to proactively review patients with early CKD, the Lawndale team were enacting for themselves a different environment of patient care and of professional autonomy compared with other practices that responded differently.

4 There is also an important methodological twist. The problem for the researcher is that when anyone, even the researcher's informant, produces an 'official' version of the way the community under study is practising, they necessarily give a codified, simplified version that shares the potential defects of the objective 'rules' that Bourdieu so derides. That is one reason why the anthropologist's informant often acts as a teacher (and therefore perhaps why JG so often had to resist slipping into trainee or medical student mode when discussing patients with the GPs). Bourdieu argues (Bourdieu 1992) that when anthropologists or sociologists have observed behaviours, customs, artefacts, rituals, classification systems and so on they have until now been caught between two extreme and equally unhelpful alternative approaches: the objective and the subjective. On the one hand the subjective approach is misleading for the obvious reason that it climbs so far inside the minds of the people under study that the scientist cannot get beyond their subjects' own interpretation of what they do and it is therefore not worthy of being called scientific study – more a gradual process of complete cultural conversion. On the other hand, the objective approach is also misleading because it strips away the very essence of a people's belief and behaviour systems by trying – like the maps of the main roads – to extract simple rules from situations that are both improvisatory (and hence happenstance) and yet conforming to the *habitus* (and hence predictable). The trick seems to be to steer away from these extremes and to study the *practices* that embody and reveal the *habitus*, rather than to search for the underlying rules. We would like to think that that is what we have tried to do here (p. 8).

5 'Half of our task is to demonstrate this [individual] cognitive process at the foundation of social order. The other half of our task is to demonstrate that the individual's most elementary cognitive process depends on social institutions' (Douglas 1987: 45). In her exploration of the way we delineate a version of the world that we can manage within the confines of our social institutions, the anthropologist Mary Douglas argues that language becomes the commonly held link between our experience of the world and the way we structure it, which becomes our 'automatic pilot' (ibid.: 63). Thus '[e]ven the simplest acts of classifying and remembering are institutionalized' (ibid.: 67), as social networks shape and constrain what is considered necessary or even permissible 'knowledge'. She concludes: 'For better or worse, individuals really do share their thoughts and they to some extent harmonize their preferences, and they have no other way to make big decisions except within the scope of institutions they build' (ibid.: 128).

6 The political 'third way' of British and US politics from the late 1990s is another ambitious compromise/synthesis, in this case between market liberalism and democratic socialism, for which this prolific thinker is well known and for which, as it happens, he was severely criticized by Bourdieu. The 'third way' politics of the Blair government was a major driving force for the changes imposed on the health service during the time of our ethnography (Klein 2001: 189–222).

7 The NHS guidance on NSAIDs and CKD are particular examples of challenges to norms, but the argument applies even to the most simple and routine of behaviours – for example the male doctors at Lawndale nearly always wore ties, whereas none of the men at Urbcester did. Any egregious challenge to that norm would raise eyebrows, and so the unspoken local dress code was upheld (even by JG when on site) without any explicit rules being laid down. If a Lawndale doctor were deliberately and consistently to refuse to conform with that dress code, it would likely be because he wanted

to make a (micro)political point, aligning himself with the more youthful, informal and politically egalitarian branches of the profession even if he might also cite as the rationale the risk of dangling ties causing cross-infection.

8   The structures and the mutually influential communities and subcommunities do not merely shape people's actions – they shape their very identities. Each Lawndale practitioner had developed a finely honed sense not only of appropriate behaviour in most conceivable circumstances, but also of their relative strengths and weaknesses and hence their capacity, freedom or ability to deal with different situations. In short, they had accumulated a sense of who and what they were, where they fitted into different hierarchies of specialist expertise, managerial clout or social influence among colleagues and patients.

9   See for example our discussion of the role of collective mindlines in establishing identity and autonomy and in enacting the clinical environment (pp. 163–4).

10 Sociologists may baulk at this broad-brush assertion, but we believe it holds true enough for present purposes. We are well aware that there are complex, esoteric debates about the strengths and weaknesses of, and the relationship between, these and other relevant social theories but these need not concern us here. (As an introduction, see, for example, King 2005.)

11 Around this time the work from the 1930s of the microbiologist and philosopher Ludwik Fleck was rediscovered (Fleck 1979 [1935]). Foreshadowing Thomas Kuhn's epoch-making (paradigm-shifting?) notion of the scientific paradigms of scientific communities (Kuhn 1964), Fleck had painstakingly linked a clear medical fact, a basic immunological test for syphilis (the Wasserman reaction), to its social origins via what he called the 'thought styles' of a 'thought community'. He had shown that only a doctor fully initiated into that community could even begin to elicit or grasp the 'facts' represented by the Wasserman reaction, which in turn were deeply imbued with centuries old concepts (such as the popular idea that syphilis was due to 'impure blood') now built into a complex modern procedure that only the initiates were capable of undertaking and interpreting. See also de Camargo (2002) for a recent attempt to understand the thought-styles of doctors. Fleck's work has been received belatedly as a classic of social constructivism (White 2002: 23–30) but it also, to our mind, foreshadows the notion of communities of practice and collective mindlines.

12 This is not the place to embark on an account of this seminal thinker, who radically altered modern perceptions of the relationship between medical power, clinical knowledge and the nature of the body. There is a whole industry of critical introductions to and exegeses of Foucault's ideas (our university library in Southampton has 212 books on the subject, not to mention all the academic journal articles). Interested readers could do worse than begin with Foucault's own *The Birth of the Clinic* (1973) but a more approachable English example of influential Foucauldian thinking is Armstrong (1983).

13 In the wider spheres of sociology and philosophy of science, the term 'social construction' has sometimes become confused, inflammatory and philosophically disreputable. Some extremist constructivists (or were they post-constructivists, who knows?) got carried away in waves of postmodernism and denied that science was different from any other type of knowledge, which in turn led others (illogically) to dismiss the whole of social construction thesis as nonsensical (see Hacking 1999 for a helpful discussion of these arguments). The term therefore appears less often nowadays in the medical sociology literature, but with or without the label of 'social construction' the underlying assumption remains that medical knowledge as well as its practice – not to mention the distribution of illness – are deeply socially contingent (Nicolson and McLaughlin 1987). For a useful critical introduction see Nettleton (2006: chapter 2).

14 Again we are well aware that there are many factional disputes between (and within) social constructionists, actor network theorists, structurationists and Foucauldians,

but we take the pragmatic view that in seeking an initial overall picture of the social origins of mindlines they all provide useful insights.

15 Star has argued that such phenomena are the result of more than just *a* network of actors, but that *many* networks interact, which is further complicated by actors usually each being a part of many different networks. Part of any such analysis, she argues, should therefore also consider how the networks interact and how that becomes stabilized over time.

> Because we are all members of more than one community of practice and thus of many networks, at the moment of action we draw together repertoires mixed from different worlds. Among other things we create metaphors – bridges between those different worlds.
>
> (Star 1991: 52)

This has implications for understanding the multiple roles of GPs who may be part of many clinical and managerial networks (Chapters 2 and 7), the interaction between doctor and patient, which we briefly discuss later in this chapter (pp. 182–91) and the role, discussed in Chapter 6, of 'boundary objects' (a term she jointly coined – see p. 120).

16 Readers who find it hard to think of hearts, budgets and guidelines as 'actors' are not alone. Ever since Michel Callon, when he coined the term 'actor-network theory', first suggested that networks bind people and inanimate objects equally (Callon 1989), that notion has been hotly debated in the literature. Even the main proponent of the theory, Bruno Latour, has suggested that the term is perfectly good except for the words 'actor', 'network', 'theory' and the hyphen (Latour 1999b)! This is not the place to enter the extensive philosophical debates in the literature, except to say that we find it difficult to escape the conclusion that people's knowledge of the world is constructed by interactions between individuals and social/organizational structures such as those we describe in the Heartshire story. The intentionality or consciousness of an action is not relevant, since unintended consequences can occur from individual human actions, organizational actions *and* the 'actions' of inanimate objects, and all can affect the outcome. (See also Giddens's [2004] views on distant influence; p. 172.) Since inanimate objects are often part of people's interactions and often constrain them, we are guardedly willing to include them in the construction 'network' (although we prefer to see them as essential nodes through which human agents operate). If the term 'actor' grates when applied to something like a heart or a leaflet, the reader may prefer to think of it as an abbreviation for 'contributing *f*Actor'.

17 Five years later as part of another study we found coincidentally that the Northton General Hospital near Lawndale was still unable to find the will or the funds to establish a direct access echocardiography service or to persuade most GPs to follow the (by now) national service framework guidance on heart failure. (Interview with Northton lead manager on cardiac services 3 November 2002). Northton's guidelines were therefore still well behind the ones that had been established in Heartshire five years earlier. It was Northton's guidelines that Jean was using to formulate the Lawndale policy for heart failure (pp. 97, 110), which meant that the inability of the actor network in her region to emulate Heartshire's had impacted on Lawndale's collective mindline for heart failure.

18 Actor-network theory sometimes has a tendency to suffocate itself with its own jargon (which is no way to irreversibilize the intéressement of sociotechnical enrollment), but sometimes it is refreshingly clear. For entertaining accounts of the method of following the development of an idea see Latour (1987) or Latour (1999a: 24–79).

19 According to an apocryphal story that we heard from several sources in the 1980s, a group of scientists and doctors met to try and set up a large drug trial on asthma. But the pharmacologists, respiratory physicians, immunologists, biochemists, trialists,

epidemiologists and others who discussed it interminably from their very different theoretical perspectives eventually gave up because they couldn't agree on exactly what they meant by asthma. For a discussion of the way in which research protocols try to render a 'political compromise' out of the 'messiness' of clinical work, see Berg (1998). This problem is also discussed philosophically in Willems (1998). See also Gabbay (1982) for an historical approach to this problem.

20 Latour (1987) would say that the place of ACE inhibitors in the management of heart failure, having been contentious and subject to change by many of the 1997 Heartshire actors, had by 1999 become 'black-boxed', that is no longer open to scrutiny but condensed and accepted as a simple, incontrovertible 'fact' (albeit, it should be added, a 'fact' subject to different interpretations and performances).

21 We use the term 'disease' to mean not just the pathology, but the entire complex of events including the pathology and its management. We recognise that the distinction between '"disease"' and "disease" is oversimplified, as indeed is the long-standing distinction between the terms 'illness' (what the patient experiences) and 'disease' (what the clinician construes the pathological problem to be). However, the only logical way to deal with our third conclusion from the Heartshire example – the infinitely variable differences of the pleomorphic disease concepts held by all the different actors at different times – is to scream and throw one's hands up in exasperation at the unmanageable complexity of it all. We prefer a more pragmatic and practical approach that calmly begins with at least this simple distinction between '"disease"' (received view), "disease" (collective mindline), and 'disease' (individual mindline) and illness–disease (single instantiation) as introduced in the next section (Table 9.1).

22 For our use of the word 'negotiation', see p. 138.

23 This may account for Freidson's observations (1988: 189) about the differences between solo, colleague-dependent and client-dependent practice, and the part those differences play in local variations in practice. Perhaps the more the clinician is exposed to colleagues, the more their practice conforms to their colleagues' norms, but the more influential the patient, the less able is the practitioner to impose the collective mindline.

24 Although we cannot enter into that question here, there is much work to be done to understand how an individual patient's view of their 'illness' relates to their collective view of the "illness" among their own communities of practice, let alone to the wider, unascertainable general view of the '"illness"'.

25 Note that Clive's mindline for 'depression' has selected some but not other elements of the received view of '"depression"' – recall for example his scepticism about the views of psychiatric 'experts' and yet his willing acceptance of the local speaker's views about there being little to choose between the available antidepressants (p. 186). Thus do the variations between '"diseases"', "diseases" and 'diseases' grow unless there is pressure to conform during the development of the collective mindline. Moreover, when the individual clinician's mindline of the 'disease' is applied in the consulting room there may be many more actors than the simple dyad of clinician and patient. Family, teachers, colleagues and others may influence what emerges as that single instantiation of the illness–disease. (See, for example, McDermott 1996 for a telling description of how a child thereby acquires a diagnosis.)

26 Of course the overlap between their constructs can be very large – especially in chronic illness when the patient has read up a great deal (as in Audrey's patient with achalasia) and the clinician has sometimes also learnt a lot from the patient over the years. On the other hand it can also be almost irreconcilably non-existent – as in the occasional patient whose whole complex and lengthy construction is ultimately reduced by the clinician to one word: 'hypochondriac'.

27 This is not to say that the received view is somehow stripped clean of social constructs only to be 'sullied' by this accretion of experience. On the contrary, there is a great deal of evidence from social studies of science that the scientific foundation of the received

view is itself socially constructed. See pp. 174–9. We will not rehearse the arguments here, still less enter into the radical critiques that charge medicine with helping to perpetrate social injustices, for example by medicalizing gender, or by maintaining a workforce with a pill to numb every social iniquity; by masking social judgements as diseases like drapetomania (the early nineteenth-century 'pathological' desire of US slaves to escape), or by colluding with the military–industrial complex to promote a reliance on expensive medications of dubious value. Suffice to say that it has long been suggested that the ways in which doctors conceive of diseases, administer treatments and interact with patients are deeply imbued with ethical and social views of which they may themselves be unaware. The argument (set out for example in Eliot Freidson 1988) is that from the time they elect to join the profession, through their strongly socializing education, through to the organizational obligations that shape their roles, clinicians absorb strong sets of values and attitudes that characterize their profession. Those values are then powerfully fed back into society through not only the professions' social roles but also the content of their knowledge and practice that we would call their mindlines.

10 Conclusions and implications

1 Actually we would also suggest that in some ways *less* research is needed. In such complex systems as healthcare organizations purely trial-based studies of the dissemination of evidence, or systematic reviews that do not look beyond randomized controlled trials of organizational interventions (both of which have been all too common within the current paradigms of EBP and 'implementation science'), are unlikely to be of much benefit.

2 For a useful analysis of the main battles around EBP see Trinder and Reynolds (2000: 212–241). For a recent skirmish see Wyer and Silva (2009) and the succeeding bout of articles in the same issue of that journal, which were sparked by Djulbegovic *et al.* (2009b).

3 Our argument does not apply, of course, to the 'bad apples' among clinicians. They are a different matter but we believe they are a small minority who should not set the tone for the wider business of implementing best practice.

4 There are many ways, not necessarily spending time in meetings, in which such a community's knowledge could be harnessed to produce a workable consensus, including nominal group technique and Delphi techniques (Hutchings *et al.* 2006). For an early example of the Delphi technique being used to change clinical practice (among a community of surgeons and anaesthetists) see Gabbay and Francis (1988).

5 We ourselves have attempted to do that with an online community of practice that we have launched for GPs, www.kasebook.com, which would need a great deal more resource, marketing and training to fulfil its potential as a forum through which colleagues and opinion leaders can influence collective mindlines. Nevertheless, with currently around 450 members it provides an opportunity for clinicians to share practical knowledge while making it easy to indicate their wide-ranging sources of evidence from personal experience through to published guidance and research.

6 See note 5 above. Face-to-face discussions are likely to be the most useful. Although KaseBook has been moderately successful it has probably also shown that clinicians prefer discussing clinical problems in live conversations, not through a computer screen.

7 'If knowledge leaks in the direction of shared practice, it sticks where practice is not shared' (Brown and Duguid 2001: 207), which suggests that if guidance does not incorporate practice and context and is not conveyed by people who share the same kind of practice it will be sticky (i.e. not spread). Ignoring 'epistemic differences' between those who provide the information and those who use it is a recipe for failure

(ibid.: 208; Carlile 2002). This is especially true of innovative knowledge, which relies more than most kinds of knowledge on social networks (Brown and Duguid 2001).

8 Features of such communities that may help them to function are their ability to work with experts and adopt the fresh perspectives that they bring to the group (an elaboration of the 'boundary spanning' benefits of communities that include members belonging to, say, expert groups). Scarborough and Swan (2002) cite the example of an NHS trust that brought together members of all the various professions involved in providing cataract services and encouraged them to share their expertise and adopt each other's perspectives in order to jointly re-engineer the service. The waiting time fell from twelve months to six to eight weeks. The key to this success included the '[t]rust and understanding [that] went hand in hand with the formation and synthesis of a new collective knowledge base' (ibid.: 17) that grew from the fostering of the community-based approach to knowledge sharing. The expertise of all those different professionals could never, they concluded, have been brought together and accepted by an IT-based system, however sophisticated.

9 This might also be a useful vehicle for helping the increasingly popular notion of illness scripts and pattern recognition to be more explicitly incorporated into clinical education as a part of a more context-sensitive and practical approach to developing clinicians' mindlines. Moreover, if learning becomes a habitually collective activity, it might help overcome the problem that clinicians tend not to accurately identify their own learning needs. A habit of collective learning would make it more likely that their colleagues would helpfully highlight (and help meet) each other's learning needs (Davis 2009).

References

Numbers in square brackets refer to pages in this book where the work has been cited. (For an explanation, see pp. 16, 216 note 16.)

Adler, P.S., Kwon, S.K., Heckscher, C. (2008) 'Professional work: the emergence of collaborative community', *Organization Science*, 19: 359–376. [130]

Agar, M. (1996) *The professional stranger: an informal introduction to ethnography.* (2nd edition) San Diego: Academic Press. [xv, 7, 8]

Ahmed, P.K., Lim, K.K., Loh, Y.E. (2002) *Learning through knowledge management.* Oxford: Butterworth Heinemann. [102, 103]

Ajjawi, R., Higgs, J. (2008) 'Learning to reason: a journey of professional socialisation', *Advances in Health Science Education*, 13: 133–150. [79, 91]

Albanese, M.A. (2006) 'Crafting the reflective lifelong learner: why, what and how', *Medical Education*, 40: 288–290. [79]

André, M. (2004) *Rules of thumb and management of common infections in general practice.* Linköping University Medical Dissertation No. 840: Linköping Faculty of Health Sciences. [58, 59]

André, M., Borgquist, L., Foldevi, M., Molstad, S (2002) 'Asking for "rules of thumb": a way to discover tacit knowledge in general practice', *Family Practice*, 19: 617–622. [58]

André, M., Borgquist, L., Molstad, S. (2003) 'Use of rules of thumb in the consultation in general practice – an act of balance between the individual and the general perspective', *Family Practice*, 20: 514–519. [58, 59]

Argyris, C. (1991) 'Teaching smart people how to learn', *Harvard Business Review*, 69: 99–109. [220n16]

Argyris, C., Schön D.A. (1974) *Theory in practice: increasing professional effectiveness.* San Francisco: Jossey-Bass. ('Classic paperback' edition, undated). [61, 197]

Aristotle (1975) [~350 BC] *Aristotle's metaphysics (translated with commentaries and glossary by Hippocrates G. Apostle).* Bloomington: Indiana University Press. [221n20]

Aristotle (2000) [~350 BC] *Nicomachean ethics.* Trans. and ed. R. Crisp. Cambridge: Cambridge University Press. [220n14]

Armstrong, D. (1983) *Political anatomy of the body: medical knowledge in Britain in the twentieth century.* Cambridge: Cambridge University Press. [190, 232n12]

Armstrong, D. (2002) 'Clinical autonomy, individual and collective: the problem of changing doctors' behaviour', *Social Science and Medicine*, 55: 1771–1777. [1, 217n12]

Asch, S.E. (1951) 'Effects of group pressure upon the modification and distortion of judgement', in H. Guetzkow (ed.) *Groups, leadership and men.* Pittsburgh, PA: Carnegie Press (reissued 1963). [229n14]

Ashburner, L., Birch, K. (1999) 'Professional control issues between medicine and nursing in primary care', in A.L. Mark and S. Dopson (ed.) *Organisational behaviour in health care: the research agenda.* Basingstoke: Macmillan. [1]

Atkinson, P. (1981) *The clinical experience: the construction and reconstruction of medical reality.* Hampshire: Gower Publishing Co. [81, 82, 176]

Atkinson, P. (1995) *Medical talk and medical work: the liturgy of the clinic.* London: Sage Publications. [176]

Baggot, R. (2004) *Health and social care in Britain.* (3rd edition) Basingstoke: Palgrave Macmillan. [218n25]

Baker, M.R., Kirk, S., (2001) (ed.) *Research and development for the NHS: evidence, evaluation and effectiveness.* Oxford: Radcliffe Medical Press. [5]

Baker, R., Robertson, N., Rogers, S., Davies, M., Brunskill, N., Khunti, K., Steiner, M., Williams, M., Sinfield, P. (2009). 'The National Institute of Health Research (NIHR) Collaboration for Leadership in Applied Health Research and Care (CLAHRC) for Leicestershire, Northamptonshire and Rutland (LNR): a programme protocol', *Implementation Science*, 4: 72. [205]

Balint, M. (1964) *The doctor, his patient and the illness.* (First edition 1957) London: Pitman. [202]

Balla, J.I., Heneghan, C., Glasziou P., Thompson, M., Balla, M. (2009) 'A model for reflection for good clinical practice', *Journal of Evaluation in Clinical Practice*, 15: 964–969. [60]

Bandura, A. (1986) *Social foundations of thought and action.* Englewood Cliffs, NJ: Prentice Hall. [223n19, 230n23, 231n3]

Barnes, B. (1974) *Scientific knowledge and sociological theory.* London: Routledge & Kegan Paul. [174]

Barnes, B., Bloor, D., Henry, J. (1996). *Scientific knowledge: a sociological analysis.* London: Athlone. [174]

Basbøll, T., Graham H. (2006) 'Substitutes for strategy research: notes on the source of Karl Weick's anecdote of the young lieutenant and the map of the Pyrenees', *Ephemera Notes: Theory & Politics in Organization*, 6: 194–204. [229n13]

Becker, H., Geer, B., Hughes, E.C., Strauss, A.L. (1976) *Boys in white: student culture in medical school.* (First edition 1961) New Brunswick, NJ: Transaction Books. [78, 83, 91]

Benner, P.E. (1984) *From novice to expert: excellence and power in clinical nursing practice.* Menlo Park, CA: Addison-Wesley. [90–5]

Benner, P., Tanner, C., Chesla, C. (1996) *Expertise in nursing practice.* New York: Springer. [115, 222n9, 223n5, 226n5]

Berg, M. (1998) 'Order(s) and disorder(s): of protocols and medical practices', in M. Berg and A. Mol (ed.) *Differences in medicine: unravelling practices, techniques, and bodies.* Durham, NC: Duke University Press. [234n19]

Berg, M., Mol, A. (1998) *Differences in medicine: unravelling practices, techniques, and bodies.* Durham, NC: Duke University Press. [181]

Berger, P.L., Luckmann, T. (1966) *The social construction of reality: a treatise in the sociology of knowledge.* London: Allen Lane, the Penguin Press. [173–4, 188, 222n10]

Blackler, F. (1995) 'Knowledge, knowledge work and organizations: an overview and interpretation', *Organization Studies*, 16: 1021–1046. [225n17]

Bloor, D. (1976) *Knowledge and social imagery.* London: Routledge & Kegan Paul. [174]

Bloor, M. (1976) 'Bishop Berkeley and the adenotonsillectomy enigma: an exploration of variation in the social construction of medical disposals', *Sociology*, 10: 43–61. [175]

Bloor, M. (2001) 'The ethnography of health and medicine', in P. Atkinson, A. Coffey,

S. Delamont, J. Lofland and L. Lofland (ed.) *Handbook of ethnography.* London: Sage Publications. [6]

Boden, D. (1994) *The business of talk: organizations in action.* Cambridge: Polity Press. [51, 196, 219n3, 228n4, 230n20]

Boshuizen, H.P.A. (2009) 'Teaching for expertise: problem-based methods in medicine and other professional domains', in K.A Ericsson (ed.) *Development of professional expertise: toward measurement of expert performance and design of optimal learning environments.* Cambridge: Cambridge University Press. [77, 92]

Boshuizen, H.P.A., Schmidt, H.G. (1992) 'On the role of biomedical knowledge in clinical reasoning by experts, intermediates and novices', *Cognitive Science*, 16: 153–184. [74]

Boshuizen, H.P.A., Schmidt, H.G. (2000) 'The development of clinical reasoning expertise', in J. Higgs and M. Jones (ed.) *Clinical reasoning in the health professions.* Oxford: Butterworth-Heinemann. [56, 92]

Bosk, C.L. (1979) *Forgive and remember: managing medical failure.* Chicago: Chicago University Press. [79, 83, 125, 222n16, 223n2]

Boström, M., Ehrenberg, A., Petter Gustavsson, J., Wallin, J. (2009) 'Registered nurses' application of evidence-based practice: a national survey', *Journal of Evaluation in Clinical Practice*, 15: 1159–1163. [217n11]

Bourdieu, P. (1992) *The logic of practice.* (First edition 1990) London: Polity Press. [168–70, 231n4]

Bourdieu, P. (2006) *Outline of a theory of practice.* (First edition 1972) Cambridge: Cambridge University Press. [168–70]

Bowen, J.L. (2006) 'Educational strategies to promote clinical diagnostic reasoning', *New England Journal of Medicine*, 355: 2217–2225. [56]

Bowker, C.B., Star, S.L.(1999) *Sorting things out: classification and its consequences.* Cambridge, MA: MIT Press. [175]

Briggs, A. (1979 reprint) *Report of the Committee on Nursing.* Cmmd.5115. London: HMSO. [215n8]

British Cardiac Society, British Hyperlipidaemia Association, British Hypertension Society, British Diabetic Association. (2000) 'Joint British recommendations on prevention of coronary heart disease in clinical practice: summary', *British Medical Journal*, 320: 705–708. [32]

Brown, J., Libberton, P. (ed.) (2007) *Principles of professional studies in nursing.* London: Palgrave. [79]

Brown, J., Chapman, T., Graham, D. (2007) 'Becoming a new doctor: a learning or survival exercise?', *Medical Education*, 41: 653–660. [93]

Brown, J.S., Duguid, P. (1991) 'Organisational learning and communities of practice: towards a unified theory of working, learning and innovation', *Organization Science*, 2: 40–55. [117]

Brown, J.S., Duguid, P. (2000) *The social life of information.* Boston: Harvard Business School Press. [vii, xv, 116–17, 217n6]

Brown, J.S., Duguid, P. (2001) 'Knowledge and organisation: a social practice perspective', *Organization Science*, 12: 198–213. [89, 202, 227n3, 235n7]

Brown, J.S, Denning, S., Groh, K., Prusak, L. (2005) *Storytelling in organizations.* Burlington, MA: Elsevier Butterworth-Heinemann. [115]

Bruner, J.S. (1986) *Actual minds, possible worlds.* Cambridge, MA: Harvard University Press. [115, 224n15]

Buchan, H., Lourey, E., D'Este, C., Sanson-Fisher, R. (2009) 'Effectiveness of strategies to encourage general practitioners to accept an offer of free access to online evidence-based information: a randomised controlled trial', *Implementation Science*, 4: 68. [28]

Byrne, D (2004) 'Evidence-based: what constitutes valid evidence?', in A. Gray and S. Harrison (ed.) *Governing medicine: theory and practice*. Maidenhead: Open University Press. [30]

Byrne, P.S., Long, B.E.L. (1976) *Doctors talking to patients*. London: HMSO. [218n23]

Callon, M. (1986) 'Some elements of a sociology of translation: domestication of the scallops and the fishermen of St Brieuc Bay', in J. Law (ed.) *Power, action and belief: a new sociology of knowledge?* Sociological Review Monograph 32. London: Routledge & Kegan Paul. [180]

Callon, M. (1989) 'Society in the making: the study of technology as a tool for sociological analysis', in W.E. Bijker, T.P. Hughes and T.J. Pinch (ed.) *The social construction of technological systems: new directions in the sociology and history of technology*. Cambridge, MA: MIT Press. [233n16]

de Camargo, K.R. (2002) 'The thought style of physicians: strategies for keeping up with medical knowledge', *Social Studies of Science*, 32: 827–855. [232n11]

de Camargo, K.R., Coeli, C.M. (2006) 'Theory in practice: why "good medicine" and "scientific medicine" are not necessarily the same thing', *Advances in Health Sciences Education*, 11: 77–89. [61]

Carley, K. (1986) 'Knowledge acquisition as a social phenomenon', *Instructional Science*, 14: 381–438. [223n4]

Carlile, P.R. (2002) 'A pragmatic view of knowledge and boundaries: boundary objects in new product development', *Organization Science*, 13: 442–455. [235n7]

Carlsen, B., Norheim, O.F. (2008) ' "What lies beneath it all?" – an interview study of GPs' attitudes to the use of guidelines', *BMC Health Services Research*, 8: 218. [27]

Carmel, S.H.M. (2003) *High technology medicine in practice: the organisation of work in intensive care*. Unpublished PhD thesis, University of London. [65]

Carrithers, M. (1992) *Why humans have cultures: explaining anthropology and social diversity*. Oxford: Oxford University Press. [176]

Chaiklin, S. (1996) 'Understanding the social and scientific practice of *Understanding Practice*', in S. Chaiklin and J. Lave (ed.) *Understanding practice: perspectives on activity and context*. Cambridge: Cambridge University Press. (Reprinted 2003). [66]

Chaiklin, S., Lave, J. (ed.) (1996) *Understanding practice: perspectives on activity and context*. Cambridge: Cambridge University Press. (Reprinted 2003). [221n18]

Chalmers, A.F. (2003) *What is this thing called science?* (3rd edition) Maidenhead: Open University Press. [66, 219n6]

Chalmers, I. (2008) 'Confronting therapeutic ignorance: tackling uncertainties about the effects of treatments will help to protect patients', *British Medical Journal*, 337: a841. [5]

Charlin, B., Boshuizen, H.P.A, Custers, E.J., Feltovich, P.J. (2007) 'Scripts and clinical reasoning', *Medical Education*, 41: 1178–1184. [56]

Charon, R. (2006) *Narrative medicine: honoring the stories of illness*. Oxford: Oxford University Press. [121]

Chatwin, B. (1998) *The songlines*. (First edition 1987) London: Vintage. [vii, 46]

Chauvet, S., Hofmeyer, N. (2007) 'Humor as a facilitative style in problem-based learning environments for nursing students', *Nurse Education Today*, 27: 286–292. [79]

Checkland, K. (2004) 'National Service Frameworks and UK general practitioners: street-level bureaucrats at work?', *Sociology of Health & Illness*, 26: 951–975. [230n22]

Checkland, K., McDonald, R., Harrison, S. (2007) 'Ticking boxes and changing the social world: data collection and the new UK General Practice Contract', *Social Policy & Administration*, 41: 693–710. [228n8]

Childs, L. (2008) 'Quality and risk management in primary care settings', in L. Coles and E. Porter (ed.) *Public health skills: a practical guide for nurses and public health practitioners*. Oxford: Blackwell Publishing. [1]

Choo, C.W. (1998) *The knowing organization: how organizations use information to construct meaning, create knowledge, and make decisions*. New York: Oxford University Press. [196, 200]

CHSRF (1999) *Issues in linkage and exchange between researchers and decision makers*. Ottawa: Canadian Health Services Research Foundation. [205]

CHSRF (2005a) *Conceptualizing and combining evidence for health system guidance*. Ottawa: Canadian Health Services Research Foundation. [101, 196, 201, 204]

CHSRF (2005b) *Weighing up the evidence: making evidence-informed guidance accurate, achievable and acceptable*. Ottawa: Canadian Health Services Research Foundation. [101, 196, 201, 202]

Cicourel, A.V. (1987) 'The interpenetration of communicative contexts: examples from medical encounters', *Social Psychology Quarterly*, 50: 217–226. [168]

Clark, J.A., Mishler, E.G. (1992) 'Attending to patients' stories: reframing the clinical task', *Sociology of Health and Illness*, 14: 344–372. [121, 123, 190]

Clase, C.M. (2006) 'Glomerular filtration rate: screening cannot be recommended on the basis of current knowledge', *British Medical Journal*, 333: 1030–1031. [153]

Cohen, M.D., March, J.G., Olsen, J.P (1972) 'A garbage can model of organizational choice', *Administrative Science Quarterly*, 17: 1–25. [137]

Coleman, J.S., Katz, E., Menzel, H. (1966) *Medical innovation, a diffusion study*. Indianapolis: Dobbs Merrill. [130]

Coles, C. (1985) *A study of the relationships between curriculum and learning in undergraduate medical education*. Unpublished PhD thesis, University of Southampton. [81, 222n12]

Coles, C. (2010) 'Curriculum development in learning medicine', in T. Dornan, K. Mann, A. Scherpbier and J. Spencer (ed.) *Medical education: theory and practice*. Edinburgh: Elsevier. [222n12]

Collins, H., Evans, R. (2007) *Rethinking expertise*. London: University of Chicago Press. [202, 224nn9,11]

Connell, N.A.D., Klein, J.H., Meyer, E. (2004) 'Narrative approaches to the transfer of organisational knowledge', *Knowledge Management Research and Practice*, 2: 184–193. [118]

Cook, D.J., Greengold N.L., Ellrodt, A.G., Scott, R.W. (1997) 'The relation between systematic reviews and practice guidelines', *Annals of Internal Medicine*, 127: 210–216. [216n2]

Cook, S.D.N., Brown, J.S. (1999) 'Bridging epistemologies: the generative dance between organizational knowledge and organizational knowing', *Organization Science*, 10: 381–400. [218n14]

Cooksey, D. (2006) *A review of UK health research funding*. Norwich: HMSO. [205]

Coresh, J., Byrd-Holt, D., Astor, B.C., Briggs, J.P., Eggers, P.W., Lacher, D.A., Hostetter, T.H. (2005) 'Chronic kidney disease awareness, prevalence, and trends among U.S. adults, 1999 to 2000', *Journal of the American Society of Nephrology*, 16: 180–188. [153]

Cox, K. (2001) 'Stories as case knowledge: case knowledge as stories', *Medical Education*, 35: 862–866. [116]

CRAP (Clinicians for the Restoration of Autonomous Practice) writing group (2002) 'EBM: unmasking the ugly truth', *British Medical Journal*, 325: 1496–1498. [3]

Crilly, T., Jashapara, A., Ferlie, E. (2010) *Research utilisation and knowledge mobilisation: a scoping review of the literature*. Southampton: NHS National Institute for Health R&D, Service Delivery and Organisation Programme. [199, 204]

Cross, R., Borgatti, S.P. (2004) 'The ties that share: relational characteristics that facilitate information seeking', in M. Huysman and V. Wulf (ed.) *Social capital and information technology*. Cambridge, MA: MIT Press. [225n21]

Cruess, R.L., Cruess, S.R., Steinert, Y. (2009) *Teaching medical professionalism*. New York: Cambridge University Press. [79]

CSAG (Clinical Standards Advisory Group) (1998) *Report on clinical effectiveness using stroke care as an example*. London: The Stationery Office. [5, 30]

Cullum, N., Ciliska, D., Haynes, B., Marks, S. (2008) *Evidence-based nursing: an introduction*. Oxford: Blackwell. [24]

Czarniawska, B. (1997) *Narrating the organization*. Chicago: University of Chicago Press. [117]

Czarniawska, B. (1998) *A narrative approach to organization studies*. Qualitative research methods volume 43. Thousand Oaks, CA: Sage Publications. [196, 221n4]

Daft, R.L., Weick, K.E. (1984) 'Towards a model of organisations as interpretation systems', *Academy of Management Review*, 9: 284–295. (Reprinted in K.E. Weick (2001) *Making sense of the organization*. Oxford: Blackwell Publishing.) [164]

Darbyshire, P. (1994) 'Skilled expert practice: is it "all in the mind"? A response to English's critique of Benner's novice to expert model', *Journal of Advanced Nursing*, 19: 755–761. [94]

Davenport, T., Prusak, L. (1998) *Working knowledge: how organizations manage what they know*. Boston: Harvard Business School Press. [102]

Davies, P., Walker, A.E., Grimshaw, J.M. (2010) 'A systematic review of the use of theory in the design of guideline dissemination and implementation strategies and interpretation of the results of rigorous evaluations', *Implementation Science*, 5: 14. [196, 214n4]

Davis, D.A. (2009) 'How to help professionals maintain and improve their knowledge and skills: triangulating best practices in medicine', in K.A Ericsson (ed.) *Development of professional expertise: toward measurement of expert performance and design of optimal learning environments*. Cambridge: Cambridge University Press. [107, 236n9]

Davis, J.H., Stasson, M., Ono, K., Zimmerman, S. (1988) 'Effects of straw polls on group decision making: sequential voting pattern, timing and local majorities', *Journal of Personality and Social Psychology*, 55: 918–926. [229n14]

Dawson, S. (1999) 'Managing, organising and performing in health care: what do we know and how can we learn?', in A.L. Mark and S Dopson (ed.). *Organisational behaviour in health care: the research agenda*. Basingstoke: Macmillan. [214n4]

Dawson, S., Sutherland, K., Dopson, S., Miller, R., with Law, S. (1998) *The relationship between R&D and clinical practice in primary and secondary care: cases of adult asthma and glue ear in children*. Unpublished report. Judge Institute of Management Studies, University of Cambridge, and Saïd Business School, University of Oxford. [5]

Denning, S. (2005) 'Using narrative as a tool for change', in J. Seely Brown, S. Denning, K. Groh and L. Prusak (ed.) *Storytelling in organizations*. Burlington, MA: Elsevier Butterworth-Heinemann. [119–20]

Department of Health (2003) *Investing in general practice: the new GMS Contract*. London: Department of Health. [216n14]

Department of Health (2005) *The National Service Framework for renal services part two: chronic kidney disease, acute renal failure and end of life care*. London: Department of Health. [153]

Department of Health (2006) *Revisions to the GMS Contract 2006/7: delivering investment in general practice*. London: Department of Health. [152, 216n14]

Di Vito-Thomas, P. (2005) 'Nursing student stories on learning how to think like a nurse', *Nurse Educator*, 30: 133–136. [79]

Djulbegovic, B., Trikalinos, T.A., Roback, J., Chen, R., Guyatt, G. (2009a) 'Impact of quality of evidence on the strength of recommendations: an empirical study', *BMC Health Services Research*, 9: 120. [216n2]

Djulbegovic, B., Guyatt, G.H., Ashcroft, R.E. (2009b) 'Epistemologic inquiries in evidence-based medicine', *Cancer Control*, 16: 158–168. [235n2]

Dobbins, M., Robeson, P., Ciliska, D., Hanna, S., Cameron, R., O'Mara, L., DeCorby, K., Mercer, S. (2009) 'A description of a knowledge broker role implemented as part of a randomized controlled trial evaluating three knowledge translation strategies', *Implementation Science*, 4: 23. [202, 205]

Dobrow, M.J., Goel, V., Upshur, R.E.G. (2004) 'Evidence-based health policy: context and utilisation', *Social Science and Medicine*, 58: 207–217. [196]

Dopson, S., Gabbay, J. (1995) *Getting research into practice and purchasing (GRiPP)*. Oxford: NHS Executive. [30, 177, 226n6]

Dopson, S., Fitzgerald, L. (ed.) (2005) *Knowledge to action? Evidence-based health care in context.* Oxford: Oxford University Press. [4, 99, 177, 199]

Dopson, S., Locock, L., Chambers, D., Gabbay, J. (2001) 'Implementation of evidence-based medicine: evaluation of the Promoting Action on Clinical Effectiveness programme', *Journal of Health Services Research and Policy*, 6: 23–31. [30, 180, 201]

Dopson, S., Locock, L., Gabbay, J., Ferlie, E., Fitzgerald, L. (2003) 'Evidence-based medicine and the implementation gap', *Health: An Interdisciplinary Journal for the Social Study of Health, Illness and Medicine*, 7: 311–330. [2]

Dopson, S., FitzGerald, L., Ferlie, E., Gabbay, J., Locock, L. (2010) 'No magic targets! Changing clinical practice to become more evidence based', *Health Care Management Review*, 35: 2–12. (First published ibid., 27: 35–47 [2002]). [5]

Dornan, T., Boshuizen, H., King, N., Scherpbier, A.J. (2007) 'Experience-based learning: a model linking the processes and outcomes of medical students' workplace learning', *Medical Education*, 41: 84–91. [88]

Douglas, M. (1987) *How institutions think*. London: Routledge & Kegan Paul. [101, 228n3, 231n5]

Doumit, G., Gattellari, M., Grimshaw, J., O'Brien, M.A. (2007) 'Local opinion leaders: effects on professional practice and health care outcomes', *Cochrane Database of Systematic Reviews*, Issue 1. Art. No.: CD000125. DOI: 0.1002/14651858.CD000125.pub3. [130]

Dowie, J., Elstein, A. (1988) *Professional judgement: a reader in clinical decision making.* Cambridge: Cambridge University Press. [55]

Dowswell, G., Harrison, S., Wright, J. (2001) 'Clinical guidelines: attitudes, information processes and culture in English primary care', *International Journal of Health Planning and Management*, 16: 107–124. [27]

Dreyfus, H.L., Dreyfus, S.E. (1986) *Mind over machine: the power of human intuition and expertise in the era of the computer.* New York: The Free Press. [90–5]

Dunning, M., Abi-Aad, G., Gilbert, D., Hutton, H., Brown, C. (1999) *Experience, evidence and everyday practice: creating systems for delivering effective health care.* London: King's Fund. [180]

Eccles, M.P., Armstrong, D., Baker, R., Cleary, K., Davies, H., Davies, S., Glasziou, P., Ilott, I., Kinmonth, A.-L., Leng, G., Logan, S., Marteau, T., Michie, S., Rogers, H., Rycroft-Malone, J., Sibbald, B. (2009) 'An implementation research agenda', *Implementation Science*, 4: 18. [214n4]

Eggly, S. (2002) 'Physician–patient co-construction of illness narratives in medical interview', *Health Communication*, 14: 339–360. [118, 122, 190]

Ellis, J., Mulligan, I., Rowe, J., Sackett, D.L. (1995) 'Inpatient general medicine is evidence based', *Lancet*, 346: 407–410. [221n17]

Elstein, A.S. (1999) 'Heuristics and biases: selected errors in clinical reasoning', *Academic Medicine*, 74: 791–794. [58]

Elstein, A.S., Schwarz, A. (2000) 'Clinical reasoning in medicine', in J. Higgs and M. Jones (ed.) *Clinical reasoning in the health professions*. Oxford: Butterworth-Heinemann. [57]

Elstein, A.S., Schwarz, A. (2002) 'Clinical problem solving and diagnostic decision making: selective review of the cognitive literature', *British Medical Journal*, 324: 729–732. [55, 220n12]

Elston, M.A. (1991) 'The politics of professional power: medicine in a changing health service', in J. Gabe, M. Calnan and M. Bury (ed.) *The sociology of the health service*. London: Routledge. [2]

Elston, M.A. (1997) *The sociology of medical science and technology*. Oxford: Blackwell Publishers. [174]

Elwyn, G. (2004) 'Arriving at the postmodern consultation', *European Journal of General Practice*, 10: 93–96. [190]

Elwyn, G., Gwyn, R., Edwards, A.G.K., Grol, R. (1999a) 'Is "shared decision-making" feasible in consultations for upper respiratory tract infection? Assessing the influence of antibiotic expectations using discourse analysis', *Health Expectations*, 2: 105–117. [168, 190]

Elwyn, G., Edwards, A., Kinnersley, P. (1999b) 'Shared decision-making in primary care: the neglected second half of the consultation', *British Journal of General Practice*, 49: 477–482. [190]

Engeström, Y., Brown, K., Engeström, R., Koistinen, K. (1990) 'Organizational forgetting: an activity-theoretical perspective', in D. Middleton and D. Edwards (ed.) *Collective remembering*. (Third reprint 1997) London: Sage Publications. [151]

Eraut, M. (2000). 'Non-formal learning and tacit knowledge in professional work', *British Journal of Educational Psychology*, 70: 113–136. [63]

Eraut, M. (2004) *Developing professional knowledge and competence*. (First edition 1994) London: Falmer Press. [62–3, 219n4]

Ericsson, K.A. (ed.) (2009) *Development of professional expertise: toward measurement of expert performance and design of optimal learning environments*. Cambridge: Cambridge University Press. [203]

Eriksen, T.H. (2001) *Small places; large issues: an introduction to social and cultural anthropology*. London: Pluto Press. [8]

Essex, B. (1994) *Doctors, dilemmas, decisions*. London: BMJ Publishing Group. [58]

Essex, B., Healy, M. (1994) 'Evaluation of a rule base for decision making in general practice', *British Journal of General Practice*, 44: 211–213. [58]

Eva, K.W. (2005). 'What every teacher needs to know about clinical reasoning', *Medical Education*, 39: 98–106. [55]

Eva, K.W., Norman, G.R. (2005) 'Heuristics and biases – a biased perspective on clinical reasoning', *Medical Education*, 39: 870–872. [58]

Evans, D., Haines, A. (2000) *Implementing changes in evidence-based health care*. Oxford: Radcliffe Publishing. [1, 204]

Evensen, A., Sanson-Fisher, R., D'Este, C., Fitzgerald, M. (2010) 'Trends in publications regarding evidence–practice gaps: a literature review', *Implementation Science*, 5: 11. [214n4]

Fairclough, N. (1992) *Discourse and social change*. Cambridge: Polity Press. [165, 225nn21,22]

Fairhurst, K., Huby, G. (1998) 'From trial data to practical knowledge: qualitative study of how general practitioners have accessed and used evidence about statin drugs in their management of hypercholesterolaemia', *British Medical Journal*, 317: 1130–1134. [225n24]

Farquhar, C.M., Kofa, E.W., Slutsky, J.R. (2002) 'Clinicians' attitudes to clinical practice guidelines: a systematic review', *Medical Journal of Australia*, 177: 502–506. [27]

Feest, K., Forbes, K. (2007) *Today's students. Tomorrow's doctors: reflections from the wards*. Oxford: Radcliffe Publishing. [91]

Ferlie, E., Ashburner, L., Fitzgerald, L., Pettigrew, A. (1996) *The new public management in action*. Oxford: Oxford University Press. [1]

Ferlie, E., Fitzgerald, L., Wood, M. (2000) 'Getting evidence into clinical practice; an organisational behaviour perspective', *Journal of Health Services Research and Policy*, 5: 1–7. [5]

Ferlie, E., Gabbay, J., Fitzgerald, L., Locock, L., Dopson, S. (2001) 'Evidence-based medicine and organisational change: an overview of some recent qualitative research', in L. Ashburner (ed.) *Organisational behaviour and organisational studies in health care: reflections on the future*. Basingstoke: Palgrave. [5]

Fetterman, D.M. (1998) *Ethnography: step by step*. Thousand Oaks, CA: Sage Publications. [6, 7]

Fish, D., Coles, C. (1998) *Developing professional judgement in health care: learning through the critical appreciation of practice*. Oxford: Butterworth Heinemann. [1, 61, 63, 91, 202]

Fish, D., Coles, C. (2005) *Medical education: developing a curriculum for practice*. Maidenhead: Open University Press. [2, 197, 204, 222n12]

Fiske, S.T., Linville, P.W. (1980) 'What does the schema concept buy us?', *Personality and Social Psychology Bulletin*, 6: 543–557. [56]

Fitzgerald, L., Ferlie, E., Wood, M., Hawkins, C. (1999) 'Evidence into practice? An exploratory analysis of the interpretation of evidence', in A.L. Mark and S. Dopson (ed.) *Organisational behaviour in health care: the research agenda*. Basingstoke: Macmillan. [99]

Fleck, L. (1979) *Genesis and development of a scientific fact*. (First edition 1935) Chicago: University of Chicago Press. [232n11]

Fondas, N., Stewart, R. (1994) 'Enactment in managerial jobs: a role analysis', *Journal of Management Studies*, 31: 83–103. [36]

Forsetlund, L., Bjørndal, A., Rashidian, A., Jamtvedt, G., O'Brien, M.A., Wolf, F., Davis, D., Odgaard-Jensen, J., Oxman, A.D. (2009) 'Continuing education meetings and workshops: effects on professional practice and health care outcomes', *Cochrane Database of Systematic Reviews*, Issue 2. Art. No.: CD003030. DOI: 10.1002/14651858. CD003030.pub2. [107]

Forsman, H., Gustavsson, P., Ehrenberg, A., Rudman, A., Wallin, L. (2009) 'Research use in clinical practice – extent and patterns among nurses one and three years postgraduation', *Journal of Advanced Nursing*, 65: 1195–1206. [217n11]

Foucault, M. (1973) *The birth of the clinic: an archaeology of medical perception*. London: Tavistock. [232n12]

Fox, N.J. (2003) 'Practice-based evidence: towards collaborative and transgressive research', *Sociology*, 37: 81–102. [205]

Fox, P. (1989) 'From senility to Alzheimer's disease: the rise of the Alzheimer's disease movement', *Milbank Quarterly*, 67: 58–102. [175]

Fox, R.C. (1988) *Essays in medical sociology: journeys into the field*. (2nd, enlarged edition) New Brunswick, NJ: Transaction. [79]

Fox, R.C. (2000) 'Medical uncertainty revisited', in G.L. Albrecht, R. Fitzpatrick and S.C. Scrimshaw (ed.) *Handbook of social studies in health and medicine*. London: Sage Publications. [79]

Fraser, S.W., Greenhalgh, T. (2001) 'Coping with complexity: educating for capability', *British Medical Journal*, 323: 799–803. [44]

Freeman, A.C., Sweeney, K. (2001) 'Why general practitioners do not implement evidence: qualitative study', *British Medical Journal*, 323: 1100. [28]

Freidson, E. (1988) *Profession of medicine: a study of the sociology of applied knowledge.* (First edition 1970) Chicago: Chicago University Press. [63–4, 80, 174, 234n23, 235n27]

French, B. (1999) 'The dissemination of research', in A. Mulhall and A. le May (ed.) *Nursing research: dissemination and implementation*. Edinburgh: Churchill Livingstone. [99]

Gabbay, J. (1982) 'Asthma attacked? Tactics for the reconstruction of a disease concept', in P. Wright and A. Treacher (ed.) *The problem of medical knowledge: examining the social construction of medicine*. Edinburgh: Edinburgh University Press. [174, 176, 234n19]

Gabbay, J. (1991) 'Courses of action: the case for experiential learning programmes in public health', *Public Health*, 105: 39–50. [83, 202, 204]

Gabbay, J., Francis, L. (1988) 'How much day surgery? Delphic predictions', *British Medical Journal*, 297: 1249–1252. [226n2, 235n4]

Gabbay, J., le May, A. (2004) 'Evidence based guidelines or collectively constructed "mindlines"? Ethnographic study of knowledge management in primary care', *British Medical Journal*, 329: 1013–1016. [vii, 15, 44, 144]

Gabbay, J., le May, A. (2009) 'Practice made perfect: discovering the roles of a community of general practice', in A. le May (ed.) *Communities of practice in health and social care*. Oxford: Wiley Blackwell. [144]

Gabbay, J., McNicol, M., Spiby, J., Davies, S., Layton, A. (1990) 'What did audit achieve? Lessons from preliminary evaluation of a year's medical audit', *British Medical Journal*, 301: 166–169. [204]

Gabbay, J., le May, A., Jefferson, H., Webb, D., Lovelock, R., Powell, J., Lathlean, J. (2003) 'A case study of knowledge management in multi-agency consumer-informed "communities of practice": implications for evidence-based policy development in health and social services', *Health: An Interdisciplinary Journal for the Social Study of Health, Illness and Medicine*, 7: 283–310. [103, 123, 137, 139, 144]

Gabbay, M.B. (ed.) (1999) *The evidence-based primary care handbook*. London: Royal Society of Medicine Press. [24]

Gabriel, Y. (2000) ' The voice of experience and the voice of the expert – can they speak to each other?', in B. Hurwitz, T. Greenhalgh and V. Skultans (ed.) *Narrative research in health and illness*. London: Blackwell Publishing. [187]

Garfinkel, H. (1967) *Studies in ethnomethodology.* (1984 edition) Cambridge: Polity Press. [xv, 159, 197, 230n20]

Gattuso, S., Fullagar, S., Young, I. (2005) 'Speaking of women's "nameless misery": the everyday construction of depression in Australian women's magazines', *Social Science and Medicine*, 61: 1640–1648. [190]

Gawande, A. (2006) 'The learning curve', in L. Prusak and E. Matson (ed.) *Knowledge management and organizational learning: a reader*. Oxford: Oxford University Press. [223n3]

Gawande, A. (2007) 'The checklist: if something so simple can transform intensive care, what else can it do?', *New Yorker Magazine*, 10 December: 86. [94]

Geertz, C. (1983) *Local knowledge: further essays in interpretative anthropology*. London: Fontana Press. [167–8]

Geertz, C. (2000) *The interpretation of cultures*. New York: Basic Books. [7, 215n5]

Gibbons, M., Limoges, C., Nowotny, H., Schwartzman, S., Scott, P., Trow, M. (1994) *The new production of knowledge: the dynamics of science and research in contemporary societies.* (2007 reprint) London: Sage Publications. [205]

Giddens, A. (2004) *The constitution of society: outline of the theory of structuration.* (First edition 1984) Cambridge: Polity Press. [171–3, 233n16]

Gigerenzer, G. (2007) *Gut feelings: the intelligence of the unconscious.* New York: Viking Penguin. [58, 94]

Gigerenzer, G., Todd, P.M., ABC Research Group (1999) *Simple heuristics that make us smart.* Oxford: Oxford University Press. [58]

Gill, P. (2006) *Body count: how they turned AIDS into a catastrophe.* London: Profile Books. [68]

Ginsburg, L.R., Lewis, S., Zackheim, L., Casebeer, A. (2007) 'Revisiting interaction in knowledge translation', *Implementation Science*, 2: 34. [205]

Glendinning, C., Dowling, B. (2003) 'Introduction: modernizing the NHS', in B. Dowling and C. Glendinning (ed.) *The new primary care: modern, dependable, successful?* Maidenhead: Open University Press. [9, 37]

Gobbi, M. (2005) 'Nursing practice as bricoleur activity: a concept explored', *Nursing Inquiry*, 12: 117–125. [116]

Goffman, E. (1959) *The presentation of self in everyday life.* (1990 reprint) London: Penguin Books. [82]

Graham, R.P., James, P.A., Cowan, T.M. (2000) 'Are clinical practice guidelines valid for primary care?', *Journal of Clinical Epidemiology*, 53: 949–954. [29]

Gray, A., Harrison, S. (2004) *Governing medicine: theory and practice.* Maidenhead: Open University Press. [5]

Gray, B. (2009) 'The emotional labour of nursing – defining and managing emotions in nursing work', *Nurse Education Today*, 29: 168–175. [79]

Gray, J.A.M. (1997) *Evidence-based healthcare: how to make health policy and management decisions.* New York: Churchill Livingstone. [2]

Greatbatch, D., Hanlon, G., Goode, J., O'Cathain, A., Strangleman, T., Luff, D. (2005) 'Telephone triage, expert systems and clinical expertise', *Sociology of Health & Illness*, 27: 802–830. [94]

Greenhalgh, J., Flynn, R., Long, A.F., Tyson, S. (2008) 'Tacit and encoded knowledge in the use of standardised outcome measures in multidisciplinary team decision making: a case study of in-patient neurorehabilitation', *Social Science and Medicine*, 67: 183–194. [228n3]

Greenhalgh, T. (1999) 'Narrative based medicine in an evidence based world', *British Medical Journal*, 318 (7179): 323–325. [121]

Greenhalgh, T. (2002) 'Intuition and evidence – uneasy bedfellows?', *British Journal of General Practice*, 52: 395–400. [52, 54]

Greenhalgh, T. (2008) 'Role of routines in collaborative work in healthcare organisations', *British Medical Journal*, 337: a2448. [230n21]

Greenhalgh, T., Worrall, J.G. (1997) 'From EBM to CSM: the evolution of context-sensitive medicine', *Journal of Evaluation in Clinical Practice*, 3: 105–108. [201, 204]

Greenhalgh, T., Hurwitz, B. (ed.) (1998) *Narrative based medicine: dialogue and discourse in clinical medicine.* London: BMJ Books. [121]

Greenhalgh, T., Robert, G., MacFarlane, F., Bate, S.P., Kyriakidou, O. (2004) 'Diffusion of innovations in service organisations: systematic review and recommendations', *Milbank Quarterly*, 82: 581–629. [196]

Greenhalgh, T., Russell, J., Swinglehurst, D. (2005a) 'Narrative methods in quality improvement research', *Quality and Safety in Health Care*, 14: 443–449. [121]

Greenhalgh, T., Robert, G., MacFarlane, F., Bate, S.P., Kyriakidou, O. (2005b). *Diffusion of innovations in health service organisations.* Oxford: Blackwell. [196]

Greenhalgh, T., Potts, H.W.W., Wong, G., Bark, P., Swinglehurst, D. (2009) 'Tensions and paradoxes in electronic patient record research: a systematic literature review using the meta-narrative method', *Milbank Quarterly*, 87: 729–788. [52]

Griffin, S., Kinmonth, A., Veltman, M., Gillard, S., Grant, J., Stewart, M. (2004) 'Effect on health-related outcomes of interventions to alter the interaction between patients and practitioners: a systematic review of trials', *Annals of Family Medicine*, 2: 595–608. [190]

Grimshaw, J.M, Shirran, L., Thomas, R., Mowatt, G., Fraser, C., Bero, L., Grilli, R., Harvey, E., Oxman, A., O'Brien, M.A. (2001) 'Changing provider behaviour: an overview of systematic reviews of interventions', *Medical Care*, 39: 8 Supplement 2: II2–II45. [4]

Grimshaw, J.M., Thomas, R.E., MacLennan, G., Fraser, C., Ramsay, C.R., Vale, L., Whitty, P., Eccles, M.P., Matowe, L., Shirran, L., Wensing, M., Dijkstra, R., Donaldson, C. (2004) 'Effectiveness and efficiency of guideline dissemination and implementation strategies', *Health Technology Assessment*, Volume 8: Number 6. [4]

Grol, R. (1997) 'Beliefs and evidence in changing practice', *British Medical Journal*, 315: 418–421. [4]

Grol, R., Dalhuijsen, J., Thomas, S., Veld, C., Rutten, G., Mokkink, H. (1998) 'Attributes of clinical guidelines that influence use of guidelines in general practice: observational study', *British Medical Journal*, 317: 858–861. [3, 27]

Hacking, I. (1999) *The social construction of what?* Cambridge, MA: Harvard University Press. [232n13]

Hage, J., Powers, C.H. (1992) *Post industrial lives: roles and relationships in the 21st century*. Newbury Park, CA: Sage Publications. [35]

Haines, A., Donald, A. (ed.) (1998) *Getting research findings into practice*. London: BMJ Books. [214n4]

Haines, A., Kuruvilla, S., Borchert, M. (2004) 'Bridging the implementation gap between knowledge and action for health', *Bulletin of the WHO*, 82: 724–732. [1]

Hamm, R.M. (2003) 'Medical decision scripts: combining cognitive scripts and judgement strategies to account fully for medical decision making', in D. Hardman and L. Macchi (ed.) *Thinking: psychological perspectives on reasoning, judgement and decision making*. Chichester: John Wiley & Sons. [219n7]

Hammersley, M. (1990) *Reading ethnographic research: a critical guide*. London: Longman. [8]

Hammersley, M., Atkinson, P. (1983) *Ethnography: principles in practice*. (1993 edition) London: Routledge. [7]

Hannes, K., Leys, M., Vermeire, E., Aertgeerts, B., Buntinx, F., Depoorter, A.-M. (2005) 'Implementing evidence-based medicine in general practice: a focus group based study', *BMC Family Practice*, 6: 37. [39]

Hanson, N.R. (1958) *Patterns of discovery – an inquiry into the conceptual foundations of science*. Cambridge: Cambridge University Press. [7]

Harrison, S. (1998) 'The politics of evidence-based medicine in the United Kingdom', *Policy and Politics*, 26: 15–31. [2, 197]

Harrison, S., McDonald, R. (2008) *The politics of healthcare in Britain*. London: Sage Publications. [1, 203, 217n10, 228–9n9]

Harrison, S., Dowswell, G., Wright, J. (2002) 'Practice nurses and clinical guidelines in a changing primary care context: an empirical study', *Journal of Advanced Nursing*, 39: 299–307. [217n11]

Hayes, B., Adams, R. (2000) 'Parallels between the process of clinical reasoning and categorization', in J. Higgs and M. Jones (ed.) *Clinical reasoning in the health professions*. Oxford: Butterworth-Heinemann. [56, 57]

Haynes, R.B. (1993) 'Some problems in applying evidence in clinical practice', *Annals of the New York Academy of Sciences*, 703: 210–224. [1]

Haynes, R.B. (2002) 'What kind of evidence is it that evidence-based medicine advocates want health care providers and consumers to pay attention to?', *BMC Health Services Research*, 2: 3. [3]

Heath, I. (1995) *The mystery of general practice*. London: Nuffield Provincial Hospitals Trust. [218n21]

Helman, C. (2000) *Culture, health and illness*. (4th edition) Oxford: Butterworth-Heinemann. [197]

Heneghan, C., Perera, R., Mant, D., Glasziou, P. (2007) 'Hypertension guideline recommendations in general practice: awareness, agreement, adoption, and adherence', *British Journal of General Practice*, 57: 948–952. [27]

Hermans, H.J.M., Hermans-Jansen, E. (1995) *Self narratives: the construction of meaning in psychotherapy*. New York: Guilford Press. [227n8]

Herxheimer, A., Ziebland, S. (2000) 'The DIPEx project: collecting personal experiences of illness and health care', in B. Hurwitz, T. Greenhalgh and V. Skultans (ed.) *Narrative research in health and illness*. London: Blackwell Publishing. [121, 187]

Higgs, J., Jones, M. (ed.) (2000) *Clinical reasoning in the health professions*. (First edition 1995) Oxford: Butterworth-Heinemann. [55]

Hojat, M., Paskin, D.L., Callahan, C.A. (2007) 'Components of postgraduate competence: analyses of thirty years of longitudinal data', *Medical Education*, 41: 982–989. [222n14]

Hunter, K.M. (1991) *Doctors' stories: the narrative structure of medical knowledge*. Princeton, NJ: Princeton University Press. [30, 82, 115, 120, 122, 123, 125, 217n13]

Hurwitz, B., Greenhalgh, T. (1999) 'Narrative based medicine: why study narrative?', *British Medical Journal*, 318: 48–50. [122]

Hurwitz, B., Greenhalgh, T., Skultans, V. (2004) *Narrative research in health and illness*. London: BMJ Publications. [121]

Hutchings, A., Raine, R., Sanderson, C., Black, N. (2006) 'A comparison of formal consensus methods used for developing clinical guidelines', *Journal of Health Services Policy and Research*, 11: 218–224. [235n4]

Jaén, C.R., Stange, K.C., Nutting, P.A. (1994) 'Competing demands of primary care: a model for the delivery of clinical preventive services', *Journal of Family Practice*, 38: 166–171. [35]

James Lind Alliance. (2010) http://www.jameslindlibrary.org/ (accessed 25 July 2010) [5]

Jamous, H., Pelloile, B. (1970) 'Professions or self-perpetuating systems? Changes in the French university hospital systems', in J.A. Jackson (ed.) *Professions and professionalization*. Cambridge: Cambridge University Press. [64, 217n12, 223n18]

Janis, I.L. (1972) *Victims of groupthink: a psychological study of foreign-policy decisions and fiascoes*. Boston: Houghton Mifflin Company. [161]

Jenkins, S.K., Thomas, M.B. (2005) 'Thought for application and application with thought: issues in theoretical thinking and practical wisdom', *Advances in Health Sciences Education*, 10: 115–123. [61]

Jha, V., Bekker, H.L., Duffy, S.R.G., Roberts, T.E. (2006) 'Perceptions of professionalism in medicine: a qualitative study', *Medical Education*, 40: 1027–1036. [79]

John, R., Webb, M., Young, A., Stevens, P.E. (2004) 'Unreferred chronic kidney disease: a longitudinal study', *American Journal of Kidney Diseases*, 43: 825–835. [153]

Johnson, T. (1972) *Professions and power*. London: Macmillan. [219n29]

Johnson, T. (1984) 'Professionalism: occupation or ideology?', in S. Goodlad (ed.) *Education for the profession: quis custodiet?* Guilford: SRHE & NFER-Nelson Publications. [219n29]

Johnston, O., Kumar, S., Kendall, K., Peveler, R., Gabbay, J., Kendrick, A. (2007)

'Qualitative study of depression management in primary care: GP and patient goals, and the value of listening', *British Journal of General Practice*, 57: 872–879. [187, 188]

Joint Specialty Committee on Renal Medicine of the Royal College of Physicians and the Renal Association, Royal College of General Practitioners. (2006) *Chronic kidney disease in adults: UK guidelines for identification, management and referral.* London: Royal College of Physicians. [153]

Jordan, M.E., Lanham, H.J., Crabtree, B.F., Nutting, P.A., Miller, W.L., Stange K.C., McDaniel R.R. (2009) 'The role of conversation in health care interventions: enabling sensemaking and learning', *Implementation Science*, 4: 15. [117]

Keller, C., Keller, J.D. (1996) 'Thinking and acting with iron', in S. Chaiklin and J. Lave (ed.) *Understanding practice: perspectives on activity and context.* Cambridge: Cambridge University Press. (Reprinted 2003). [61]

King, A. (2005) 'Structure and agency', in A. Harrington (ed.) *Modern social theory: an introduction.* Oxford: Oxford University Press. [232n10]

Kitson, A.L. (2008) 'The need for systems change: reflections on knowledge translation and organizational change', *Journal of Advanced Nursing*, 65: 217–228. [199]

Kitson, A.L., Bisby, M. (2008) *Speeding up the spread: putting KT [knowledge translation] research into practice and developing an integrated KT collaborative research agenda.* Edmonton: Alberta Heritage Medical Foundation. [196, 205]

Klein, J.G. (2005) 'Five pitfalls in decisions about diagnosis and prescribing', *British Medical Journal*, 330: 781–784. [58]

Klein, J.H., Connell, N.A.D., Meyer, E. (2005) 'Knowledge characteristics of communities of practice', *Knowledge Management Research and Practice*, 3: 106–114. [144, 227–8n7]

Klein, R. (2001) *The new politics of the NHS.* (4th edition) Harlow: Prentice Hall. [1, 231n6]

Kleinman, A. (1988) *The illness narratives: suffering, healing, and the human condition.* New York: Basic Books. [79, 187]

Kleinman, A., Eisenberg, L., Good, B. (1978) 'Culture, illness and care: clinical lessons from anthropologic and cross-cultural research', *Annals of Internal Medicine*, 88: 251–258. [188, 197]

Kolb, D.A. (1984) *Experiential learning.* Englewood Cliffs, NJ: Prentice Hall. [108, 223n16, 225n28]

Kroll, L., Singleton, A., Collier, J., Rees-Jones, I. (2008) 'Learning not to take it seriously: junior doctors' accounts of error', *Medical Education*, 42: 982–990. [79]

KT08 Forum (2008) *Knowledge translation: forum for the future: forum report.* http://www.uofaweb.ualberta.ca/kusp/pdfs/KT08_Final_Report_Dec2008.pdf (accessed 17 April 2010). [196]

Kuhn, T. (1964) *The structure of scientific revolutions.* Chicago: University of Chicago Press. [174, 232n11]

Lacasse, J.R., Leo, J. (2005) 'Serotonin and depression: a disconnect between the advertisements and the scientific literature', *PLoS Medicine*, 2: e392. [221–2n6]

Lakatos, I. (1970) 'Falsification and the methodology of scientific research programmes', in I. Lakatos and A. Musgrave (ed.) *Criticism and the growth of knowledge.* Cambridge: Cambridge University Press. [220n10]

Lakatos, I., Musgrave, A. (ed.) (1970) *Criticism and the growth of knowledge.* Cambridge: Cambridge University Press. [174, 219n6]

Lam, A. (2000) 'Tacit knowledge, organizational learning and societal institutions: an integrated framework', *Organizational Studies*, 21: 487–513. [196]

Langley, C., Faulkner, A., Watkins, C., Gray, S., Harvey, I. (1998) 'Use of guidelines in primary care: practitioners' perspectives', *Family Practice*, 15: 105–111. [27]

Lathlean, J., le May, A. (2002) 'Communities of practice: an opportunity for interagency working', *Journal of Clinical Nursing*, 11: 394–398. [137, 144]

Lathlean, J., Myall, M. (2009) 'Developing dermatology outpatient services through a community of practice', in A. le May (ed.) *Communities of practice in health and social care.* Oxford: Wiley Blackwell. [137]

Latour, B. (1987) *Science in action: how to follow scientists and engineers through society.* Milton Keynes: Open University Press. [66, 180, 181, 221n4, 233n18, 234n20]

Latour, B. (1999a) *Pandora's hope: essays on the reality of science studies.* Cambridge, MA: Harvard University Press. [14, 180, 233n18]

Latour, B. (1999b) 'On recalling ANT', in J. Law and J. Hassard (ed.) *Actor network theory and after.* Oxford: Blackwell. [233n16]

Latour, B. (2005) *Reassembling the social: an introduction to actor-network-theory.* Oxford: Oxford University Press. [180, 197]

Launer, J. (2002) *Narrative-based primary care: a practical guide.* Oxford: Radcliffe Publishing. [121, 122, 190, 202]

Launer, J. (2003) 'Narrative-based medicine: a passing fad or a giant leap for general practice?', *British Journal of General Practice*, 53: 91–92. [121]

Launer, J. (2006) 'New stories for old: narrative based primary care in Great Britain', *Families, Systems and Health*, 24: 336–344. [121, 190]

Lave, J. (1986) 'The values of quantification', in J. Law (ed.) *Power, belief and action: a new sociology of knowledge?* London: Routledge & Kegan Paul. [64–5]

Lave, J. (1996) 'Introduction: the practice of learning', in S. Chaiklin and J. Lave (ed.) *Understanding practice: perspectives on activity and context.* Cambridge: Cambridge University Press. (Reprinted 2003). [30, 82]

Lave, J., Wenger, E. (1991) *Situated learning: legitimate peripheral participation.* London: Cambridge University Press. [82–3, 94–5, 134, 142, 223n20]

le May, A. (1999) *Evidence based practice.* Nursing Times Clinical Monograph No. 1. London: EMAP. [24, 101]

le May, A. (2009a) 'Generating patient capital: the contribution of story telling in communities of practice designed to develop older people's services', in A. le May (ed.) *Communities of practice in health and social care.* Oxford: Wiley Blackwell. [123, 137]

le May, A. (2009b) 'Introducing communities of practice', in A. le May (ed.) *Communities of practice in health and social care.* Oxford: Wiley Blackwell. [145, 164, 165, 200]

le May, A., Gabbay, J. (2010) 'Evidence based practice: more than research needed?', in G. Lewith, J. Cousins and H. Walach (ed.) *Clinical research in complementary therapies.* Edinburgh: Elsevier. [111]

le May, A., Mulhall, A., Alexander, C. (1998) 'Bridging the research practice gap: exploring the research cultures of practitioners and managers', *Journal of Advanced Nursing*, 28: 428–437. [5]

Lemieux-Charles, L., Champagne, F. (2008) *Using knowledge and evidence in health care: multidisciplinary perspectives.* Toronto: University of Toronto Press. [199]

Lesser, E., Prusak, L. (1999) *Communities of practice, social capital and organizational knowledge.* Cambridge, MA: Institute of Knowledge Management. [164]

Levi-Strauss, C. (1966) *The savage mind.* London: Weidenfeld & Nicolson. [116]

Li, L.C., Grimshaw, J.M., Nielsen, C., Judd, M., Coyte, P.C., Graham, I.D. (2009) 'Use of communities of practice in business and health sectors: a systematic review', *Implementation Science*, 4: 27. [227n1]

Lindblom, C.E. (1959) 'The science of "muddling through"', *Public Administration Review*, 19: 79–88. [137]

Links, M. (2006) 'Analogies between reading of medical and religious texts', *British Medical Journal*, 333: 1068–1070. [29]

Lipman, T., Murtagha, M.J., Thomson, R. (2004) 'How research-conscious GPs make decisions about anticoagulation in patients with atrial fibrillation: a qualitative study', *Family Practice*, 21: 290–298. [27]

Lipsky, M. (1980) *Street level bureaucracy: dilemmas of the individual in public services*. New York: Russell Sage Foundation. [230n22]

Little, P., Gould, C., Williamson, I., Warner, G., Gantley, M., Kinmonth, A.L. (1997) 'Re-attendance and complications in a randomised trial of prescribing strategies for sore throat: the medicalising effect of prescribing antibiotics', *British Medical Journal*, 315: 350–352. [160, 164]

Locock, L., Dopson, S., Chambers, D., Gabbay, J. (2001) 'Understanding the role of opinion leaders in improving clinical effectiveness', *Social Science and Medicine*, 53: 745–757. [130, 201]

Loewe, R., Schwartzman, J., Freeman, J., Quinn, L., Zuckerman, E. (1998) 'Doctor talk and diabetes: towards an analysis of the clinical construction of chronic illness', *Social Science and Medicine*, 9: 1267–1276. [118]

Lomas, J. (1997) *Improving research dissemination and uptake in the health sector: beyond the sound of one hand clapping*. Policy Commentary C97–1. Hamilton, ON: McMaster University Centre for Health Economics and Policy Analysis. [1, 205]

Lomas, J. (2000) 'Using "linkage and exchange" to move research into policy at a Canadian foundation', *Health Affairs*, 19: 236–240. [205]

Lomas, J. (2007) 'The in-between world of knowledge brokering', *British Medical Journal*, 334: 129–132. [130, 202, 205]

Lord, C.G., Ross, L., Lepper, M.R. (1979) 'Biased assimilation and attitude polarization: the effects of prior theories on subsequently considered evidence', *Journal of Personality and Social Psychology*, 37: 2098–2109. [220n11]

Lugtenberg, M., Zegers-van Schaick, J.M., Westert, G.P., Burgers, J.S. (2009) 'Why don't physicians adhere to guideline recommendations in practice? An analysis of barriers among Dutch general practitioners', *Implementation Science*, 4: 54. [3, 28]

Lutfey, K.E., Campbell, S.M., Renfrew, M.R., Marceau, L.D., Roland, M., McKinlay J.B. (2008) 'How are patient characteristics relevant for physicians' clinical decision making in diabetes? An analysis of qualitative results from a cross-national factorial experiment', *Social Science and Medicine*, 67: 1391–1399. [218n24]

McAlister, F.A., van Diepen, S., Padwal, R.S., Johnson, J.A., Majumdar, S.R. (2007) 'How evidence-based are the recommendations in evidence-based guidelines?', *PLoS Medicine*, 4: e250. [216n2]

McCormack, B., Kitson, A., Harvey, G., Rycroft-Malone, J., Titchen, A., Seers, K. (2002) 'Getting evidence into practice: the meaning of "context"', *Journal of Advanced Nursing*, 38: 94–104. [196, 204]

McDermott, R.P. (1996) 'The acquisition of a child by a learning disability', in S. Chaiklin and J. Lave (ed.) *Understanding practice: perspectives on activity and context*. Cambridge: Cambridge University Press. (Reprinted 2003). [234n25]

McDonald, C.J. (1996) 'Medical heuristics: the silent adjudicators of clinical practice', *Annals of Internal Medicine*, 124: 56–62. [58]

McDonald, R. (2002) 'Street-level bureaucrats? Heart disease, health economics and policy in a primary care group', *Health and Social Care in the Community*, 10: 129–135. [228n3]

McDonald, R., Harrison, S. (2004) 'The micropolitics of clinical guidelines: an empirical study', *Policy and Politics*, 32: 223–239. [39, 216n2]

McGrath, K. (2002) 'The Golden Circle: a way of arguing and acting about technology in the London Ambulance Service', *European Journal of Information Systems*, 11: 251–266. [180]

MacNaughton, J. (1998) 'Anecdote in clinical medicine', in T. Greenhalgh and B. Hurwitz (ed.) *Narrative based medicine: dialogue and discourse in clinical medicine*. London: BMJ Books. [115, 116]

McVicar, A., Clancy, J., Mayes, N. (2010) 'An exploratory study of the application of biosciences in practice, and implications for pre-qualifying education', *Nurse Education Today*, 30: 615–622. [221n5]

Magala, S.J. (1997) 'Book review essay', *Organizational Studies*, 18: 317–338. [229n11]

Malinowski, B. (1922) *Argonauts of the Western Pacific: an account of native enterprise and adventure in the archipelagoes of Melanesian New Guinea*. London: Routledge. [9]

Mann, K.V., Ruedy, J., Millar, N., Pantelis, A. (2005) 'Achievement of non-cognitive goals of medical education: perceptions of medical students, residents, faculty and other health professionals', *Medical Education*, 39: 40–48. [79]

Marinker, M. (1973) 'The doctors' role in prescribing', *Journal of the Royal College of General Practitioners*, Supplement 23: *The medical use of psychotropic drugs*. London: Royal College of General Practitioners. [175]

Marshall, M., Roland, M. (2002) 'The new contract: renaissance or requiem for general practice?', *British Journal of General Practice*, 52: 531–532. [216n14]

Martin, J. (2002) *Organizational culture: mapping the terrain*. Thousand Oaks, CA: Sage Publications. [80]

Massoud, F.A., Havranek, E.P., Wolfe, R., Gross, C.P., Rathore, S.S., Steiner, J.F., Ordin, D.L., Krumholz, H.M., Cobley, U.T. (2003) 'Most hospitalized older persons do not meet the criteria for clinical trials in heart failure', *American Heart Journal*, 146: 250–257. [221n19]

Mattingly, C. (1994) ' The concept of therapeutic "emplotment" ', *Social Science and Medicine*, 38: 811–822. [227n8]

May, C. (2006) 'Mobilising modern facts: health technology assessment and the politics of evidence', *Sociology of Health & Illness*, 28: 513–532. [101]

May, C. (2007) 'The clinical encounter and the problem of context', *Sociology*, 41: 29–45. [30]

May, C., Rapley, T., Moreira, T., Finch, T., Heaven, B. (2006a) 'Technogovernance: evidence, subjectivity, and the clinical encounter in primary care medicine', *Social Science and Medicine*, 62: 1022–1030. [30]

May, C., Rapley, T., Kaner, E. (2006b) 'Clinical reasoning, clinical trials and risky drinkers in everyday primary care: a qualitative study of British general practitioners', *Addiction Research & Theory*, 14: 387–397. [103]

Minsky, M. (1975) 'A framework for representing knowledge', in P.H. Winston (ed.) *The psychology of computer vision*. New York: McGraw-Hill. (Reprinted in A. Collins, E.E. Smith (ed.) (1992) *Cognitive science*. San Mateo, CA: Morgan-Kaufmann.) http://web.media.mit.edu/~minsky/papers/Frames/frames.html (accessed 11 September 2010) [55]

Mishler, E.G. (1981) 'Viewpoint: critical perspectives on the biomedical model', in E.G Mishler (ed.) *Social contexts of health, illness, and patient care*. Cambridge: Cambridge University Press. [66]

Mol, A. (2002a) *The body multiple: ontology in medical practice*. Durham, NC: Duke University Press. [181]

Mol, A. (2002b) 'Cutting surgeons, walking patients: some complexities involved in comparing', in J. Law and A. Mol (ed.), *Complexities: social studies of knowledge practices*. Durham, NC: Duke University Press. [181]

Montgomery, K. (2006) *How doctors think: clinical judgement and the practice of medicine*. Oxford: Oxford University Press. [30, 59, 63, 67, 217nn12,13, 221n20]

Moreira, T., May, C., Bond, J. (2009) 'Regulatory objectivity in action: mild cognitive impairment and the collective production of uncertainty', *Social Studies of Science*, 39: 665–690. [175]

Mulhall, A., le May, A. (ed.) (1999) *Nursing research dissemination and implementation*. Edinburgh: Churchill Livingstone. [4]

Mulhall, A., le May, A. (2004). 'Reviewing the case for critical appraisal skills training', *Clinical Effectiveness in Nursing*, 8: 101–110. [2]

Mulhall, A., le May, A., Alexander, C. (1996) 'The utilisation of nursing research: a phenomenological study involving nurses and managers', in Foundation of Nursing Studies, *Reflection for action*. London: Foundation of Nursing Studies. [30]

Mutch, A. (2003) 'Communities of practice and *habitus*: a critique', *Organization Studies*, 24: 383–401. [170]

Nahapiet, J., Ghoshal, S. (1998) 'Social capital, intellectual capital, and the organisational advantage', *Academy of Management Review*, 23: 242–266. [164, 225n21]

Nettleton, S. (2006) *The sociology of health and illness*. (2nd edition) Cambridge: Polity Press. [174, 232n13]

Newell, S., Edelman, L., Scarborough, H., Swan, J., Bresnen, M. (2003) ' "Best practice" development and transfer in the NHS: the importance of process as well as product knowledge', *Health Services Management Research*, 16: 1–12. [225n23]

Newman, M., Papadopolous, I., Sigsworth, J. (1998) 'Barriers to evidence-based practice', *Intensive and Critical Care Nursing*, 14: 231–238. [4]

Newton, J., Knight, D., Woolhead, G. (1996) 'General practitioners and clinical guidelines: a survey of knowledge, use and beliefs', *British Journal of General Practice*, 46: 513–517. [27]

Nicolson, M., McLaughlin, C. (1987) 'Social constructionism and medical sociology', *Sociology of Health and Illness*, 9: 107–126. [232n13]

Nightingale, F. (1860) *Notes on nursing: what it is and what it is not*. London: Harris and Sons. [116]

NIHR (National Institute for Health Research) (2010) *Research for patient benefit*. http://www.nihr-ccf.org.uk/site/programmes/rfpb/default.cfm (accessed 19 April 2010). [205]

Nonaka, I. (1994) 'A dynamic theory of organizational knowledge creation', *Organization Science*, 5: 14–37. [99, 117]

Nonaka, I., Takeuchi, H. (1995) *The knowledge-creating company*. New York: Oxford University Press. [99]

Norman, G. (2005) 'Research in clinical reasoning: past history and current trends', *Medical Education*, 39: 418–427. [55]

Norman, G., Young, M., Brooks, L. (2007) 'Non-analytical models of clinical reasoning: the role of experience', *Medical Education*, 41: 1140–1145. [55]

Nowotny, H., Scott, P., Gibbons, M. (2001) *Re-thinking science: knowledge and the public in an age of uncertainty*. Cambridge: Polity Press. [218n17]

Nutley, S.M., Walter, I., Davies, H.T.O. (2007) *Using evidence: how research can inform public services*. Bristol: Policy Press. [199, 200, 201, 202]

Oliver, S., Harden, A., Rees, R., Shepherd, J., Brunton, G., Garcia, J., Oakley, A. (2005) 'An emerging framework for including different types of evidence in systematic reviews for public policy', *Evaluation*, 11: 428–446. [201]

Oliver, S.R., Rees, R., Clarke-Jones, L., Milne, R., Oakley, A., Gabbay, J., Stein, K., Buchanan, P., Gyte, G. (2007) 'A multidimensional conceptual framework for analysing public involvement in health services research', *Health Expectations*, 11: 72–84. [205]

O'Neil, M. (2009) 'CHSRF knowledge transfer: politics, policy and practice: research for change in Canadian healthcare', *Healthcare Quarterly*, 12: 18–21. [205]

O'Neill, E.S. (1995) 'Heuristic reasoning in diagnostic judgement', *Journal of Professional Nursing*, 11: 239–245. [58]

Orr, J.E. (1997) 'Sharing knowledge, celebrating identity: community memory in a service culture', in D. Middleton and D. Edwards (ed.) *Collective Remembering*. (First edition 1990) London: Sage Publications. [116, 126, 151, 196]

Osler, W. (1905) *Counsels and ideals from the writings of William Osler*. Oxford: Henry Frowde. [116]

Oswald, N., Bateman, H. (1998) 'Applying research evidence to individuals in primary care: a study using non-rheumatic atrial fibrillation', *Family Practice*, 16: 414–419. [30]

Oswald, N., Bateman, H. (2000) 'Treating individuals according to evidence: why do primary care practitioners do what they do?', *Journal of Evaluation in Clinical Practice*, 6: 139–148. [30]

Outhwaite, W. (2005) ' Interpretivism and interactionism', in A. Harrington (ed.) *Modern social theory: an introduction*. Oxford: Oxford University Press. [229n18]

Patel, V.L., Kaufman, D.R. (2000) 'Clinical reasoning and biomedical knowledge: implications for teaching', in J. Higgs and M. Jones (ed.) *Clinical reasoning in the health professions*. Oxford: Butterworth-Heinemann. [56]

Patel, V.L., Evans, D.A., Groen, G.J. (1989) 'Biomedical knowledge and clinical reasoning', in D.A. Evans and V.L. Patel (ed.) *Cognitive science in medicine*. Cambridge, MA: MIT Press. [74]

Patton, J.R. (2003) 'Intuition in decisions', *Management Decision*, 41: 989–996. [52]

Pawson, R. (2006) *Evidence-based policy: a realist perspective*. London: Sage Publications. [197]

Payer, L. (1996) *Medicine and culture: varieties of treatment in the United States, England, Germany and France*. New York: Henry Holt & Co. [197, 222n15]

Peckham, S., Exworthy, M. (2003) *Primary care in the UK: policy organisation and management*. Basingstoke: Palgrave Macmillan. [1, 9, 37]

Pendleton, D., Schofield, T., Tate, P., Havelock, P. (1984) *The consultation: an approach to learning and teaching*. Oxford: Oxford University Press. [40]

Polanyi, M. (1958) *Personal knowledge*. London: Routledge & Kegan Paul. [72, 75–6, 93, 219n1, 224n14]

Polanyi, M. (1967) *The tacit dimension*. Gloucester, MA: Peter Smith. [72]

Pope, C.J. (2003) 'Resisting evidence: the study of evidence-based medicine as a contemporary social movement', *Health: An Interdisciplinary Journal for the Social Study of Health, Illness and Medicine*, 7: 267–282. [2, 197]

Pope, C.J., le May, A., Gabbay, J. (2007) 'Chasing chameleons, chimeras and caterpillars: evaluating and organisational innovation in the National Health Service', in L. McKee, E. Ferlie and P. Hyde (ed.) *Organizing and reorganizing: power and change in health care organizations*. Basingstoke: Palgrave Macmillan. [215n9]

Popper, K.R. (1975) *The logic of scientific discovery*. (First edition 1959) London: Hutchinson. [220n10]

Presseau, J., Sniehotta, F., Francis, J., Campbell, N. (2009) 'Multiple goals and time constraints: perceived impact on physicians' performance of evidence-based behaviours', *Implementation Science*, 4: 77. [35]

Prout, A. (1996) 'Actor-network theory, technology and medical sociology: an illustrative analysis of the metered dose inhaler', *Sociology of Health and Illness*, 18: 198–219. [180]

Prusak, L., Matson, E. (2006) *Knowledge management and organizational learning: a reader*. Oxford: Oxford University Press. [225n17]

Pugh, D.S., Hickson, D.J. (1996) *Writers on organisations*. (5th edition) London: Penguin. [159]

Putnam, R. (2000) *Bowling alone: the collapse and revival of American community*. New York: Simon & Schuster. [164]

Rabindranath, K.S., Anderson, N.R., Gama, R., Holland, M.R. (2002) 'Comparative evaluation of the new Sheffield table and the modified joint British societies coronary risk prediction chart against a laboratory based risk score calculation', *Postgraduate Medical Journal*, 78: 269–272. [65]

Rademakers, J.J.D.J.M., de Rooy, N., ten Cate, O.T.J (2007) 'Senior medical students' appraisal of CanMEDS competencies', *Medical Education*, 41: 990–994. [79]

Raine, R., Sanderson, C., Hutchings, A., Carter, S., Larkin, K., Black, N. (2004) 'An experimental study of determinants of group judgments in clinical guideline development', *Lancet*, 364: 429–437. [216n2]

Rapley, T. (2008) 'Distributed decision making: the anatomy of decisions-in-action', *Sociology of Health and Illness*, 30: 429–444. [163]

Revans, R.W. (1998) *ABC of action learning: empowering managers to act and to learn from action*. (First edition 1982) London: Lemos and Crane. [83, 202, 204]

Rich, R. (1991) 'Knowledge creation, diffusion and utilization: perspectives of the founding editor', *Science Communication*, 12: 319–337. [202]

Ridderikhoff, J. (1991) 'Medical problem-solving: an exploration of strategies', *Medical Education*, 25: 196–207. [57]

Ridderikhoff, J. (1993) 'Problem-solving in general practice', *Theoretical Medicine*, 14: 343–363. [57]

Rikers, R.M., Loyens, S.M., Schmidt, H.G. (2004) 'The role of encapsulated knowledge in clinical case representations of medical students and family doctors', *Medical Education*, 38: 1035–1043. [75]

Rogers, E.M. (2003) *Diffusion of Innovations*. (First edition 1995) New York: Free Press. [98–9, 130, 225n21]

Rothwell, P. (2005) 'External validity of randomised controlled trials: "To whom do the results of this trial apply?"', *Lancet*, 365: 82–93. [30]

Rycroft-Malone, J. (2006) 'The politics of the evidence-based practice movements: legacies and current challenges', *Journal of Nursing Research*, 11: 95–108. [2]

Rycroft-Malone, J., Seers, K., Titchen, A., Harvey, G., Kitson, A., McCormack, B. (2003) 'What counts as evidence in evidence-based practice?', *Journal of Advanced Nursing*, 47: 81–90. [101]

Rycroft-Malone, J., Fontenla, M., Bick, D., Seers, K. (2008) 'Protocol-based care: impact on roles and service delivery', *Journal of Evaluation in Clinical Practice*, 14: 867–873. [217n11]

Sackett, D.L, Straus, S.E. (1998) 'Finding and applying evidence during clinical rounds: the "Evidence Cart"', *Journal of the American Medical Association*, 280: 1336–1338. [80]

Sackett, D.L., Rosenberg, W.M.C., Gray, J.A.M., Haynes, R.B., Richardson, W.S. (1996) 'Evidence-based medicine: what it is and what it isn't', *British Medical Journal*, 312: 71–72. [3]

Sackett, D.L., Richardson, W.S., Rosenberg, W.M.C., Haynes, R.B. (1997) *Evidence-based medicine: how to practice and teach EBM*. New York: Churchill Livingstone. [2–3]

Säljö, R., Wyndhamn, J. (1996) 'Solving everyday problems in the formal setting: an empirical study of the school as context for thought', in S. Chaiklin and J. Lave (ed.)

Understanding practice: perspectives on activity and context. Cambridge: Cambridge University Press. (Reprinted 2003). [66]

Sanjek, R. (1996) 'Ethnography', in A. Barnard and J. Spencer (ed.) *Encyclopaedia of social and cultural anthropology.* Oxford: Routledge. [7]

Satterfield, J.M., Hughes, E. (2007) 'Emotion skills training for medical students: a systematic review', *Medical Education*, 41: 935–941. [79]

Scarborough, H., Swan, J. (2002) 'Knowledge communities and innovations', *Trends in Communication*, 8: 7–20. [203, 230–1n2, 236n8]

Schank, R.C., Abelson, R.P. (1995) 'Knowledge and memory: the real story', in R.S. Wyer (ed.) *Knowledge and memory: the real story.* Advances in social cognition, Volume 8. Hillsdale, NJ: Lawrence Erlbaum Associates. [115–16, 119]

Schein, E.H. (1992) *Organizational culture and leadership.* (2nd edition) San Francisco: Jossey-Bass Publishers. [80]

Schmidt, H.G., Rikers, R.M.J.P. (2007) 'How expertise develops in medicine: knowledge encapsulation and illness script formation', *Medical Education*, 41: 1133–1139. [75]

Schmidt, H.G., Norman, G., Boshuizen, H.P.A. (1990) 'A cognitive perspective on medical expertise: theory implications', *Academic Medicine*, 65: 611–621. [57]

Schön, D.A. (1991) *The reflective practitioner: how professionals think in action.* (First edition 1983) Aldershot: Ashgate Arena. [61–3]

Seeleman, C., Suurmond, J., Stronks, K. (2009) 'Cultural competence: a conceptual framework for teaching and learning', *Medical Educational*, 43: 229–237. [79]

Sharf, B.F. (1990) 'Physician–patient communication as interpersonal rhetoric: a narrative approach', *Health Communication*, 2: 217–231. [123, 190]

Sheaff, R. (2008) 'Medicine and management in English primary care: a shifting balance of power?', in L. McKee, E. Ferlie and P. Hyde (ed.) *Organizing and reorganizing: power and change in health care organizations.* Basingstoke: Palgrave Macmillan. [9]

Silva, S.A., Wyer, P.C. (2009) 'Where is the wisdom? II: Evidence-based medicine and the crisis in clinical medicine. Exposition and commentary on Djulbegovic, B., Guyatt, G.H. & Ashcroft, R.E. (2009) *Cancer control*, 16: 158–168', *Journal of Evaluation in Clinical Practice*, 15: 899–906. [214n2]

Silverman, D. (1983) 'The clinical subject: adolescents in a cleft-palate clinic', *Sociology of Health and Illness*, 5: 253–274. [175, 188]

Silverman, D. (1987) *Communication and medical practice: social relations in the clinic.* London: Sage. [188]

Simon, H. (1957) *Models of man, social and rational: mathematical essays on rational human behavior in a social setting.* New York: Wiley. [219n2, 220n11]

Simon, H. (1983) *Reason in human affairs.* Oxford: Basil Blackwell. [220n11]

Simon, H. (1991) 'Bounded rationality and organizational learning', *Organization Science*, 2: 125–134. [220n11]

Siriwardena, A.N. (1995) 'Clinical guidelines in primary care: a survey of general practitioners' attitudes and behaviour', *British Journal of General Practice*, 45: 643–647. [27]

Smith, A., Goodwin, D., Mort, M., Pope, C. (2003) 'Expertise in practice: an ethnographic study exploring acquisition and use of knowledge in anaesthesia', *British Journal of Anaesthesia*, 91: 319–328. [93]

Smith, D.G. (2008) 'Viewpoint: envisioning the successful integration of EBM and humanism in the clinical encounter: fantasy or fallacy?', *Academic Medicine*, 83: 268–273. [93, 214n2]

Smith, P., Gray, B. (2001) 'Reassessing the concept of emotional labour in student nurse education: role of link lecturers and mentors in a time of change', *Nurse Education Today*, 21: 230–237. [79]

Soper, B., Hanney, S.R. (2007) 'Lessons from the evaluation of the UK's NHS R&D Implementation Methods Programme', *Implementation Science*, 2: 7. [214n4]

Spence, D. (2006) 'Who put CKD in the new GP contract?', *BMJ Rapid Responses*, 8 November 2006. http://www.bmj.com/cgi/eletters/333/7577/1047#148805 (accessed 25 July 2010) [153]

Spradley, J.P. (1979) *The ethnographic interview*. Fort Worth: Harcourt Brace Jovanovich. [45]

Star, S.L. (1991) 'Power, technology and the phenomenology of conventions: on being allergic to onions', in J. Law (ed.) *Sociology of monsters: essays on power, technology and domination*. Sociological review monograph 38. London: Routledge. [233n15]

Star, S.L., Griesemer, J.R. (1989) 'Institutional ecology, "translations", and boundary objects: amateurs and professionals in Berkeley's Museum of Vertebrate Zoology, 1907–1939', *Social Studies of Science*, 19: 387–420. [226n7]

Stead, L.F., Bergson, G., Lancaster, T. (2008) 'Physician advice for smoking cessation', *Cochrane Database of Systematic Reviews*, Issue 2. Art. No.: CD000165. DOI: 10.1002/14651858. CD000165.pub3. [41]

Stewart, M., Brown, J.B., Weston, W.W., McWhinney, I.R., McWilliam, C.L., Freeman, T.R. (1995) *Patient-centred medicine: transforming the clinical method*. Thousand Oaks, CA: Sage Publications. [40]

Stewart, R. (1999) 'Foreword', in A.L. Mark and S. Dopson (ed.) *Organisational behaviour in health care: the research agenda*. Basingstoke: Macmillan. [214n4]

Straus, S.E., Sackett, D.L. (1998) 'Using research findings in clinical practice', *British Medical Journal*, 317: 339–342. [3]

Strauss, A. (1978) *Negotiations: varieties, processes, contexts and social order*. San Francisco: Jossey-Bass Publishers. [138]

Strauss, A., Fagerhaugh, S., Suczek, B., Wiener, C. (1985) *Social organization of medical work*. Chicago: University of Chicago Press. [138]

Strong, P.M. (1979) *The ceremonial order of the clinic: parents, doctors and medical bureaucracies*. London: Routledge & Kegan Paul. [188]

Summerskill, W. (2005): 'Evidence-based practice and the individual', *Lancet*, 365: 13–14. [30]

Summerskill, W.S.M., Pope, C. (2002) 'I saw the panic rise in her eyes and evidence-based medicine went out of the door: an exploratory qualitative study of the barriers to secondary prevention in the management of coronary heart disease', *Family Practice*, 19: 605–610. [41]

Surender, R., Locock, L., Chambers, D., Dopson, S., Gabbay, J. (2002) 'Closing the gap between research and practice in health: lessons from a clinical effectiveness initiative', *Public Management Review*, 4: 45–61. [30]

Swick, H.M., Szenas, P., Danoff, D., Whitcomb, M.E. (1999) 'Teaching professionalism in undergraduate medical education', *Journal of the American Medical Association*, 282: 830–832. [79]

Tanenbaum, S.J. (1994) 'Knowing and acting in medical practice: the epistemological politics of outcomes research', *Journal of Health Politics, Policy & Law*, 19: 27–44. [222n7]

Teunissen, P., Schele, F., Scherpbier, A.J.J.A., van der Vleuten, C.P., Boor, K., van Luijk, S.J., van Diemen-Steenvoorde, J.A.A.M. (2007) 'How residents learn: qualitative evidence for the pivotal role of clinical activities', *Medical Education*, 41: 763–770. [81]

Thompson, C., Dowding, D. (2009) *Essential decision making and clinical judgement for nurses*. Edinburgh: Churchill Livingstone. [55]

Timmermans, S., Berg, M. (1997) 'Standardization in action: achieving local universality through medical protocols', *Social Studies in Science*, 27: 273–305. [180]

Timmermans, S., Angell, A. (2001) 'Evidence-based medicine, clinical uncertainty, and learning to doctor', *Journal of Health and Social Behaviour*, 42: 342–359. [220n12]

Timmermans, S., Berg, M. (2003) *The gold standard: the challenge of evidence-based medicine and standardization in health care*. Philadelphia: Temple University Press. [2, 103, 197, 202, 217n4, 218n16, 227n6]

Titchen, A. (2009) 'Developing expertise through nurturing professional artistry in the workplace', in S. Hardy, A. Titchen, B. McCormack and K. Manley (ed.) *Revealing nursing expertise through practitioner inquiry*. Oxford: Wiley-Blackwell. [91]

Tomlinson, S. (2001) *Education in a post-welfare society*. Milton Keynes: Open University Press. [197]

Trinder, L., Reynolds, S. (2000) *Evidence-based practice: a critical appraisal*. Oxford: Blackwell. [3, 197, 235n2]

Tsoukas, H., Vladimirou, E. (2001) 'What is organizational knowledge?', *Journal of Management Studies*, 38: 973–993. [217n12]

Turner, B.S. (1995) *Medical power and social knowledge*. (2nd edition) London: Sage Publications. [175]

Turner, M.E., Pratkanis, A.R. (1998) 'Twenty-five years of groupthink theory research: lessons from the evaluation of a theory', *Organizational Behavior and Human Decision Processes*, 73: 105–115. [229n15]

Tversky A., Kahneman, D. (1974) 'Judgment under uncertainty: heuristics and biases', *Science*, 185: 1124–1131. (Reprinted in D. Kahneman, P. Slovic, A. Tversky (ed.) (1982) *Judgment under uncertainty: heuristics and biases*. Cambridge: Cambridge University Press). [58]

Upshur, R.E.G. (2000) 'Seven characteristics of medical evidence', *Journal of Evaluation in Clinical Practice*, 6: 93–97. [196]

Upshur, R.E.G. (2001) 'If not evidence, then what? Or does medicine really need a base?', *Journal of Evaluation in Clinical Practice*, 8: 113–119. [196]

van Deemter, K. (2010) *Not exactly: in praise of vagueness*. Oxford: Oxford University Press. [44]

Van de Ven, A.H (2007) *Engaged scholarship: a guide for organizational and social research*. Oxford: Oxford University Press. [205]

Van de Ven, A.H., Schomaker, M.S. (2002) 'Commentary: the rhetoric of evidence-based medicine', *Health Care Management Review*, 27: 89–91. [201]

Van de Ven, A.H., Jonson, P.E. (2006) 'Knowledge for theory and practice', *Academy of Management Review*, 31: 802–821. [205]

Van de Ven, A.H., Polley, D.E., Garud, R., Venkataraman, S. (1999) *The innovation journey*. Oxford: Oxford University Press. [99, 199]

van de Wiel, M.J.W., Boshuizen, H.P.A., Schmidt, H.K., Schaper, N.C. (1999) 'The explanation of clinical concepts by expert physicians, clerks and advanced students', *Teaching and Learning in Medicine*, 11: 153–163. [75]

van Hell, E.A., Kuks, J.B.M., Schönrock-Adema, J., van Lohuizen, M.T., Cohen-Schotanus, J. (2008) 'Transition to clinical training: influence of pre-clinical knowledge and skills, and consequences for clinical performance', *Medical Education*, 42: 830–837. [222n11]

Vogt, F., Armstrong, D., Marteau T.M. (2010) 'General practitioners' perceptions of the effectiveness of medical interventions: an exploration of underlying constructs', *Implementation Science*, 5: 17. [218n24]

Vygotsky, L.S. (1978). *Mind in society: development of higher psychological processes*. Ed. M. Cole, V.

John-Steiner, S. Scribner, E. Souberman. Cambridge, MA: Harvard University Press. [223n19]

Watkins, C., Harvey, I., Langley, C., Gray, S., Faulkner, A. (1999) 'General practitioners' use of guidelines in the consultation and their attitudes to them', *British Journal of General Practice*, 49: 11–15. [27]

Weick, K.E. (1995) *Sensemaking in organizations*. Thousand Oaks, CA: Sage Publications. [54, 124, 159–64, 229n13]

Weick, K.E. (2001) *Making sense of the organization*. Oxford: Blackwell Publishing. [116, 162, 164, 229n12]

Weick, K.E., Roberts, K.H. (1993) 'Collective mind in organizations: heedful inter-relating on flight decks', *Administrative Science Quarterly*, 38: 357–381. [162, 188]

Wenger, E. (1998) *Communities of practice: learning, meaning and identity*. New York: Cambridge University Press. [134, 142–4, 226–7n7, 227n3, 228n2]

Wenger, E., McDermott, R., Snyder, W. (2002) *Cultivating communities of practice*. Boston: Harvard Business School. [133–4, 145]

West, E., Barron, D.N., Dowsett, J., Newton, J.N. (1999) 'Hierarchies and cliques in the social networks of health care professionals: implications for the design of dissemination strategies', *Social Science and Medicine*, 48: 633–646. [130]

White, K. (1991) 'The sociology of health and illness', *Current Sociology*, 39: 1–134. [174]

White, K. (2002) *An introduction to the sociology of health and illness*. London: Sage. [232n11]

Willems, D. (1998) 'Inhaling drugs and making worlds: the proliferation of lungs and asthmas', in M. Berg and A. Mol (ed.) *Differences in medicine: unraveling practices, techniques, and bodies*. Durham, NC: Duke University Press. [234n19]

Williams, R.G., Klamen, D.L., Hoffman, R.M. (2008) 'Medical student acquisition of clinical working knowledge', *Teaching and Learning in Medicine*, 20: 5–10. [75]

Wilson, J.M.G., Jungner, G. (1968) *Principles and practice of screening for disease*. Geneva: WHO. [112]

Witteman, C.L.M., Harries, C., Bekker, H.L., Van Aarle, E.J.M. (2007) 'Evaluating psychodiagnostic decisions', *Journal of Evaluation in Clinical Practice*, 13: 10–15. [227n9]

Wittgenstein, L. (1953) *Philosophical investigations*. Trans. G.E.M. Anscome and R. Rhees. (1976 edition) Oxford: Basil Blackwell. [219n5]

Wittgenstein, L. (1974) *Tractatus logico-philosophicus*. Trans. D.F Pears and B.F. McGuiness. (First edition 1922) London: Routledge & Kegan Paul. [195]

Woods, N.N. (2007) 'Science is fundamental: the role of biomedical knowledge in clinical reasoning', *Medical Education*, 41: 1173–1177. [74, 75]

Woods, N.N., Brooks, L., Norman, G.R. (2007) 'It all makes sense: biomedical knowledge, causal connections and memory in the novice diagnostician', *Advances in Health Science Education*, 12: 405–415. [75]

Wright, P., Treacher, A. (ed.) (1982) *The problem of medical knowledge: examining the social construction of medicine*. Edinburgh: Edinburgh University Press. [174]

Wyer, P.C., Silva, S.A. (2009) 'Where is the wisdom? 1: a conceptual history of evidence-based medicine', *Journal of Evaluation in Clinical Practice*, 15: 891–898. [1, 214n2, 235n2]

Young, R.M. (1977) 'Science *is* social relations', *Radical Science Journal*, 5: 65–129. [174]

Zhu, Z. (2006) 'Nonaka meets Giddens: a critique', *Knowledge Management Research and Practice*, 4: 106–115. [225n17]

Index

For author index, see References. See also 16, 216n16, 237 for an explanation.

acculturation 79–81; *see also* socialization
actor network theory 177–82, 227n6, 233nn16,18
advanced beginner *see* beginner
anecdote 15, 112–17, 123–5, 128, 132, 135, 137, 140, 224n8; *see also* narrative; stories; storytelling
anthropology 6–7, 168, 196, 214n5, 215, 231; *see also* ethnography
antibiotics, use of 35, 36, 49–51, 59, 60–2, 94, 106–7, 120, 127–29, 149, 160, 164, 171, 183
antidepressants *see* depression
appraisal, 2, 3, 108, 198; *see also* critical appraisal
apprenticeship 2, 64, 75–84, 100, 223nn16,19; *see also* beginner; learning; legitimate peripheral participation; teaching; trainee
artistry, professional 61, 63, 91, 202; *see also* practical knowledge
asthma 5, 176, 183, 188, 190, 216n14, 218nn15,26, 233n19
audit, clinical 2, 12, 15, 23, 24, 27, 28, 35, 42, 43, 107, 108, 109, 110, 112, 113, 125, 128, 135, 142, 147–9, 160–1, 166, 168, 178–80, 203, 204, 226n29, 226n3
authority *see* autonomy; expertise; experts
autonomy 2, 5, 43, 163, 203, 217n12, 218n15, 228–9n9, 230n22, 231n3, 232n9; see also clinical freedom; power, professional

Ba 226n3
beginner 62, 217n9, 224n10; advanced 92; *see also* apprenticeship, novice, transition
biomedical science 57, 69, 73–5, 92, 222n7, 228n9; *see also* encapsulation theory
boundary objects 202, 226–7n7, 233n15; *see also* community of practice; cross boundary flow; stories as boundary objects
boundary spanning *see* cross-boundary flow
bounded rationality 220n11; *see also* rationalism; satisficing
bricolage 116; *see also habitus*
bureaucracy 1, 4, 5, 163, 203, 230n22
bureaucratic-scientific model 203, 217n10

Canadian Health Services Research Foundation (CHSRF) 205
capability 44; *see also* competence, craft, knowledge-in-practice-in-context
capital: collective 164; human, 164–5, organizational; 164–5; patient 23on24; professional 165, 168, 170, 230n25; social, 118, 124, 170
categorization theory 56, 57
checklist 45, 94, 105; *see also* protocol
cholesterol 22, 31, 32, 33, 34, 40, 41, 50, 64, 95, 147, 148, 150, 158, 162
chronic kidney disease 101, 103, 104, 228n9; collective mindlines and 153–7, 230n20; enactment 163,

231n3;GP views; 104, 140, 141, 153, 156; guidelines 31, 103, 110, 211; QOF requirements152–3, 229n10; renegotiation; 154–7; sensemaking and 157–63; social construction of 152–7, 170, 180, 230n20

CKD *see* chronic kidney disease

clinical education *see* learning

clinical experience 23, 28, 32, 33, 42, 44–5, 48, 57, 59–66, 70–5, 88–103, 109–11, 117, 125, 133, 165, 186, 225n27

clinical freedom 1,171–2, 203, 228n9, 232n8*; see also* autonomy; power, professional

clinical judgement 2, 3, 19, 30–2, 43, 48–51, 57, 63, 66–8, 92, 138, 144, 154, 155, 159, 170, 217n12; *see also* artistry; autonomy; knowledge-in-practice-in-context; wisdom

clinical practice guidelines *see* guidelines

clinical reasoning 48, 51, 55–60, 66, 93–4, 219n5, 227n9; *see also* pattern recognition; hypothetico-deductivism; knowledge-in-practice-in-context; mindlines

clinical trial 1, 3, 4, 30–1, 34, 67–8 95, 96, 181, 186, 197, 205, 222n7, 233n19, 235n1

clinical uncertainty 5, 29, 63, 79, 159, 221n20

Cochrane Collaboration 3–4, 20, 68, 182

co-construction: of collective mindlines 148–164; of 'disease' 177–82; of illness–disease 182–91; *see also* narrative, shared

codified knowledge 61–64, 66, 99 101, 169, 173, 181, 184, 191, 193, 195, 201, 205, 222n16, 230n2; *see also* formal knowledge; textbook

codified structures 172–3, 80*; see also* structuration

coffee room *see* discussions, informal

collective mindlines *see* mindlines

college *see* Royal College of General Practitioners

combination (of information) 99–103; *see also* SECI spiral

common sense vi, 20, 33, 134, 151, 167–8, 173, 186

community of practice 83, 135, 136–46, 204, 224n8, 233n15, 236n8; artificial; 137; criteria 142, 144–5; collective

mindlines and 164; collective capital and 164–5; cross-boundary flow 143 *see also* boundary; cross-boundary flow of knowledge; identity and 143–5; information/knowledge flows in 137–9, 141; joint enterprise 142–3; learning 15, 130–42, 149–51; legitimate peripheral participation in 142; meaning and 143; non-involvement in 227n4; on-line 235n5; patients 188; properties of 142; reification 142, 217n7, 228n2; shared domain 145; storytelling in 137, 151; *see also* social life of knowledge

competence 4, 9, 80, 90, 92–3, 143, 168, 199, 204; cultural 79; *see also* capability

competencies 2, 52, 90, 93, 197, 198, 204; *see also* learning, skills

competent practitioner *see* competence

complexification 35

computer *see* information technology

congestive heart failure *see* heart failure

connoisseurship 93, 224n11

consensus 161, 162, 235m4; *see also* collective mindlines

construct ('disease' or 'illness') 184–90; *see also* social construction; social constructivism

constructivism *see* social constructivism

constructuralism 223n4

consultation, clinical 29, 35, 39–40, 182–90, 218nn18,23; *see also* illness–disease; patient

contacts (professional) *see* networks

context xv, 7, 16, 30, 52, 62–6, 81, 91, 95, 101, 108, 143, 150, 165, 170, 174, 176–82, 200–5, 218n17, 223n19, 224n9, 225n18, 230n2, 235n7; *see also* contextual adroitness; contextualization; knowledge-in-practice-in-context; local knowledge

contextual adroitness 90, 91, 94–5, 108, 224n9; *see also* practical knowledge

contextualization 7, 30, 101–2, 13, 132, 182, 198, 200, 205, 218n17

continuing professional development 2, 12, 15, 23, 42, 45, 50, 103–8, 132, 204; *see also* learning

contract *see* Quality and Outcomes Framework

co-presence 172, 180; *see also* structuration

CPD *see* continuing professional development

craft 61, 65, 66, 67, 77, 81, 82, 107, 220n14, 227n3; *see also* practical knowledge

critical appraisal 24, 68, 95, 133, 139, 162, 198, 201–4, 217n10

cross-boundary flow (of knowledge) 141, 202, 227n3, 236n8; *see* also community of practice

culture 6–8, 168, 171, 197, 203, 204, 214n5, 222n15; clinical 79, 81–2, 176; organizational 80–1; student 78–9, 173, 222n13

curriculum 52, 75, 77, 78, 79, 90, 204, 221n12

decision making, clinical 8, 15, 18, 27, 38, 39, 42, 43, 51–64, 77, 93–5, 102, 107, 202, 216n1, 218n24, 219nn2,3, 220n11, 228n4, 229n12, 220nn22,23; apparent lack of 35; 51; collective mindlines and 137, 154–6, 160–4, construction of 168–70

decontextualization *see* context

democratization *see* autonomy

Department of Health (England and Wales) 19, 102, 110, 119, 144, 152, 216n14, 229n10

depression, 21, 22, 49, 70, 71, 81, 83, 96, 114, 118–19, 122–4, 186, 222n6, 228n7, 234n25; concepts of 187–90

deprofessionalization *see* autonomy

diabetes 26, 89, 104, 105, 107; and collective mindlines 148, 149, 150, 156, 165; and sensemaking 160–1; local guidelines 26, 161

diagnosis: missed 132; narrative and 122; process of 48, 49, 50, 56–60, 75–6, 92, 234n25; sensemaking and 157, 159–61; social construction of 234n15

diffusion of innovations 98–9, 199, 200, 201, 202, 225nn23,24, 235n7; *see also* implementation

discourse analysis 165, 168, 219n3, 225nn21,22, 228n4, 230n20

discussions, informal 15, 27, 29, 89, 95, 96, 98, 102, 105–6, 111–26, 127–33, 134, 135, 143, 150, 200, 225n28, 230n25; *see also* stories

disease concept 68, 121, 154–6, 174–91, 195–6, 233–4n19, 234nn21,25, 234–5n27; *see also* illness–disease; social construction

disease construct *see* disease concept

disease prevention 36, 40–1, 43, 119, 155, 158, 218nn25,26

distant influence 172, 233n16; *see also* structuration

domain knowledge 56, 60

domain, shared *see* community of practice

duality 172; *see* also structuration

dyad (patient–clinician) 182, 185, 234n25; *see also* patient; illness–disease

education *see* learning

education, continuing *see* continuing professional development

eminence–based practice 2, 94

enactment 163–4, 217n12, 231n3, 232n9; *see also habitus*; sensemaking

encapsulation theory 75, 76, 81, 92, 222n7

engaged scholarship 205

enterprise *see* joint enterprise

epistemology 196; *see also* disease concept

ethics 44, 60, 79; *see also* values

ethnography *see* methods

ethnomethodology 159, 162, 197, 219n3, 230

evidence: colloquial 201; context-free; 201, 203, 204; context-specific 201, 205; experiential *see* experiential knowledge; hierarchy of 110; research-based 1–4, 6, 10, 27, 30, 34, 38, 61; 66–8, 102, 103, 104–5, 107, 109, 137, 138, 198–205, 216n2, 221n17 *see also* canonical knowledge; variety of sources 19–25, 27–28, 33, 46, 57, 78, 95–8, 101–11, 117, 130–3, 137, 141, 151, 198, 200–4; *see also* knowledge sources, research evidence

evidence-based medicine *see* evidence-based practice

evidence-based practice: benefits 3–4; critiques 2–5, 41, 106–7, 195, 198, 199, 201, 214n2, 220n12, 235nn1,2; definition 2–3; model 3, 181; policy-making group's use of 138–9

experiential knowledge vi, vii, 23, 32, 34, 42, 44, 45, 46, 48, 57–65, 70, 71, 73, 75, 77, 78, 82, 86, 88, 92, 97, 102, 109, 117, 120, 124, 137–8, 164, 186, 191, 201, 222n16, 225n27, 226n5

expert 56, 58, 64, 74, 76, 85–96, 103–11, 174, 223n6; local 23, 24, 53, 95–7, 110, 128–32, 147, 148, 198, 201; *see also* opinion leader

expert system 2, 20, 24–9, 203, 236n8

expertise 42, 54, 63, 77, 85–95, 144–5, 186, 224n11; interactional 202, 224,11; *see also* expert

externalization (of tacit knowledge) 99–102, 140, 151, 225n18; *see also* SECI spiral

face, presentation of 82

fieldwork 7, 11–14, 72, 196

flowcharts 87–8, 93, 94, 216n3

formal knowledge 25, 28, 29–31, 36, 61–6, 91, 99–100, 101, 110, 117, 123–4, 151, 168–9, 173, 181, 182, 184, 186, 191, 197, 201–5, 222n16, 224n15, 230n2, 231n4; *see also* evidence, context-free; evidence, research-based; knowledge, canonical; textbook; theory, clinical

frame theory 55–6, 219n8, 220n13

garbage-can theory of decision making 137, 193

General Medical Services contract *see* Quality and Outcomes Framework

generalization vs. specificity (in clinical science) 30, 34, 44, 68, 124, 205, 217n12, 221n20; *see also* medicine as a science

GMS contract *see* Quality and Outcomes Framework

goals, multiple 31–45, 57, 59, 61, 94–5, 119, 150, 154, 182, 201, 228n4; *see also* roles, multiple

GP contract *see* Quality and Outcomes Framework

groupthink 161–2, 203–4, 229nn14,15,16

guardian (of professional standing) 38, 42–3

guidelines: attitudes to 19–31; 218n16; critiques of 3, 103, 216n2; discussion of 57; 105–6, 127–9, 140–1, 153–5, 235nn4,5,6; limitations of 3, 19–24, 28–31, 33, 35, 38, 40, 42, 43–7, 49, 60, 61–4, 68, 89, 98, 153–5, 158–9, 169, 181, 216n4; non-use of 3, 5, 22–5, 32, 71, 94, 103, 108; reification of 142, 146; usefulness of 19, 20, 97, 98, 101–3, 109–10, 147, 148, 153, 157, 178–9, 189, 191, 217n12, 224n13, 226n29, 227n6, 228n9; *see also* protocol

habitus 168–70; and collective mindlines 169–70, 231n4

health promotion 31, 36, 38, 40–1, 43, 104, 148, 218nn25,26

healthcare system 1–4, 38, 52

heart failure 33, 97–8, 110, 141, 148, 150, 177–81, 226n29, 233n17, 234n20

heedful interaction 162–3, 188; *see also* sensemaking

heuristics: in clinical thinking 56–61, 73, 94, 220nn11,12 *see also* illness scripts; information seeking 109, 111, 202; *see also* knowledge sources

history (recent history of health professions) 1–2

hypothesis 12, 55, 57, 115, 122

hypothetical situations 70, 97

hypothetico-deductivism 55, 57, 60, 219n6 220n9, 220n10; *see also* clinical reasoning; hypothesis

identity: community of practice and 134, 143–4, 151, 163; learning and 89; professional 35, 134, 143, 163, 170, 232n8; stories and 126, 151

illness scripts 56–7, 60, 73, 81, 92, 99, 124, 181, 219n7, 236n9; *see also* heuristics; maxims; pattern recognition; rules of thumb; schemata

illness–disease 185, 188–91, 195, 196, 203, 228n6, 234nn21,25, *see also* co-construction, disease concept

implementation (of research-based evidence) 4–6, 30, 63, 177–9, 195, 198–206

implications (of mindlines), policy/practical 210–16

improvisation 61–2, 65, 82, 168, 227n8, 231n4

information technology 1, 2, 20, 25, 27, 28, 32, 33, 34, 37, 39, 54, 87, 89, 97, 109–10, 113, 114, 130, 135, 136, 140, 141, 142, 146, 148, 149, 150, 153, 154, 157, 200, 217n7, 217n8, 226, 235nn5,6, 236n8; *see also* expert system; internet

information-seeking heuristics *see* heuristics

innovations *see* diffusion of innovations

institutional thinking 228n3, 231n5

interactionism 38, 52, 111, 126, 130, 133, 137, 142, 162, 176, 181, 188, 219n3, 223n4, 225n18, 229n18, 230nn20,22, 233n16; *see also* negotiation; social constructivism

internalization (of explicit knowledge) 168, 99–103, 110–11, 123, 138, 151, 199, 223n19, 225n23; *see also* SECI spiral

internet *see* information technology

intuition 22, 52, 54–5, 61, 90, 94, 102

IT system *see* information technology

Joanna Briggs Institute 68, 412n3
joint enterprise 134, 136, 142, 145 *see* community of practice
judgement *see* clinical judgement
justification, retrospective 159–61, 229n12, 230n20; *see also* sensemaking

KaseBook 236nn5,6
knowing-in-action 62, 220n16; *see also* knowledge-in-practice-in-context; situated knowledge
knowledge management 6, 7, 99, 102, 116, 204, 225nn16,17
knowledge sources 15, 19–25, 28, 37, 44, 46, 57–8, 69–84, 87, 95–111, 113, 115–17, 130–3, 135–6, 137–41, 144, 150–1, 153, 198, 200–5, 217n6, 227n6; *see also* evidence, variety of sources; heuristics, information seeking
knowledge spiral 99–103
knowledge systems *see* expert system
knowledge transfer 63, 64, 146, 195, 196, 198, 199, 200, 204, 225n23; *see also* implementation; knowledge, utilization; knowledge transformation
knowledge transformation vii, 6, 101–3, 111, 126, 137–9, 181, 199, 200, 225nn18,24, 230n2; *see also* implementation; SECI spiral
knowledge translation *see* knowledge transfer
knowledge: canonical *see* codified knowledge; formal knowledge; textbook; experiential *see* experiential knowledge; explicit 3, 61, 99–102, 138–41, 146, 150, 154, 198, 230n2 *see also* formal knowledge; external influences *see* context; enactment; social construction; formal *see* formal knowledge; in practice 61–5 *see also* practical knowledge; local *see* local knowledge; nurturing (vs. sharing) 227n7; overload 78, 159, 222n11; peer group 77–9, 109, 126, 220n11 *see also* apprenticeship; community of practice; personal 72, 92, 111, 130, 221n3 *see also* practical knowledge; practical *see* practical knowledge; professional 61–4 *see also* practical knowledge; propositional *see* formal knowledge; rule-based 217n12; sources of *see* knowledge sources; 'sticky'

202, 235n7; tacit *see* tacit knowledge; textbook *see* codified knowledge; formal knowledge; transfer *see* knowledge transfer; translation *see* knowledge transfer; utilization 199, 214n4 *see also* knowledge transformation; versus information 101–3
knowledge-in-practice-in-context 64–8, 72, 82, 101, 102, 127, 142, 151, 166, 171, 182, 198, 199, 202, 204; *see also* practical knowledge; practical reasoning

language 174, 232n3; and clinical learning 76, 80, 165, 225nn21,22; *see also* acculturation; learning; socialization
learning: action 83, 204; attitudes *see* socialization, secondary; bedside 82–4; biomedical sciences 73–5 *see also* biomedical sciences; collective 236n9 *see also* community of practice; community of practice 15, 130–42, 149–50; cycle 222n16; decontextualized 62–3, 77; experiential 57, 62–3; foundations of mindlines 69–84; inter-professional 2; loop, single and double 220n16; new information 95–103, 109–11, 136–41 *see also* community of practice; pattern recognition 55–61; peer group 70, 77–9, 81–4, 91, 109, 116, 126, 135, 160, 228n7 *see also* community of practice; practical, 61, 64–6, 75–7, 85–95, 108, 223n3, 225n28 *see also* community of practice; craft; problem-based 2, 77; shared histories of; 143, 165 *see also* community of practice; situated 59, 61–66, 82; skills 69–71, 75–7, 81; soft skills 78–81; story-based 112–26; styles 108, 223n16, 225n28; word-of-mouth *see* learning; community of practice; learning, story-based; *see also* apprenticeship; continuing professional development; *habitus*; socialization; stories
lectures 69, 71, 74, 96, 101, 103, 104, 105, 106, 107, 132, 184, 186, 222n12, 225n27; *see also* continuing professional development; teaching
legitimate peripheral participation 82–3, 142; *see also* apprenticeship; community of practice
linear–rational thinking *see* rationalism
lingua franca see stories as boundary objects
local knowledge 38, 39, 41, 52, 53–4, 73,

88, 103, 108, 112–4, 118, 123, 132, 138, 140, 165, 201; *see also* context; contextual adroitness
logico-scientific mode (vs narrative mode of thinking) 115, 224n15; *see also* rationalism; technical-rational

manager: clinician as 31–9, 41–3, 54, 89, 104, 108, 119, 134, 144, 146, 154–5, 170, 216n14, 228n7; practice manager 10, 12, 31, 33, 54, 135–6, 140, 145, 148, 149, 165, 167
managerialism 1, 2, 4
masters *see* apprenticeship; learning; old hands
Max Planck Institute 58
maxims 58, 67, 93, 173; *see also* rules of thumb
medicine: as a science 29–30, 66–8, 73–4; 174–7, 221nn20,6, 234n27; epistemology of *see* research evidence, clinical role of; disease concept; narrative *see* narrative medicine; social construction of *see* social constructivism
meetings clinical 11–12, 15, 22, 23, 33, 43, 103, 106, 107, 112, 114–15, 124, 125, 131–2, 135–41, 143–5, 148–9, 153–4, 219n3, 227nn2,4,7, 229n11, 235n4; *see also* community of practice; continuing professional development; discussions, informal; quality practice award; Quality and Outcomes Framework
memory, collective 151
metaphor 80, 101, 117, 184, 233n15
methods: ethnography 6–16, 231n4; theoretical underpinnings 14–18
mindlines, clinical: challenges to; 116, 143, 152, 159–60, 229n10, clinical reasoning and 48–61; collective; 15, 44, 46, 101–2, 118, 120, 125, 138, 146–165, 169–70, 177–82, 184, 188–91, 198, 200, 203, 205; community of practice and 128–46; content 73; definition 43–5; development 69–94; EBP and 195–206; multiple roles and flexibility of 31–44, 46; negotiation of *see* negotiation; practical knowledge and 61–66; research implementation and 198–206; research programme on 196–7, 234n24; sharing 95–126; social origins/social construction of 147–91; sources 46; updating 95–111
modernization 4, 10
muddling through 61, 137
multidisciplinary teams 1, 33, 43, 137, 146,

162, 200, 202; *see also* community of practice
multiple cues *see* knowledge sources
mutual engagement 134, 136, 145; *see also* community of practice

narrative 115–24, 130, 159, 176, 185, 190, 224n15, 226n1, 227nn8,9; mode of thinking 115; medicine 121–2; patient 121–5, 184–5, 227n8; shared 114, 119–26, 185, 190, 227n8; *see also* anecdotes; boundary objects; stories
National Institute for Health Research 205
National Institute of Health and Clinical Excellence (NICE) 4, 5, 19, 20, 36, 138, 213, 216n3, 226n29
National Service Frameworks (NSF) 4, 33, 54, 110, 138, 153, 154, 224n13, 233n17
negotiating space *see* illness–disease; patients, negotiation
negotiation 218n19; of collective mindlines 102, 134, 138–9, 141, 143–6, 152, 154, 179, 181 *see also* mindlines, collective; of decisions 52, 161–2, 165, 200; of illness–disease 182–91 *see also* patient negotiation; of meaning 6, 139, 142–3, 154, 166, 169, 176, 182–91, 227n5; of roles 38, 138, 143; of social order 138; *see also* interactionism
networking *see* networks, professional
networks (professional) 33, 37, 95, 98, 107, 109, 113, 130–3, 135–6, 144, 145, 154, 156, 160, 164–5, 170, 185, 201, 204, 225n21, 231n5, 233n15, 235n7; *see also* actor-network theory; community of practice; semantic networks
NICE *see* National Institute of Health and Clinical Excellence
normalization 103
novice 52, 58, 85–92, 224n9; *see also* beginner; student
nursing 1, 5, 11, 12, 22, 23, 25, 33, 34, 35, 58, 72–3, 74, 77, 79, 89, 90–5, 109, 113, 127, 133, 135, 140, 149, 165, 167, 214n1, 215n8, 217n11, 218n26, 221n5, 222n9, 223n6, 226n5, 230n22; *see also* community of practice; medicine as a science; multidisciplinary teams

old hands/old timers 81, 83, 225n18; *see also* apprenticeship
ontology (of disease) 196; *see also* illness–disease
opinion leaders 15, 44, 46, 53, 95, 96, 98,

109, 130, 178–9, 181, 198, 200–2, 204, 226n2, 235n5; *see also* expert, local
organization theory 6, 16–17, 36, 80, 99, 117, 133, 137, 159–65, 198, 201, 204, 217n18, 219n3, 220n16, 225n17, 226n3, 227nn3,7, 228n4, 229n11, 230n20 235n7; *see also* theory
organizational culture *see* culture
OT *see* goals, multiple

paradigm 124, 174, 175, 232n11
participation *see* legitimate peripheral participation
pathway, clinical care 4, 20, 22, 45, 52, 109, 120, 154; *see also* guidelines
patients: negotiation (influence on decisions) 19, 24, 31–2, 36, 39, 41, 45, 51, 53, 70, 97, 100, 162, 182–91, 234nn25,26; views of illness 182–9, 234n24; *see also* negotiation of illness–disease
pattern recognition 55–61, 74–5, 92–5, 116, 124, 236n9; *see also* illness scripts
PCT *see* primary care trust
performing (a 'disease' or illness–disease) 181, 190
pharmaceutical adviser 19, 20, 37, 49, 106, 110
pharmaceutical industry 19, 23, 39, 95, 96, 102, 171, 175, 178, 180, 181, 200, 201, 222n6
pharmaceutical representative 37, 51, 69, 74, 96–7, 105, 109, 110, 130, 133, 179, 227n6
phronesis 193, 220n14
pinball machine analogy 180–1, 196; *see also* epistemology
policy makers 6, 7, 16, 30, 102, 137, 138, 172, 181, 185, 199, 200, 205, 215n8, 227n5
political economy of clinical knowledge 197; *see also* power and knowledge; social construction
power: professional 2, 36, 38, 64, 163, 164, 165, 170, 188, 219n29, 223n18; and knowledge 40, 82, 138, 161, 165, 170–3, 174, 175, 188, 197, 201, 225n22, 232n12; *see also* autonomy; clinical freedom
practical consciousness 173; *see* also structuration
practical knowledge *see* artistry, professional; contextual adroitness; craft; knowledge, in practice;

knowledge, personal; knowledge, professional; knowledge-in-practice-in-context
practical reasoning 64; *see also* practical knowledge; reflective practice
practical skills 62–4, 73, 75, 77, 78, 88, 101, *see also* apprenticeship; expertise; learning
practice guidelines *see* guidelines
practice management *see* manager
practice policy 15, 25, 43, 101, 105, 110, 141, 147, 148, 153, 154, 163
practice-based evidence 18, 197, 198, 205
prevention *see* health promotion
primary care trust 34, 36, 37, 106–7, 110, 158, 160, 167, 180
probability 30, 43, 58, 68, 222n7; *see also* medicine as a science
professional artistry *see* artistry, professional
professional capital *see* capital
professional contacts *see* networks
professional standing 39, 41, 42–3, 144, 155, 165, 169, 217n11, 219n29
professionalism 79
proficiency 93; *see also* expertise
proletarianization *see* autonomy
propositional knowledge *see* formal knowledge
protocol 92, 95, 117, 131, 141–2, 158, 163, 165, 179–80, 211–13, 217n11, 218n26; *see also* guidelines

Quality and Outcomes Framework (QOF) 43, 141, 152–6, 163, 180, 213, 215n10, 216n14, 217n10, 218n27, 226n29, 228nn7,8, 230nn20,1
quality of care 9, 10, 42, 43, 98, 112, 121, 142, 144, 146, 152, 161, 166, 197, 215n2, 216n14, 216n1, 219n29, 228n7, 230n21
quality practice award (QPA) 10, 12, 22, 23, 41, 112, 136

randomized controlled trial *see* clinical trial
rationalism vi, 2, 5, 6, 52, 55, 57, 58, 59–60, 61, 63, 64, 67, 68, 90, 92–4, 115, 137, 159, 198, 199, 220n11, 222n7, 224n15; *see also* evidence-based practice; formal knowledge
rationalization, retrospective 159–60, 229n12, 230n20; *see* sensemaking
reasoning *see* clinical reasoning
recursive 162, 230n19; *see also* recursivity
recursivity 162, 230n19; *see also* recursive

referencing 16, 17, 216n16, 221n4, 237
reflection-in-action *see* reflective practice
reflective commentary studies 159, 197; *see also* think-aloud studies
reflective practice 61, 62, 220n16; *see also* knowledge, professional; practical reasoning
reification *see* community of practice, reification; social construction
rep *see* pharmaceutical representative
repertoire, shared *see* shared repertoire
research evidence: clinical role of vii, 5, 29–31, 38, 57, 61–2, 66–8, 99, 101–3, 107–11, 123–5, 133, 137–8, 160, 178, 181–2, 184, 195, 198–205, 215n11, 217n10, 221nn17,6, 226nn29,2, 234n19; *see also* evidence, research-based; guidelines; implementation; medicine as a science; protocol; systematic reviews
research world (vs. clinical practice world) vi, 61–2, 102, 124, 153, 198, 199, 200
research–practice gap *see* implementation
respect 82, 95, 97, 110, 116, 126, 128, 130, 131, 132, 135, 137, 138, 143, 160, 164, 169, 179, 186, 188, 200; *see also* trust
ritual 80, 96, 168, 176, 188, 197, 201, 231n4
role: conflict *see* roles, multiple; model 73, 79, 82, 116, 119; scripts 35, 100; sending 36; set 36, 44
roles, multiple 31–45, 59–60, 90–1, 95, 107, 131, 141, 143, 144, 150, 153–4, 156, 170, 182, 201, 233n15, 235n27; *see also* goals, multiple
routines 19, 35, 45, 48, 50, 73, 88, 92, 97, 134, 141, 142, 149, 150, 158, 164, 171, 173, 184, 186, 198, 204, 217n4, 228n2, 230n21; *see also* practice policy; SOPHIEs
Royal College of General Practitioners (RCGP) 10, 24, 36, 52, 107, 119, 136,144, 153, 178, 180
rules of thumb 49, 56, 58–60, 73, 86, 117; *see also* illness scripts

satisficing 51, 219n2
schemata 56, 60, 82, 86, 99; *see also* illness scripts
science: biomedical, 73–77, 221n5; Modes 1 and 2 205, 218n17; of individuals *see* generalization vs. specificity; philosophy of 14, 173–7, 219n6, 232n13, 234n27; *see also* medicine as a science; social

construction, of medicine; social construction, of science
scientific bureaucratic model *see* bureaucratic, scientific
scientific evidence *see* research evidence
scripts, illness: role 35: *see also* illness scripts
SECI spiral 99–103, 108, 111, 120, 138, 151, 152, 202, 224n15, 225n17; *see also Ba*; knowledge management; social life of knowledge
semantic networks 219n7
sensemaking: collective 101, 137–8, 157–64, 200, 229n11; generic 162; individual 60, 71, 74, 76, 86, 168, 181–2, 185; 223n17, 225n18, 229n12; narrative and 101, 116–8, 121–4, 137; organizational 229n11; retrospective 48, 60, 159–61, 229n12, 230n20; *see also* enactment; heedful interacting
shared enterprise *see* joint enterprise
shared histories of learning 143, 165; *see also* community of practice
shared repertoire 136, 142; *see also* community of practice
situated learning 84; *see also* context; knowledge-in-practice-in-context; learning
skills *see* learning, skills
social capital *see* capital
social cognitive theory 223n19, 230n23, 231n3
social construction: of chronic kidney disease 152–7; of heart failure *see* actor network theory; of medicine 166–7, 175–7, 223n17, 232n11, 234nn23,27; of mindlines 45, 46, 147–91, 225n18; of science 174; of society 173; *see also* co-construction; disease concept, epistemology of; social constructivism
social constructivism 173–7, 232nn10,13,14; soft 174; strong 175–6; *see also* disease concept; epistemology; interactionism; social construction
social control 86, 125, 175, 186, 223n2
social embeddedness of knowledge 222n9
social life of knowledge vii, 6, 117; *see also* community of practice
social origins of medical knowledge *see* social construction
social principles 173; *see also* structuration
social theory 167–73
socialization: primary 172, 173–4, 188, 189; secondary 70, 77–84, 189, 221n3, 222nn13,15, 223n21, 225n20,

235n27; SECI spiral 99–102; *see also* apprenticeship; common sense; learning, soft skills

soft skills *see* learning, soft skills

songlines vii–viii, 46

SOPHIE 25, 26, 149; as reification 142, 146, 150

specificity vs. generalization (in clinical science) *see* generalization vs. specificity

spread of innovations *see* diffusion

standards 146, 198, 203, 216nn14,1, 226n29, 229n10; *see also* targets

stories: as boundary objects 114, 120, 121–4, 190, 226n7; as persuasion 116, 124–5, 188, 203, 226nn2,5,6; knowledge flow and 56, 82, 86, 95–7, 101, 105, 109, 111, 112–26, 132, 135, 137–43, 151, 184–5, 191, 203, 226n2; learning and 70, 79, 82, 86, 117, 125, 226n5; main elements of 118–19; practical knowledge and 44, 116–17; relational properties of 119–20; sensemaking and 117, 121, 159, 227n9; status and 125–6; teaching and 116; vs. anecdotes 226n1; *see also* anecdotes; community of practice; discussions, informal; mindlines, collective; narrative; SECI spiral; songlines

story telling *see* stories

street level bureaucrats 228n3, 230n22

structuration 171–3, 180, 232n14, 233n16

student, clinical 11–13, 49, 55, 56, 69–93, 116, 128, 176, 222n11&16, 223nn17,21, 224n8; *see also* novice; trainee

symbolic interactionism 219n3, 228n4

systematic reviews 1, 24, 31, 61, 68, 109, 184, 231n1; *see also* Cochrane collaboration; research evidence

tacit knowledge 55, 60–4, 67, 70–2, 73, 88, 92–4, 99–103, 11, 117, 120, 131, 133, 138, 151, 168, 171, 173, 184,198, 203, 219n1, 220n14, 224nn11,14,15, 225n18, 228n3, 230n2; *see also* knowledge, personal; practical knowledge

targets 1, 2, 25, 33, 35, 37, 41, 43, 45, 146, 156, 167, 178–9, 181, 198, 203; *see also* standards

teaching 2,10, 11, 46, 49, 62–4, 70, 71, 73, 74, 77, 79, 81, 82–4, 86–7, 88,

89, 91, 93, 96, 104, 109, 113, 116, 160, 204, 219n4, 222n12, 223n17, 225n27, 234n25; *see also* apprenticeship; learning; student; trainee

technical rational 63; *see also* logico-scientific mode; rationalism

textbook 21, 25, 27, 43, 46, 52, 61–3, 79, 82, 87, 101, 109, 133, 169, 184–5, 186, 188, 190

theory, clinical 6, 7, 44, 59–66, 71, 77, 81, 92, 109, 117, 119, 124; *see also* formal knowledge

theory: educational 223n19; espoused 220n16; in practice 197; in use 220n16; *see also* actor-network theory; categorization theory; constructuralism; encapsulation theory; frame theory; garbage-can theory; learning cycle; methods; social cognitive theory; social construction; social theory

think-aloud studies 56–7, 74, 218n24; *see also* reflective commentary studies

thought community/thought collective 232n11

thumbnails 85–8, 94, 223n17

trainee 27, 36, 37, 38, 48, 55, 73, 80, 81–3, 88–91, 127–8, 142; *see also* apprenticeship; learning; legitimate peripheral participation; novice; student; teaching

training (clinical) *see* trainee

transformation of knowledge *see* knowledge transformation

transition (from novice to expert) 85–95, 223nn5,6

trials *see* clinical trial

trust 15, 29, 35, 45, 63, 83, 95, 96, 102, 104, 106, 108, 110–11, 130–3, 135, 141–4, 164, 170, 198, 200, 202, 224n10, 225n21, 228n1; *see also* respect

tutoring *see* teaching

uncertainty *see* clinical uncertainty

values 2, 44, 46, 73, 78–81, 91, 95, 165, 169, 170, 173–7, 201, 222n15, 225n22, 230n20, 235n27

web/websites *see* ethics: information technology

wisdom 2, 59, 86, 101, 173, 203, 220n14; *see also* clinical judgement

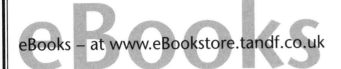

.